Fetal Growth

Edited by

F. Sharp, R.B. Fraser and R.D.B. Milner

With 71 Figures

Springer-Verlag
London Berlin Heidelberg New York
Paris Tokyo Hong Kong

F. Sharp, MD, FRCOG
R.B. Fraser, MD, FRCOG, DCH
Department of Obstetrics and Gynaecology, Clinical Sciences Centre,
Northern General Hospital, Herries Road, Sheffield S5 7AU

R.D.G. Milner, MA, ScD (Cantab), MD (Lond), FRCP (Lond)
Department of Paediatrics, University of Sheffield,
Children's Hospital, Sheffield S10 2TH

ISBN-13: 978-1-4471-1709-4 e-ISBN-13: 978-1-4471-1707-0
DOI: 10.1007/ 978-1-4471-1707-0

British Library Cataloguing in Publication Data
Royal College of Obstetricians and Gynaecologists Study Group (20th: 1988)
Fetal growth. 1. Man. Foetuses. Development I. Sharp, F. (Frank), *1938–*
II. Fraser, R.B. (Robert Bruce), *1948–* III. Milner, R.D.G., *1937–*
612'. 647

Library of Congress Cataloging-in-Publication Data
Fetal Growth edited by F. Sharp, R.B. Fraser, and R.D.G. Milner
p. cm. Includes bibliographies and index.
1. Fetus—Growth. 2. Fetus—Growth retardation. 3. Growth disorders. I. Sharp, F. (Frank), 1938— II. Fraser, R.B. (Robert Bruce), 1948— III. Milner, R.D.G. [DNLM: Fetal Development. WQ 210 F4185] RG613. F473 1989 612'.647 dc20.
DNLM/DLC for Library of Congress 89-6434
CIP

Softcover reprint of the hardcover 1st edition 1989

Typeset and Printed by the Peacock Press Ltd., Ashton-under-Lyne, Lancashire England.

2128/3916-543210

Preface

This book is based on the 20th Study Group of the Royal College of Obstetricians and Gynaecologists, which concerned the important topic of fetal growth. Basic scientific, and both obstetric and paediatric aspects of the subject were addressed in contributions from many different disciplines, and we are greatly indebted to all the international experts who took part in this workshop at the RCOG in London in November 1988.

The deliberations covered the broad topics of normal fetal growth, fetal overgrowth and undergrowth. Clinical implications of these entities, especially fetal undergrowth, played a large part in the proceedings as dictated by clinical concerns. Definitions, epidemiology, aetiology and screening were covered, as were technological developments, with special reference to blood flow and volume flow measurements, both fetal and placental. Other aspects of clinical fetal monitoring, including fetal activity measurement, and biophysical evaluation were rationalised and placed in context, and the important newly emerging areas of cordocentesis and therapy in IUGR addressed. Finally, neonatal management of the SGA baby, mortality and long-term morbidity were considered.

This volume represents the edited proceedings of an important study group, along with a much-edited transcript of the discussion periods which followed the formal presentations. We are very grateful to all the participants who gave us a valuable three days of their time and also to Sally Barber, Postgraduate Education Secretary, and Diane Morgan, Publications Officer of the RCOG, without whose unstinting input this publication could not have been produced so rapidly. We hope they feel their efforts have been worthwhile.

London
March 1989

Frank Sharp
R.D.G. Milner
R.B. Fraser

Participants

PROFESSOR E.D. ALBERMAN
Department of Clinical Epidemiology, The London Hospital Medical College, London E1 1BB

MR J.M. BRUDENELL
73 Harley Street, London W1N 1DE

PROFESSOR S. CAMPBELL
Professor and Head, Department of Obstetrics and Gynaecology, King's College School of Medicine and Dentistry, Denmark Hill, London SE5 8RX

PROFESSOR T. CHARD
Professor of Reproductive Physiology, St Bartholomew's Hospital Medical College, West Smithfield, London EC1A 7BE

PROFESSOR J.F. CLAPP III
Department of Obstetrics and Gynecology, The University of Vermont, College of Medicine, Given Building, Burlington, VT 05405, USA

PROFESSOR F. COCKBURN
Samson Gemell Professor of Child Health, University Department of Child Health, Royal Hospital for Sick Children, Yorkhill, Glasgow G3 8SJ

MR J.O. DRIFE
Department of Obstetrics and Gynaecology, Clinical Sciences Building, Leicester Royal Infirmary, P.O. Box 65, Leicester LE2 7LX

PROFESSOR S.H. EIK-NES
Department of Obstetrics and Gynaecology, Ultrasound Section, University Hospital Clinic, Trondheim N-7006, Norway

MR R.B. FRASER
Department of Obstetrics and Gynaecology, Clinical Sciences Centre, Northern General Hospital, Sheffield S5 7AU

MR M.D.G. GILLMER
Consultant Obstetrician and Gynaecologist, Maternity Department, John Radcliffe Hospital, Headington, Oxford OX3 9DU

DR M.H. HALL
Consultant Obstetrician and Gynaecologist, Aberdeen Maternity Hospital, Cornhill Road, Aberdeen AB9 2ZA

DR V.K.M. HAN
Department of Paediatrics, Lawson Research Institute, University of Western Ontario, London, Ontario N6A 4V2, Canada

PROFESSOR W.W. HAY JR
Professor of Pediatrics, Division of Perinatal Medicine, University of Colorado School of Medicine, 4200 East Ninth Avenue, Denver, CO 80262, USA

PROFESSOR D.J. HILL
Professor of Diabetes Research, Lawson Research Institute, St Joseph's Health Centre, 268 Grosvenor Street, London, Ontario N6A 4V2, Canada

PROFESSOR P.W. HOWIE
Department of Obstetrics and Gynaecology, University of Dundee Medical School, Ninewells Hospital, Dundee DD1 9SY

PROFESSOR M.I. LEVENE
Department of Paediatrics and Child Health, Leeds University School of Medicine, Clarendon Wing, The General Infirmary of Leeds, Leeds LS1 3EX

PROFESSOR T. LIND
Consultant Obstetrician and Gynaecologist, MRC Human Reproduction Group, Princess Mary Maternity Hospital, Great North Road, Newcastle upon Tyne NE2 3BD

DR K. MARŠÁL
Department of Obstetrics and Gynaecology, University of Lund, S-214 01 Malmö, Sweden

PROFESSOR R.D.G. MILNER
Department of Paediatrics, University of Sheffield, Children's Hospital, Sheffield S10 2TH

MR K. H. NICOLAIDES
Harris Birthright Centre for Fetal Medicine, Department of Obstetrics and Gynaecology, King's College School of Medicine and Dentistry, Denmark Hill, London SE5 8RX

DR N. PATEL
Department of Obstetrics and Gynaecology, Ninewells Hospital, Dundee DD1 9SY

PROFESSOR P.-H. PERSSON
Erikslustvagen 22, Box 20037, 20074 Malmö, Sweden

MR G.D. PINKER
President, Royal College of Obstetricians and Gynaecologists, 27 Sussex Place, Regent's Park, London NW1 4RG

PROFESSOR D. RUSH
Head, Epidemiology Program, Human Nutrition Research Center on Aging, Tufts University, 711 Washington Street, Boston, MA 02111, USA

PROFESSOR F. SHARP
Department of Obstetrics and Gynaecology, Clinical Sciences Centre, Northern General Hospital, Herries Road, Sheffield S5 7AU

DR M.H.L. SNOW
MRC Mammalian Development Unit, Wolfson House, University College London, 4 Stephenson Way, London NW1 2HE

MR P.J. STEER
Senior Lecturer, Department of Obstetrics and Gynaecology, St Mary's Hospital Medical School, Praed Street, London W2 1PG

DR A. STEWART
Senior Lecturer in Perinatal Medicine, Departments of Obstetrics and Paediatrics, University College and Middlesex School of Medicine, The Rayne Institute, University College London, University Street, London WC1E 6JJ

DR M.J. WHITTLE
Consultant Obstetrician/Perinatologist, The Queen Mother's Hospital, Yorkhill, Glasgow G3 8SH

PROFESSOR J.S. WIGGLESWORTH
Professor of Perinatal Pathology, Departments of Histopathology and Paediatrics, Royal Postgraduate Medical School, Du Cane Road, London W12 0HS

Additional Contributors

MR D.L. ECONOMIDES
Harris Birthright Research Centre for Fetal Medicine, Department of Obstetrics and Gynaecology, King's College Hospital, London SE5 8RX

MRS F.A. FORD
Research Dietician, Department of Obstetrics and Gynaecology, Clinical Sciences Centre, Northern General Hospital, Sheffield S5 7AU

DR R.J.S. HOWELL
Departments of Reproductive Physiology, and Obstetrics and Gynaecology, St Bartholomew's Hospital Medical College and the London Hospital Medical College, London EC1A 7BE

MR G. THORPE-BEESTON
Harris Birthright Research Centre for Fetal Medicine, Department of Obstetrics and Gynaecology, King's College Hospital, London SE5 8RX

DR P.G. WHITTAKER
Department of Obstetrics and Gynaecology, University of Newcastle, Princess Mary Maternity Hospital, Great North Road, Newcastle upon Tyne NE2 3BD

Contents

SECTION 1

NORMAL FETAL GROWTH

Effect of genome on size at birth

Dr M. H. L. Snow

INTRODUCTION

Size at birth is the outcome of length of gestation and rate of embryo/fetal growth. Among mammals there is a wide range in gestation length although for any particular species pregnancy is of characteristic duration. Fetal growth rate also varies and it seems that mammals can be divided into a small number of groups on the basis of their intrauterine growth rate.[1,2] The maintenance of these characteristics is under genetic control although there is an impact of environmental factors such as maternal health, nutrition, hormonal status and the presence of drugs etc. In this consideration of the effect of genome on size at birth these variable environmental influences will not be discussed, although it is clear that their impact on the maternal/fetal unit varies at least in part because of variations in maternal genotype. The potential effect of the environment on embryonic development is discussed elsewhere in this volume (Section 2).

The successful growth and development of the embryo/fetus requires the interaction between two genomes, those of the embryo and the mother. Two aspects of the genomes will be discussed, sex differences (XX versus XY), and presumptive gene differences resulting from genetic selection for adult body size. A third aspect, aneuploidy and polyploidy will not be considered because such variations in the chromosomal composition of the organism are invariably associated with abnormal development in which growth and size may be compromised as a secondary effect.

It should be borne in mind that birthweight is a difficult parameter to analyse since gestation length is variable in most species, including man, and it is not always made clear whether adequate allowance is given for this variability. In experimental animals such as the mouse there is the added complication that the observer seldom records birthweight data before it is compromised by food intake by the pups. A better measure is the fetal weight on the day before birth but as this often means sacrificing the mother in order to obtain such fetuses this data is seldom available in studies which include observation of post-natal development, or which require breeding studies to be done.

MATERNAL VERSUS EMBRYONIC GENOTYPE

Although XY females are identified in the human population,[3] and in the mouse,[4] where they may be fertile there are no data describing the effect, if any, that this novel maternal genotype may have on fetal development. Our knowledge of maternal-fetal interaction therefore derives only from conventional XX females. The maternal genotype may act on the embryo in two ways. There may be an effect on the development of the oocyte which is subsequently manifested in development of the zygote by virtue of a cytoplasmic interaction with the paternal genome of the fertilising sperm. Two such cytoplasmic effects have been identified, *hairpin-tail (T^{hp})* and *ovum mutant (O_m)*, both in the mouse, and both are embryonic lethals.[5-7] If there are other maternal effects whose action results in altered growth rate and changed birthweight they have not been identified as such.

The second level of maternal influence lies in the ability of the pregnant female to support embryonic/fetal development. This is generally referred to as a uterine effect as this is the interface between mother and fetus. However the differences between females may lie elsewhere in the body as variations in biochemistry or physiology. Teratologists have long recognised strain differences in the response to teratogens and have in some instances linked this to differences in metabolism.[8] In the context of normal fetal development however, experimental analysis has focussed on the effect of maternal size. The pioneering experiments were done 50 years ago but have since been refined and extended in various ways.

In the early 1930s it was known that in rabbits birthweight was inversely related to litter size and that litter size increased with the average size of the strain. It was supposed that the mother exerted a growth-limiting constraint, probably through production of some endogenous metabolite. The observation that in donkey–horse hybrids the mule, born to a mare, is heavier than the hinny whose mother is a donkey seemed to support that notion, but could also be due to interspecific factors. Walton and Hammond[9] sought more reliable data in a study of hybrids between Shire horses and Shetland ponies in which there is approximately a fourfold

Table 1. Effect of uterine environment on fetal weight

Species	Genotype	Large dam	Fetal weight* Control**	Small dam
Horse[9]	Shire	71(2)	–	–
	Hybird	50(2)	–	18(3)
	Shetland	–	–	20(4)
Cattle[10]	S. Devon	43(?)	–	–
	Hybird	33(3)	–	26(3)
	Dexter	–	–	24(?)
Sheep[12]	Border Leicester	6.4(3)	–	5.0(5)
	Welsh Mountain	4.6(3)	–	3.6(4)
Mouse[15]	Large	–	1.74(31)	1.36(32)
	Small	1.31(37)	1.43(58)	–
Mouse [16]	Large	1.67(49)	–	1.57(79)
	Small	1.43(75)	–	1.34(88)
Mouse[17]	Large	0.639(57)	0.624(54)	–
	Small	–	0.524(67)	0.554(63)

* Weight in grams for mice, kilograms for others.
** Control is the uterus of the unselected stock.
Figures in parentheses are the number of fetuses analysed.

difference in weight of the mares. The birthweight of the hybrid foals from Shetland mares was very like that typical of the breed, whereas in Shire mares they achieved a birthweight some three times greater. In the latter instance the hybrids were still some way short of the normal Shire birthweight. If it is deemed unlikely that the hybrid in the Shire uterus would experience growth-limiting conditions, although there may be a maternal effect in which an oocyte borne factor subsequently interacts with the homotypic uterus to modulate embryonic growth, then these classical experiments illustrate an intrinsic limit to growth set by the embryonic/fetal genotype, and also a growth-limiting effect of the smaller maternal genotype. Similar results were obtained from comparable studies on cattle(10,11) and sheep.(12) In the sheep study, embryo transfer techniques were used to place large or small genotype embryos into a uterus of opposite genotype and thus eliminate cytoplasmic effects. These data are summarised in Table 1.

Also in Table 1 are the results of similar embryo transfer studies carried out on mice, in strains in which sublines have been selected for body weight at 6 weeks of age.(13,14) The difference in growth rate that underlies these weight differences originates early in embryogenesis and is clear at birth. The studies in which pregnancy was allowed to go to term lead to similar conclusions to those described above for large, monotocus herbivores, but with one(15) concluding that the major influence on fetal weight is the uterine environment, whilst the other(16) suggests that greater control is exerted by the embryonic genotype. Aitken *et al.*(17) analysed their embryos at 16 days' gestation (mid-fetal stage, 3 days before birth) and found that fetal size was determined solely by embryonic genotype at this stage. The implication that the constraining influence of the uterus on fetal growth is a function of late gestation is supported by other data. In the mouse there is a negative correlation between fetal weight and litter size at birth and on the two days preceding birth;(18-20) reducing litter size consequently tends to increase fetal weight. In my laboratory we have attempted to exploit this in order to explore the relationship between growth rate and morphogenesis (see Section 2) but whilst we have achieved highly significant increases in fetal weight at birth we fail to alter fetal weight at 14.5 days of pregnancy, indeed our data indicate a slight depression in weight (Table 2).(21) In several separate studies carried out some years ago I recorded 14.5 d fetal weight data in 29 litters of Q strain mice and those data are also set in Table 2; there is no correlation between litter size and fetal weight. Consequently I conclude that the uterine constraint to fetal growth is a function of late gestation and probably brought about by fetal mass reaching a critical level that the mother finds progressively harder to maintain. It is not known if the constraint in fetal growth of monotocus species described above is also a late gestation phenomenon. Although comparisons between species should be regarded with care, human twin pregnancies have been claimed to show a decline in fetal growth over the last 10 weeks from a situation where they were the same size as singletons in the second trimester (see Section 2, for references).

A rather more covert uterine effect can be demonstrated in the mouse which is probably related to early embryonic growth rate, but it has not been convincingly correlated with birthweight. There is variation in the number of presacral vertebrae

Table 2. Fetal weight in Q strain mice at 14.5 dpc and birth in control and experimentally-reduced litters.

Group	Age	No. of litters	Litter size	log(10) Fetal weight
Control	14.5 d	12	11.3 ± 0.65	2.324 ± 0.007
	birth	32	8.5 ± 0.63	3.127 ± 0.004
Fallopian tube removed	14.5 d	12	4.8 ± 0.60	2.307 ± 0.01
	birth	32	6.3 ± 0.54	3.183 ± 0.005**
Ovary removed	14.5 d	11	6.9 ± 1.1	2.282 ± 0.005*
	birth	32	6.8 ± 0.65	3.165 ± 0.005**

* Significantly different from controls $p < 0.05$
** Significantly different from controls $p < 0.001$
Relationship between litter and fetal weight at 14.5 d.
29 litters analysed, mean litter size 10.89 ± 0.43, range 8–16.
Mean fetal weight (mg) 251.2. Regression of fetal weight on litter size $y = 239.3 \pm 1.001x$. Correlation coefficient $r = 0.11$. Not significant

(p.s.v.) in different strains of mice, with some strains exhibiting fairly stable proportions of individuals with either 26 or 27 p.s.v.[22] The different phenotypes may reflect the presence of 13 or 14 thoracic, or 5 or 6 lumbar vertebrae. The incidence of a particular phenotype was found to be different in reciprocal crosses between C57B1 and C3H strain mice,[23] an effect shown by embryo transfer to be mediated through uterine environment.[24] A convincing argument was made that the skeletal variation was unrelated to the birthweight of individual fetuses, but it was suggested that early embryonic growth rate may be important. On the other hand it should be noted that the C57B1 mouse is the bigger strain and shows the higher vertebral number and that the hybrid in the C57B1 uterus, which shows a significant increase in lumbar vertebrae is larger than when in the C3H uterus. In a subsequent study on mice selected for body size a correlation was found between birthweight and skeletal type.[25] The possible relationship between embryonic/fetal growth and variation in skeletal phenotype is discussed in Section 2.

Antigenic differences

There is antigenic disparity between the mother and her fetus. In outcrossed matings the differences may be considerable by virtue of the contribution made by the paternal genome. This is the situation in man. Even in closely inbred laboratory animal stocks there will be disparity due to the expression of Y-chromosome specific genes in male fetuses, and maybe some due to mutation that has occurred and is present and expressed in particular embryos. The fact that a fetus is not rejected as an allograft, in the same way that skin grafts would be rejected, has been the subject of intensive study. It is clear that the fetus expresses antigens and that the mother reacts to them. Indeed wide ranging changes in the maternal immunological and endocrinological physiology are identified as reactions to "foreign" fetal tissue.[26,27] The mechanism(s) whereby the fetus avoids rejection are not precisely known, and several possibilities are discussed, including placental filtration of antigens, modification of fetal antigens and modification of maternal responses, perhaps mediated by special "blocking" antibodies.

With respect to an impact on fetal growth it is unclear whether antigenic differences are important in other than pathological circumstances. In mice fetal and placental weight are positively correlated and it has been suggested that placental size can be related to the antigenic dissimilarity between mother and fetus.[28,29] It has been shown that maternal preimmunisation can influence the decidual cell reaction following implantation,[30] but the impact on subsequent placental development and on fetal weight is less well defined.[31-33] Ounsted[34] reports a small change in birthweight of Holstein-Friesian calves related to the degree of in-breeding, and comments that if antigenic differences were to enhance fetal growth then this could help account for the increase in human birthweight with parity.

Very recent observations on gender differences in growth rate in mice suggest that this growth differential at least is unlikely to have an immunological basis. These data are discussed in the next section.

EMBRYONIC GENOTYPE

As indicated above the embryonic genotype as a whole is probably instrumental in governing embryonic/fetal growth until the maternal uterine size becomes limiting. In this section the influence of sex will be discussed, and the impact that genetic selection for size has on various components of growth.

XX versus XY

In most mammals males tend to be larger than females, and in general the difference is observable at birth. The basis for this is obscure, although two possible mechanisms are frequently discussed. Firstly, the enhanced growth of the male fetus has been ascribed to the anabolic effect of male gonadal hormones. Secondly, as outlined above, it has been suggested that the greater antigenic differences between mother and her male fetuses would result in larger placentas, and there is generally a good positive correlation between placental and fetal weight.

In a study on rats,[35] in which male fetuses on the day before birth were found to be on average over 5% heavier than their female litter mates, both these mechanisms were considered. The difference in placental weight between male and female was found to be insufficient to account for the dimorphism, and the authors discounted antigenic factors. They also suggested that if gonadal hormones were involved they too should have affected placental weight, which clearly was not the case. In support of their dismissal of an endocrinological explanation they point out that the sex differences are present even in anencephalic fetuses, in which hormone levels would be low or non-existent.

Surprisingly, the mouse does not show a sexual dimorphism in fetal weight at birth but recent studies have revealed such differences in embryonic/early fetal stages. Seller and Perkins-Cole[36] found that in mice at neurulation stages males were developmentally more advanced than females. The difference seems small, about two somites, equivalent to about 2.5 hours, but set against the speed of mouse development is significant. Two earlier studies on XO mice[37,38] had shown that XO fetuses are smaller than their XX litter mates, both at birth and in very early embryonic stages. The authors' unpublished data show that XY male fetuses from the analysed litters are even larger than XX females. Again the difference is about two somites. Burgoyne (personal communication) has followed up these observations analysing stocks of mice carrying a normal Y or a small Y chromosome (the result of a deletion), and a Y chromosome carrying the gene *sex reversal*, *sxr*, together with a stock segregating the *sxr* gene on one of the X chromosomes. The data show that the effect on growth is a positive influence by the Y chromosome (and probably of the region involved in the *sxr* translocation) rather than a growth retardation associated with carrying two X chromosomes. Previously it was thought likely that difficulties associated with inactivating one X in females might have produced this growth differential.

These data demonstrate that the growth advantage of the XY embryo is present at the earliest stages of organogenesis and thus rules out involvement of endogenous hormones. The developmental state of the placenta at these early times is so immature that it seems unlikely that materno-fetal interaction via this organ is involved either. The observation that transfer of early cavitating blastocysts, grown *in vitro* results in a preponderance of males whilst transfer of late cavitators gives more females[39] effectively locates the growth-controlling function to the embryo itself and obviates the need to invoke hormonal or immunological explanations.

The developmental advantage of the XY embryo/fetus seems to remain at a steady 2-3 h through implantation and well into organogenesis. If this is presumed to continue to birth then the difference in fetal weight between male and female mice would be small. The mouse fetus grows at a rate of less than 10 mg per hour over the two days preceding birth, so the difference expected is around 25 mg, or about 2% of birthweight. A large study would be required to establish this as significant at this time point although the XY advantage is so clear in early organogenesis.

Effect of selection for size

The large and small Q strain mice[14] have been used in an attempt to determine the factors involved in the size difference and to search for a 'growth-controlling' organ should one exist. It has been shown for several organs that large mice have more and larger cells than unselected controls, and that small mice have fewer and smaller cells.[40] The relative contribution of cell number and cell size differs according to organ. For example in spleen and lungs about 70% of the difference could be accounted for by cell number, whereas in liver and kidney cell size and cell number contributed about equally. It was concluded that selection operated more to change cell number than cell size. Furthermore, comparison of mice at several different ages postnatally indicated an increase in cell size with age, and suggested that the differences between large and small mice was the result of a change in the relationship between developmental age and chronological age. When compared at the same body weight but different ages the selected mice were found to have cells roughly equal in size and number. Thus variation in both these parameters was seen as a result of selection for some other aspect of growth rate.

The rate of growth *in vitro* of embryonic/fetal tibias from the selected lines has been shown to be influenced by an unidentified humoral factor,[41] and the utilisation of food[42] and processing of amino acids and protein[43] is increased in larger mice.

Chimaeras have been made between large and small mice and the relative contribution of each line to the overall development and to the development of different organs has been analysed. The anticipation was that if the growth-controlling factor(s) emanate from a single organ (as a circulating hormone or growth factor) then the size of the chimaera should reflect more closely the composition of that organ than any other. Eleven organs were analysed[44,45] but no consistent correlation was found that would identify such a growth-controlling organ. I have previously discussed this data[46] and suggested that neural crest or connective tissue, which were not analysed, might be good candidates even though Falconer and his colleagues could account for all the variance expected from genetic differences between the selected lines. These two tissues have the advantage of being widely distributed throughout the embryo and of arising very early in development, thus permitting their involvement in the growth regulation that is clearly possible in isolated parts of embryos at the onset of organogenesis.[46,47] Some of this data is discussed in Section 2.

The selection for size carried out by Falconer[14] illustrates an interesting interaction between maternal size, litter size and birthweight in alternate generations. Whilst the overall trend in the selection for high body weight is upwards the curve is not smooth, but pursues a zig-zag path with alternating high and not-so-high weights. The explanation for this lies in the following relationships: (i) ovulation rate is positively correlated with female body weight, (ii) birthweight is inversely proportional to litter size and (iii) adult body weight reflects birthweight. Thus a large female tends to have a large litter, which tends to depress the birthweight of those pups. This in turn results in a lower adult weight of the females, a smaller litter size and increased birthweight in the next generation.

REFERENCES

1. Huggett ASt.G, Widdas WF. The relationship between mammalian foetal weight and conception age. *J Physiol* 1951; **114**: 306-317.
2. McCance RA, Widdowson EM. Glimpses of comparative growth and development. In: *Human Growth*, 2nd edition, Vol 1. Eds: F Falkner, JM Tanner. New York, London: Plenum Corporation, 1986: pp.145-166.
3. Ferguson-Smith MA, Affara NA, Magenis RE. The ordering of Y–specific sequences by deletion mapping and analysis of X–Y interchange males and females. *Development* 1987: **101**, Supplement: 41-50.
4. Washburn LL, Eicher EM, Sex reversal in XY mice caused by dominant mutation on chromosome 17. *Nature* 1983; **303**: 338-340.

5. Johnson DR. Hair-pin tail: a case of post-reductional gene action in the mouse egg? *Genetics* 1974; **76**: 795-805.
6. Johnson DR. Further observations on the hair-pin tail *(T^{hp})* mutation in the mouse. *Genet Res* 1975; **24**: 207-213.
7. Wakasugi N. A genetically determined incompatibility system between spermatozoa and eggs leading to embryonic death in mice. *J Reprod Fert* 1974; **41**: 85-96.
8. Clarke Fraser F. Interactions and multiple causes. In: *Handbook of Teratology*. Ed. JG Wilson, F Clarke Fraser. New York, London: Plenum Press, 1977: pp.445-463.
9. Walton A, Hammond J. The maternal effects on growth and conformation in Shire horse–Shetland pony crosses. *Proc R Soc*, Ser B 1938; **125**: 311-335.
10. Joubert DM, Hammond J. Maternal effect on birthweight in South Devon x Dexter cattle crosses. *Nature* 1954; **174**: 647-651.
11. Dickinson AG. Some genetic implications of maternal effects. An hypothesis of mammalian growth. *J Agric Sci* 1960; **54**: 378-390.
12. Hunter GL. The maternal influence on size in sheep. *J Agric Sci* 1956; **48**: 36-60.
13. White JM, Legates JE, Eisen EJ. Maternal effects among lines of mice selected for body weight. *Genetics* 1968; **60**: 395-408.
14. Falconer DS. Replicated selection for bodyweight in mice. *Genet Res* 1973; **22**: 291-321.
15. Brumby PJ. The influence of the maternal environment on growth in mice. *Heredity* 1960; **14**: 1-18.
16. Moore RW, Eisen EJ, Ulberg LC. Prenatal and postnatal maternal influences on growth in mice selected for body weight. *Genetics* 1970; **64**: 59-68.
17. Aitken RJ, Bowman P, Gauld I. The effect of synchronous and asynchronous egg transfer on foetal weight in mice selected for large and small body size. *J Embryol Exp Morphol* 1977; **37**: 59-64.
18. Healy MJR, McLaren A, Michie D. Foetal growth in the mouse. *Proc R Soc*, Ser B 1960; **153**: 367-379.
19. McCarthy JC. Genetic and environmental control of foetal and placental weight in the mouse. *Animal Prod* 1965; **7**: 347-361.
20. McLaren A. Genetic and environmental effects on foetal and placental growth in the mouse. *J Reprod Fertil* 1965; **9**: 79-98.
21. Gregg BC. *An investigation of the relationship between pattern formation and growth in the mouse vertebral column*. Ph.D. Thesis. University of London, 1985.
22. Green EL. Genetic and non-genetic factors which influence the type of the skeleton in an inbred strain of mice. *Genetics* 1941; **26**: 192-222.
23. McLaren A, Michie D. Factors affecting vertebral variation in mice. 3. Maternal effects in reciprocal crosses. *J Embryol Exp Morphol* 1956; **4**: 161-166.
24. McLaren A, Michie D. Factors affecting vertebral variation in mice. 4. Experimental proof of the uterine basis of a maternal effect. *J Embryol Exp*

Morphol 1958; **6**: 645-659.
25. Truslove GM. The effect of selection for body-weight on the skeletal variation of the mouse. *Genet Res* 1976; **28**: 1-10.
26. Carter J. The maternal immunological response during pregnancy. In: *Oxford Reviews of Reproductive Biology*, Vol 6. Ed. JR Clarke. Oxford: Clarendon Press, 1984: pp.47-128.
27. Billington WD. Immunological aspects of implantation and fetal survival: the central role of trophoblast. In: *Current Topics in Developmental Biology*, Vol 23. Ed. A McLaren, G Siracusa. New York, London: Academic Press, 1987: pp.209-232.
28. James DA. Some effects of immunological factors on gestation in mice. *J Reprod Fertil* 1967; **14**: 265-272.
29. Beer AE, Scott JR, Billingham RE. Histoincompatibility and maternal immunological status as determinants of fetoplacental weight and litter size in rodents. *J Exp Med* 1975; **142**: 180-196.
30. Clarke AG, Hetherington CM. Effects of maternal preimmunisation on the decidual cell reaction in mice. *Nature* 1971; **230**: 114-115.
31. Clarke AG. The effects of maternal preimmunisation on pregnancy in the mouse. *J Reprod Fertil* 1971; **24**: 369-378.
32. Blakley A. Maternal and embryonic gene effects on placental weight in mice. *J Reprod Fertil* 1978; **54**: 301-307.
33. Hetherington CM, Fowler H. Effect of tolerance to paternal antigens on placental and fetal weight in the mouse. *J Reprod Fertil* 1978; **52**: 113-117.
34. Ounsted M. Concepts and criteria of fetal growth. In: *Abnormal Fetal Growth: Biological Bases and Consequences*. Ed. F Naftolin. West Berlin: Dahlem Konferenzen, 1978: pp.21-48.
35. Bruce NW, Norman N. Influence of sexual dimorphism on foetal and placental weights in the rat. *Nature* 1975; **257**: 62-63.
36. Seller MJ, Perkins-Cole KJ. Sex difference in mouse embryonic development at neurulation. *J Reprod Fertil* 1987; **79**: 159-161.
37. Burgoyne PS, Evans EP, Holland K. XO monosomy is associated with reduced birthweight and lowered weight gain in the mouse. *J Reprod Fertil* 1983; **68**: 381-385.
38. Burgoyne PS, Tam PP, Evans EP. Retarded development of XO conceptuses during early pregnancy in the mouse. *J Reprod Fertil* 1983; **68**: 387-393.
39. Tsunoda Y, Tokunaga T, Sugie T. Altered sex ratio of live young after transfer of fast- and slow-developing mouse embryos. *Gamete Res* 1985; **12:** 301-304.
40. Falconer DS, Gauld IK, Roberts RC. Cell numbers and cell sizes in organs of mice selected for large and small body size. *Genet Res* 1978; **31**: 387-301.
41. Blakley A. Embryonic bone growth in lines of mice selected for large and small body size. *Genet Res* 1979; **34**: 77-85.
42. Roberts RC. The growth of mice selected for large and small size in relation to food intake and the efficiency of conversion. *Genet Res* 1981; **38**: 9-24.
43. Priestley GC, Robertson MSM. Protein and nucleic acid metabolism in organs from mice selected for large and small body size. *Genet Res* 1973; **22**: 255-278.

44. Falconer DS, Gauld IK, Roberts RC. Growth control in chimeras. In: *Genetic Mosaics and Chimeras in Mammals*. Ed. LB Russell. New York: Plenum Press, 1978: pp.39-49.
45. Falconer DS, Gauld IK, Roberts RC, Williams DA. The control of body size in mouse chimeras. *Genet Res* 1981; **38**: 25-46.
46. Snow MHL. Control of embryonic growth rate and fetal size in mammals. In: *Human Growth*, 2nd edition Vol 1. Ed. by F Falkner, JM Tanner. New York, London: Plenum Corporation, 1986: pp.67-82.
47. Snow MHL. Restorative growth in mammalian embryos. In: *Issues and Reviews in Teratology*, Vol 1. Ed. H Kalter. New York: Plenum Corporation, 1983: pp.251-284.

Fetal growth curves

Professor P.-H. Persson

INTRODUCTION

Recording birthweights of newborn infants is a relatively new procedure. The French obstetrician, François Mauriceau was perhaps the first to record an infant's birthweight. The first apparently accurate report on birthweights was published in Göttingen in 1753 by the German obstetrician Johannes Roederer. He found the average birthweight of male infants to be 3050 g and of females 2860 g.(1) One of the first investigators to point out that all babies with a low birthweight were not necessarily premature was Raymond D McBurney. In 1946, he presented cases of "undernourished full-term infants" thus introducing the concept of restricted intrauterine growth.(2) Low birthweight, due to premature birth, undernourishment or a combination of both, is associated with a high rate of perinatal mortality and morbidity.(3,4) Consequently, intrauterine growth retardation, true or suspected, is one of the major clinical dilemmas today. In Sweden diagnosis and treatment of intrauterine growth retardation demands approximately 10% of the total resources for obstetric care. Since the beginning of the 60s a large number of articles have been published on the classification of newborn infants according to their birthweight and length, as well as standard curves for intrauterine growth. Due to the inaccessibility of the fetus *in utero*, most growth curves were based on the endpoint observations of birthweight and are by their nature cross-sectional. It is seldom known whether a low birthweight is the result of a continuously low, but otherwise normal, growth velocity for that particular fetus or if it is due to deviation from the predetermined growth rate. It has also been repeatedly pointed out that a birthweight falling within the normal limits can nonetheless constitute a deviation from the predetermined growth rate. Futhermore, preterm births probably do not reflect true intrauterine growth.

Almost all published growth curves are typically sigmoid-shaped with a flattening of the curve towards and past term. Most growth charts show a positively skewed distribution. Naeye and Dixon, as well as Milner and Richards thought this to be due to a large proportion of the babies being born with gestational age wrongly assessed.(5,6) The British birth study of 1970 showed the terminal flattening of the weight curve to be less pronounced when gestational age could be considered reliable.(7) It seems that the inability to assess gestational age correctly is one of the major problems with cross-sectional growth charts and one of the reasons for the numerous different standard charts published in the literature.

In 1958, Ian Donald introduced diagnostic ultrasound into clinical medicine. This new invention gave us a unique instrument for direct observation of the fetus. In 1964, Willcocks *et al.* showed a correlation between fetal biparietal diameter measured by ultrasound and birthweight.(8) In 1965, Thompson *et al.* suggested that fetal trunk dimensions could be measured by ultrasound in order to estimate fetal weight.(9) Since then many publications on the growth of various fetal dimensions, mainly linear, have been published. Many longitudinal studies on fetal growth have also been published. The important new contribution of ultrasound to perinatology was the possibility of an objective assessment of gestational age.(10,11) These two possibilities have been utilised in rather extensive studies on the Malmö population regarding fetal growth. Some results will be briefly presented here.

Longitudinal growth curves

Serially derived studies of growth *in utero* have the drawback that some of the individual series will be interrupted by inappropriate early delivery, causing a dropout of observations towards term. Another weakness is represented by the ultrasound method that is used for weight estimation. Most formulae for estimation of fetal weight have been developed for measurements in late pregnancy and are not valid in the second trimester or early third trimester. When developing a formula, it is important to use a stratified sample with equal numbers of observations in each weight class in the range for which the formula is intended. Using a multiple regression analysis, we evolved a formula, valid for second and third trimester, for estimating fetal weight *in utero* based on fetal biparietal (BPD), abdominal diameters (AD) (mean of two orthogonal readings) and femur length

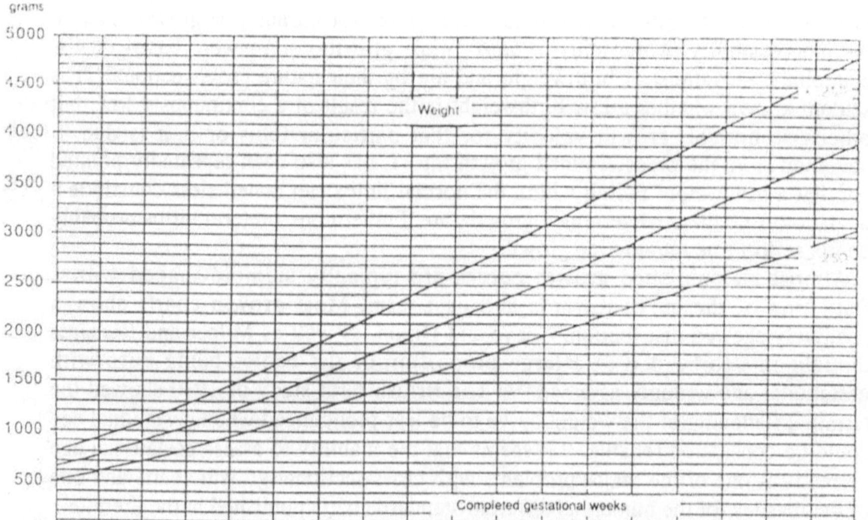

Figure I.
Reference growth curve (mean ± 2SD) serially derived from ultrasound weight estimations. (n=177).

(FL). Measurements were done by ultrasound within 48 hours before delivery or legal abortion in a stratified sample of 89 pregnancies, approximately 10 in each 500 g weight class up to 5000 g. Tested on 135 neonates of varying birthweights, the formula evolved as:

$$\text{weight} = \text{BPD}^{0.972} \times \text{AD}^{1.743} \times \text{FL}^{0.367} \times 10^{-2.647}$$

which neither under- nor over-estimated weight in any weight class, the error in estimates having an SD of 7.1% and the maximum error being 18% of true weight.

This formula was applied to 177 longitudinal measurements in 19 normal pregnancies. None of these had gestational age corrected. The data of estimated weights against gestational age (GA) were best fitted to a third degree equation (weight = $1443.4 - 32.32 \times GA + 0.203 \times GA^2 - 0.000215 \times GA^3$). The residual around the curve line corresponds to an SD of 11%. The growth standard thus obtained is shown in Figure 1. The procedure has been reported in detail elsewhere.[12]

Table 1. Longitudinal growth in late pregnancy.

Gestational day at delivery (mean and range)	n	Weight (g) (mean and SD) and deviation from the mean of reference curve (%) 225 days	261 days	delivery	Growth between day 225 and 261	day 261 and birth
295 (293 – 297)	22	2010±261 +1.2	3135±384 +1.1	3960±450 −1.4	30.3±5.8	25.6±12.0
289 (286 – 292)	140	1988±245 −0.2	3066±371 +0.7	3760±451 −1.4	29.3±3.5	25.9±10.0
282 (279 – 285)	290	2025±235 +0.8	3046±389 +1.2	3613±459 −0.5	28.0±4.2	26.3±11.2
275 (272 – 278)	226	1947±244 −1.7	2964±379 −1.7	3398±416 −1.2	27.8±4.9	26.0±13.1
268 (265 – 271)	122	1980±314 −0.6	2984±403 −2.0	3190±520 −2.0	28.2±5.4	27.0±17.0
All 280 (265 – 297)	800	1990±252 −0.2	3020±380 −0.2	3520±454 −0.8	28.2±4.6	26.2±12.1

Fetal weight was estimated at 32 and 37 weeks of gestation. Daily growth was calculated between 37 weeks and delivery. The material was divided into 5 groups according to the interval between the 37 week ultrasound examination and delivery, e.g. delivery in the 42nd, 41st, 40th, 39th and 38th completed week.

In the series presented above it was not possible to evaluate growth beyond 39 completed weeks. For the purpose of studying fetal growth around and post term, 800 pregnancies, representing an unselected part of the total population examined on a routine basis alone, were sampled. All women were examined by ultrasound at 32 and 37 weeks of pregnancy. Weight was estimated using the above formula. At delivery, which occurred 3–40 days after the 37 week examination, the infant's birthweight was recorded. The 800 deliveries were divided into 5 groups to the period elapsing between the last examination and delivery: 7, 14, 21, 28 and 34 days; 22 fetuses of the group were born large for gestational age (LGA)(mean + 2SD of the reference population) and 20 were born small for gestational age (SGA)(mean – 2SD of the reference population). In each group the daily growth rate was calculated for the period 32–37 weeks and 37 weeks to delivery.

The results of this series are shown in Table 1. No difference was found at 32 and 37 weeks in the estimated mean weight between the five groups who were

Table 2 Longitudinal growth in late pregnancy.

± 4.0		Gestatational age at examination (mean+SD)				Gestational age at delivery	
		225±4.0		261±4.4		265–279	280–296
Size at birth	n	weight (g) and % dev	growth g/day	weight(g) and % dev	growth g/day	birthweight (g) and % deviation	
LGA	12	2330 ±5.1%	→ 37.8 →	3660 +20.4%	→ 37.6 →	4370 +30.4%	
	10				→ 42.6 →		4650 +30.0%
AGA	316	1980 –0.2%	→ 29.2 →	3040 –0.2%	→ 27.5 →	3320 –0.2%	
	442				→ 26.3 →		3680 –1.3%
SGA	20	1860 –13.4%	→ 19.4 →	2420 –20.5%	→ 1.7 →	2490 –29.1%	
All	348	1990 –0.2%	→ 28.2 →	3020 –0.2%	→ 26.3 →	3320 –08%	
	452				→ 26.1 →		3700 –1.2%

Same material as in Table 1 but divided according to birthweight: Large for gestational age (LGA) above mean + 2SD of birthweight for GA, adequate for gestational age (AGA) between mean ± 2SD for GA and small for gestational age (SGA) mean –2SD for GA.

delivered at various intervals after 37 weeks, e.g. at 38, 39, 40, 41 and 42 completed weeks. No systematic over- or underestimation in mean weights compared with the longitudinal study on 19 fetuses was found. The birthweights were on the average 1% below that of the reference population. The average daily weight gain between 32 and 37 weeks was 28.2 g and between 37 weeks and delivery 26.2 g. In pregnancies where a longer period elapsed between the 37 week examination and delivery, the growth rate decreased. The daily weight gained for post-term deliveries was 25.6 g. Table 2 shows that the LGA infants had a daily weight gain between 32 and 37 weeks and between 37 weeks and term delivery of 37.8 g. LGA infants who were born post-term had a higher weight gain (42 g/day) after 37 weeks. The growth of the infants who were delivered small for gestational age was below that of the average between 32 and 37 weeks (19 g per day) and after the 37 week examination, the growth almost ceased, and about 50% of the infants actually decreased their weight between 37 weeks and delivery compared with 6% in the appropriate-for-gestational-age (AGA) group.

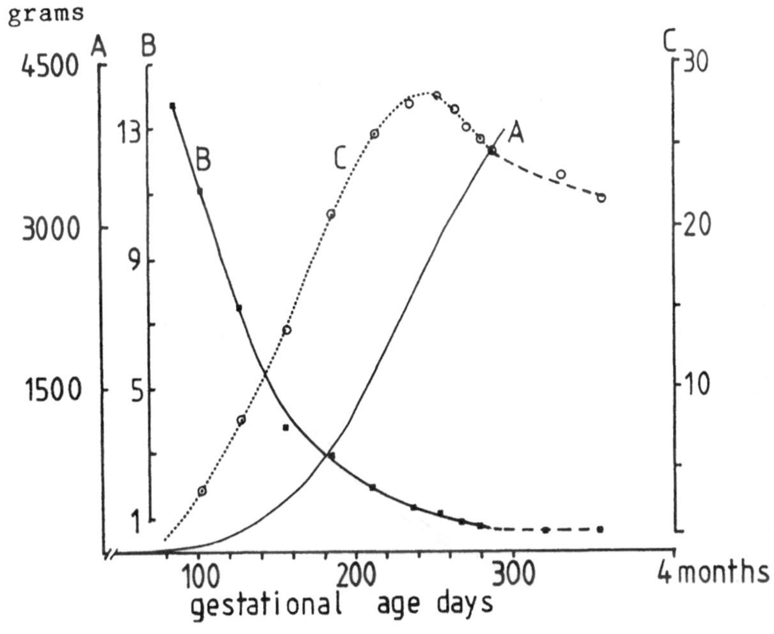

Figure II
Combination of two longitudinal ultrasound growth studies. (n=179+800)
Curve A represents ultrasound estimated fetal weights in grams on gestational age. Curve B represents the daily weight increase in percent of estimated weight. Curve C represents the daily weight growth in g/day. The B and C curves are extended to 4 months, postnatally. Values were obtained from Swedish reference curve for children.

In Figure II, the two longitudinal studies have been combined in order to calculate firstly the daily weight increment in absolute values (g per day), secondly the relation of daily weight increase in relation to the fetal weight (% per day) and the intrauterine growth over time. The daily weight increment has a maximum of ± 28 g per day ~ 250 days gestation. There is a slight decrease in weight gain to about 26 g per day ~ 280 days and an even further reduction to 24 g per day post-term. A daily growth in absolute figures directly continuous into the daily growth during the neonatal period as judged from the Swedish reference curve for children.

In a group of 59 twin pregnancies (25 monozygotic and 34 dizygotic) appearing in the Malmö population from 1982–1984, ultrasound examination was performed as a mean 4.5 times (3–6) during pregnancy. Fetal weight was estimated using the above presented formula. Zygosity was determined by blood grouping in all like-sexed babies. The weight data were fitted to equations by polynomial regressional analysis. Figure III shows the growth curves for mono- and dizygotic twins in comparison with the singleton growth curve. Previous works comparing the growth of twin and singleton birthweights suggested that the maternal organism is

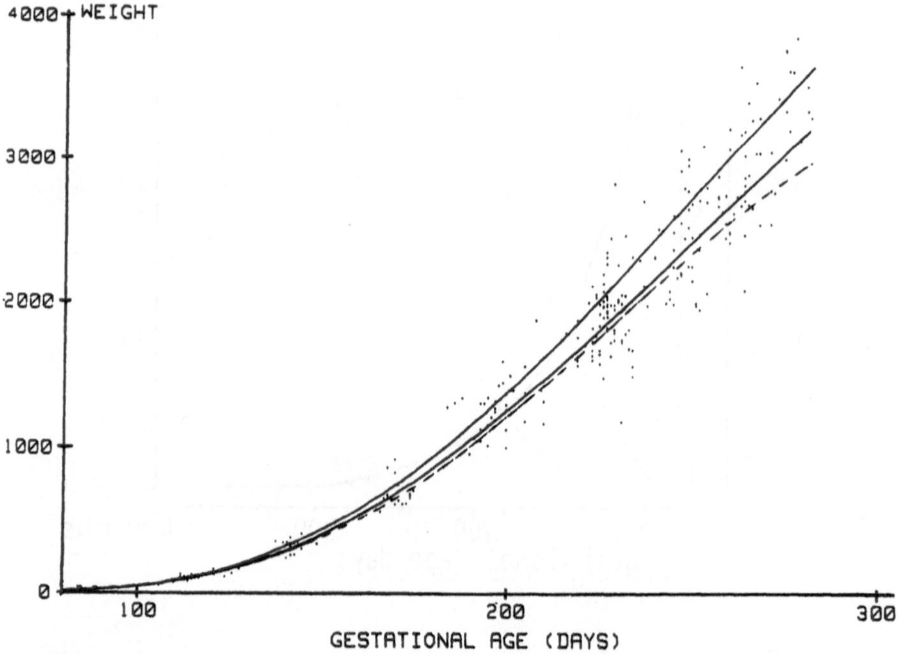

Figure III
Longitudinal ultrasound estimated fetal weight curves from 25 monozygotic and 34 dizygotic twins in comparison with the reference curve for singletons.

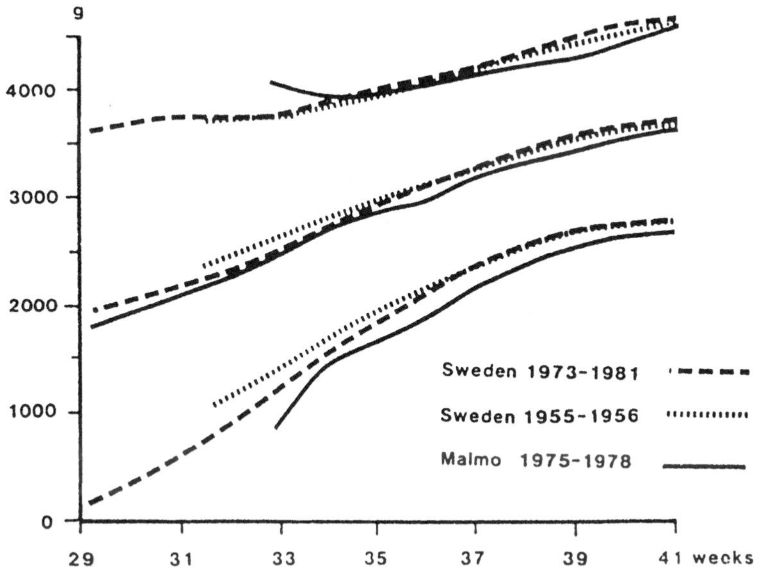

Figure IV. Birthweight curves obtained without objective assessment of GA illustrating their lack of difference. Sweden 1955/56 (n=59 984), representing a sample with regular menstrual periods; Sweden 1973–81 (n=823 000), raw data; Malmö 1975 (n=9 785) all liveborn infants.

capable of supporting fetal growth in multiple pregnancy until the total fetal weight reaches ~ 3.2 kg and that growth was restricted in multiple pregnancy from ~ 30 weeks' gestation.[13] However, when intrauterine growth is assessed longitudinally, a continuously slow growth rate can be found in twins compared with singletons, the difference between twins and singletons being significant already at 16 weeks and between mono- and dizygotic twins at 20 weeks.

Cross-sectional birthweight curves

Sterky *et al.* presented the first Swedish growth chart based on birthweights in 1956. Their basic material included all singleton births during 1955/56. Thirty-eight percent of the pregnancies were excluded from the material to obtain reliable information of gestational length at delivery. From the Swedish Medical Birth Register (by courtesy of Professor Bengt Källén) the birthweights of 825 550 singleton deliveries were obtained for the period 1973–1981. Figure IV compares the birthweight standards from Sweden 1955/56 and 1973–1981 and for the Malmö population 1975–1977. There appears to be no difference between the

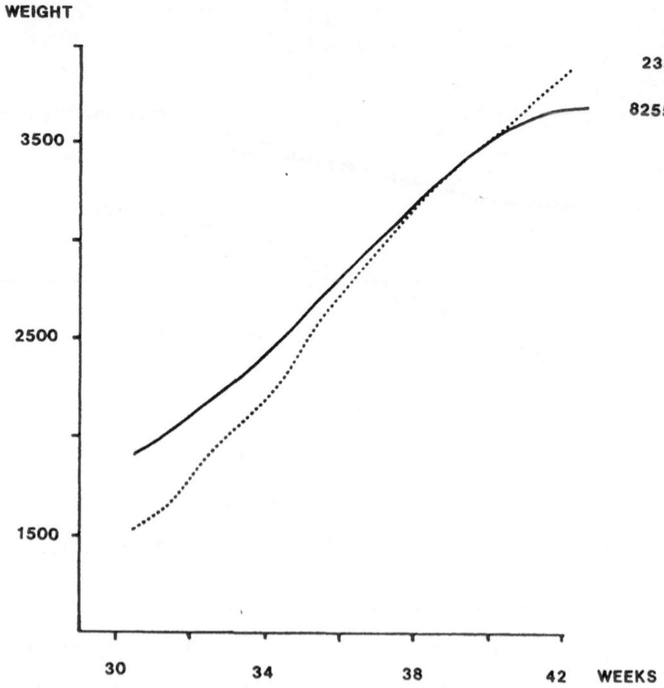

Figure V
Mean birthweight of all liveborn singletons in Sweden 1973–81 (825 000) compared with all liveborn singletons in Malmö 1979–87 (23 571).

three standard curves although the Sterky material was highly selected to obtain "normality".[14]

Partly from the same national register, all 23 000 deliveries from the city of Malmö during 1978–1987 were reviewed. In 97% of all Malmö pregnancies, gestational age is assessed and corrected according to BPD measurements in the first half of pregnancy. Figure V shows the difference between the mean values of birthweights by gestational age in two populations: the total Swedish population where gestational age is usually assessed based on the woman's statement of her menstrual period and by clinical examination in early pregnancy, and in the Malmö population where gestational age is objectively assessed by ultrasound on a routine basis. From 35 weeks' gestation and onward, there is a good agreement between the cross-sectional growth curve (with correction for gestational age by ultrasound) and the longitudinal growth curve. Between 28 and 35 weeks' gestation, the mean values of the cross-sectional growth curve were significantly below the mean values of the longitudinal growth curve with a maximum difference of 200 g at 32 weeks (Figure V).

Table 3 Frequency of birthweights below or equal to mean –2 SD and –3 SD of intrauterine growth. (n=12 000)

Gestational age(weeks)	≤ mean –2SD %	≤ mean –3SD %
≤28	3.3	
29	10.0	
30	29.4	11.5
31	36.4	2.9
32	23.3	3.3
33	17.7	6.0
34	14.3	2.9
35	5.7	2.4
36	5.4	0.0
37	2.3	0.7
38	1.9	0.5
39	2.0	0.1
40	2.7	—
≤41	3.2	—

Limits of normal fetal growth

Growth is a process over time. In the individual case, the birthweight tells us very little about intrauterine growth in the weeks just before delivery. The lack of longitudinal growth studies has reduced the problem of defining fetal growth to a problem of defining normal fetal size at delivery. In Scandinavian countries, it has been assumed that the distribution of birthweights is symmetrical. Normal fetal growth has therefore been defined as a birthweight within ±2 SD of mean weight for gestational age. The large Swedish studies presented above as well as most other growth charts, have an asymmetrical distribution with, in most cases, a positive skew. Application of a non-parametrical method to describe the dispersion of fetal growth is therefore considered a necessity, and consequently the distribution is expressed in centiles. The 5th or the 10th centile is usually taken as the cut-off limit for normal fetal size at birth. This limit indicates that 5–10% of all neonates have suffered poor intrauterine growth. However, when the weight charts are based on an objective assessment of gestational age, the distribution before 36 weeks and after 41 weeks becomes negatively skewed. The standard growth curve obtained from our two longitudinal intrauterine studies had a distribution that was quite symmetrical. The distribution was found to be proportional to the mean birthweight for gestational age and the dispersion of the weights around the mean had an SD of 11–12%. The same distribution was found in the cross-sectional material with correction for gestational age by ultrasound. The negative skew in the preterm period of the birthweight material is probably due to a relatively large proportion of growth retarded fetuses born during this gestation. Table 3 shows the proportion of birthweights below mean –2 and –3 SD of the intrauterine standard

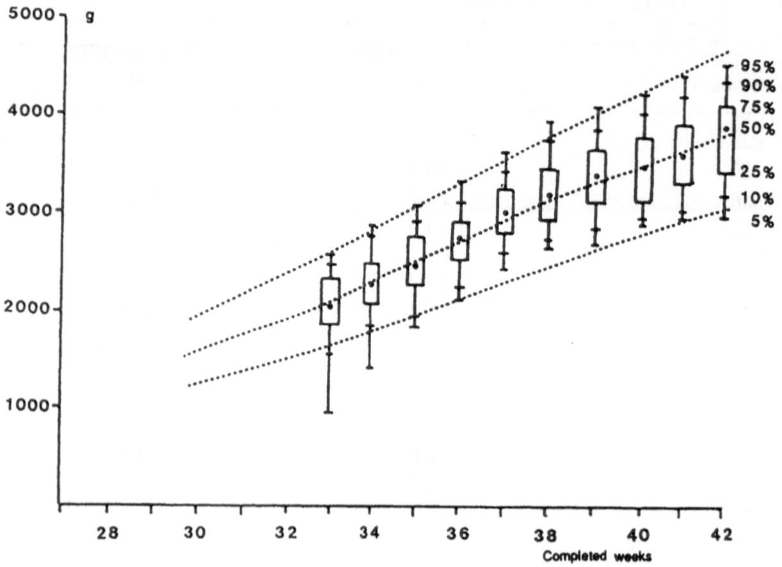

Figure VI.
Comparison of the longitudinal intrauterine weight curve (broken lines, mean ± 2SD) and birthweight distribution (dots, boxes and bars representing percentiles as indicated) illustrating the negatively skewed distribution pre- and post-term when GA is objectively assessed by ultrasound.

curve for the Malmö population over a period of 7 years. At 31 weeks' gestation as many as one third of the deliveries resulted in a birthweight below or equal to mean –2 SD of the intrauterine standard curve. In total, as many as 10% of all babies born before 37 completed weeks had weight below mean –2 SD.

Assessment of gestational age

The British birth study of 1970[7] showed the terminal flattening of the weight curve to be less pronounced when gestational age could be considered reliable, which is in consonance with the data presented here. The completely different growth curve obtained when gestational age is based on an objective assessment stresses the importance of a correct estimation of gestational age. The reliability of ultrasound fetometry for estimation of gestational age in the second trimester has been evaluated in several studies.[11,15] Measurements of fetal variables such as the biparietal diameter, femur length or crown-rump length have been shown to estimate gestational age with an error of about 3 days (SD) with a maximum error of ± 10 days.[11] Due to the shape of the growth curves, ultrasound fetometry is less accurate for estimation of gestational age in the second trimester of pregnancy. In unselected populations gestational age is unknown in at least 25% of cases. In the Malmö population 15% of mothers have gestational age corrected by more than 14 days at the routine ultrasound examination in the first half of pregnancy. In as many as 12% of the women who are certain of their last menstrual period, the date of delivery is corrected by more than 14 days. There appears to be no way of selecting a group of women, by careful anamnesis or by symptoms, where a fetometry examination in the first half of pregnancy would be less worthwhile than in other women. In our experience, it is necessary to examine all women to be able to correct gestational age in the population at large. The impact of an organised examination in the first half of pregnancy can be well demonstrated in the Swedish population. Date of delivery is predicted with an error (SD) of 13 days in the unselected population. For the Malmö population where a screening has been performed for more than a decade, the date of delivery is predicted with an error of 7 days. Today almost all pregnant Swedish women are examined by ultrasound in the first half of pregnancy. This has resulted in an improvement of the prediction of date of delivery in cases where the women cannot state a reliable last menstrual period. In cases with reliable dates, corrections are not performed unless the discrepancy is more than 7–10 days. The result of the ultrasound examination, however, in most cases is not used to influence determination of gestational age.

Therefore, in the unselected population of Swedish women with reliable dates no improvement in the prediction of date of delivery has been recorded over the last 10-year period. Unless a correction on a day-by-day basis is performed, ultrasound examination seems to be without clinical consequences for the assessment of gestational age. A day-by-day correction seems to be necessary; otherwise the diagnosis of intrauterine growth deviation will be imprecise. If an error of 7 days in the estimate of gestational age is accepted generally, a given estimated fetal size will be an uncertainty of 0.7 SD in the reference curve.

DISCUSSION

The cross-sectional growth chart based on birthweight versus gestational age after objective assessment of gestational age, as well as the longitudinal growth curve, is best described as a curve with a weak sigmoid-shape. In such curves, there appears to be no physiological constraint towards term or post term. The flattening of the growth curve found in most cross-sectional materials seems to be a finding confounded by our inability to assess gestational age by conventional clinical methods. In the longitudinal series, the daily weight increment was increased throughout pregnancy to ~ 28 g per day around 250 days' gestation. The growth rate thereafter decreased to ~ 24 g per day at 42 weeks' gestation compared to 20 g per day at 4 months postnatal age. This is in contrast to most other published growth charts. The daily weight gain was calculated by Thompson in 1970 for Aberdeen infants.(16) They found the daily weight gain to be 36 g between 32 and 36 weeks, then falling to 25 g per day between 36 and 38 weeks and to 14 g per day between 38 and 40 weeks. After 40 weeks' gestation the weight gain went down to 3.5 g per day. It has been supposed that the almost negligible fetal growth after the growth spurt at 36 weeks is imposed on the fetus by maternal or placental factors restraining growth. In my opinion it is merely a consequence of our inability to assess gestational age. It can be concluded that the intrauterine growth standard is different from the birthweight standard, at least in the preterm period. If the birthweight standard is chosen as the reference, a non-parametrical definition of the limits must be chosen, and percentiles seem logical. If the intrauterine weight is chosen as the standard, it seems logical to use standard deviations as the basis for the definition of normal growth. It must be pointed out that because of the negative skew the 5th centile of birthweight corresponds to 4.5 SD below the mean of intrauterine weights at 33 weeks' gestation. At 39 weeks' gestation, the 5th centile equals 1.8 SD below the mean. The longitudinal study on weight gain showed that infants born small for gestational age had almost no weight gain after 37 weeks' gestation. This finding might prompt more active management in the care of intrauterine growth retarded infants with a liberal attitude towards preterm induction of delivery. However, if an active attitude is adopted, one must be very careful with the identification of the growth retarded fetus. A necessary prerequisite is objective assessment of gestational age based on its correction at the time of the early screening examination to prevent adverse effect to the baby by clinical intervention in false positive cases.

REFERENCES

1. Cone TE. Pediatric history: the history of weighing the newborn infant. *Pediatrics* 1961; **28**:490-498.
2. McBurney RD. The undernourished fullterm infant. *West J Surg* 1947; **55**: 363-370.
3. Jones RA, Roberton NRC. Problems of the small-for-dates baby. *Clin Obstet Gynaecol* 1984; **11**:499-524.
4. Heinonen K, Matilainen R, Koski H, Launiala K. Intra-uterine growth retardation (IUGR) in preterm infants. *J Perinat Med* 1985; **13**:171-178.
5. Naeye L, Dixon JB. Distortions in fetal growth standards. *Pediatr Res* 1978; **12**:987-991.
6. Milner RD, Richards B. An analysis of birth weight by gestational age of infants born in England and Wales, 1967 to 1971. *J Obstet Gynaecol* 1974; **81**:956-967.
7. Chamberlain R. (ed.) *British Births 1970*. London: William Heinemann Medical Books Ltd., 1975; pp.48-88.
8. Willcocks J, Donald J, Duggan TC, Day N. Foetal cephalometry by ultrasound. *J Obstet Gynaecol Brit Comm* 1964; **71**:11-20.
9. Thompson HE, Holmes JH, Gottesfeld KR, Taylor ES. Fetal development as determined by pulsed echo techniques. *Amer J Obstet Gynec* 1965; **92**:44-49.
10. Campbell S, Warsof SL, Little D, Cooper DJ. Routine ultrasound screening for the prediction of gestational age. *Obstet Gynecol* 1985; **65**:613-620.
11. Persson PH, Weldner BM. Reliability of ultrasound fetometry in estimating gestational age in the second trimester. *Acta Obstet Gynecol Scand* 1986; **65**:481-483.

12. Persson PH, Weldner BM. Intra-uterine weight curves obtained by ultrasound. *Acta Obstet Gynecol Scand* 1986; **65**:169-173.
13. McKeown T, Record RG. Observations on foetal growth in multiple pregnancy in man. *J Endocrinol* 1952; **8**:386-401.
14. Sterky G. Swedish standard curves for intra-uterine growth. *Pediatrics* 1970; **46**:7-8.
15. Persson PH, Grennert L, Gennser G, Gullberg B. Normal range curves for the intrauterine growth of the biparietal diameter. *Acta Obstet Gynecol Scand* 1978; **Suppl 78**:15-20.
16. Tanner JM, Thomson AM. Standards for birthweight at gestation periods from 32 to 42 weeks allowing for maternal height and weight. *Arch Dis Child* 1970; **45**:566-569.

Discussion

Chairman: Professor R. D. G. Milner

CAMPBELL: You said that your cross-sectional birthweight graph corrected for gestational age was linear. But that is to some extent dominated by the 42 week readings. How many values do you have at 42 weeks?

PERSSON: It was 10 years ago, but I think that there were 400 to 500. It is true that it is not a straight line; it is a curve. What we see here is the inexactness in pregnancy dating. This error means that we underestimate gestational age with two or three dates which can be seen in the curve.

RUSH: Could you tell us whether maternal weight gain is also linear in the third trimester in your population — especially in the last month?

PERSSON: I don't know.

MILNER: If we accepted a constant rate of weight gain over that period we might be thinking of a background of a stable maternal nutrient intake.

RUSH: One of the characteristics that distinguishes Third World pregnancies from those in the developed countries is a marked falloff in weight gain towards term among economically deprived women. Sweden, in our thinking, represents the limiting case of affluence and provision. I wondered if this corollary measure was parallel.

PERSSON: It is only the case if you correct gestational age. If you live with the old method of determining gestational age it is exactly the same as it has been for the last 40 years; there is no change whatsoever.

WIGGLESWORTH: There is a slight contradiction between what you are saying and what Dr Snow said. This was in the time at which there was evidence of growth retardation in multiples. You are saying that in humans you could recognise it by ultrasound at 15 weeks or so. It fitted in with the growth charts. But in humans, that would seem not too dissimilar to Dr Snow's data. I think he mentioned 14 days in the rat which would be around organogenesis, and in the mouse 10 days. Is there a contradiction there, and why should that be?

PERSSON: I am not sure that there is any contradiction. But we are talking about human fetuses. We have the work done by McKeown and Record.[1] They state some 28-30 weeks, but this is not the case. Growth retardation is definite already at 15 weeks, and that is after organogenesis in man.

SNOW: I find it very difficult indeed to make inter-species comparisons. In straight anatomical terms my 10 $^1/_2$ days stage would be something like 36 to 40 days in man — very early indeed in clinical terms. This afternoon I will mention some data on twinning studies in the mouse, where people have made monozygotic twins. In such pregnancies there is a very early catch-up in size which takes place during organogenesis. So they are of a normal singleton size from about half way through organogenesis into the fetal period. But then their weight declines, and that is true even though there are not a lot of individuals in the litter. Only one study shows this, but there are other studies in the mouse which show similar unexplained decline in fetal growth towards the end of pregnancy.

MILNER: That is a fascinating concept. Is there something about total fetal load that may optimise fetal environment to produce the best expression of genetic growth potential? Will a pair of twins provide too little of whatever factor 'x' is for the environment to optimise their genetic potential?

SNOW: It is probably something like that. The published data on the relationship between litter size and fetal weight in the mouse show a negative correlation, suggesting that total fetal mass influences individual fetal growth towards birth. The observation of a decline in growth in circumstances where fetal mass would not be expected to depress growth suggests some other feedback interaction between fetus and mother. We have wondered whether *corpus luteum* function, perhaps through progesterone levels in early gestation may be involved in setting up this aspect of the materno-fetal relationship. In this context it may be significant that in the examples discussed the embryo is known to have been small during early organogenesis when placental development is also in its early stages.

MILNER: Thank you very much. That kind of information can only come from a polytocous species.

HALL: I want to ask Dr Persson about the problem of fetuses which would disappear from the study by being delivered. One of the problems of longitudinal studies is that you always lose some cases. Have you looked at your data including only the people who could be studied all the way through?

PERSSON: That is a problem. This study is too small and needs to be repeated; only 30 fetuses were followed throughout pregnancy. But there was no constraint towards delivery. Fifty percent of the pregnancies were delivered before 39 weeks and 6 days, and the rest continued.

HALL: But you could look at them separately.

PERSSON: Yes, we did so. We made curves for eight individuals separately, but there was no difference between them.

CLAPP: We have recently completed a series of longitudinal observations, before, during and after pregnancy and have found that average weight gain is about 14.5 kg in our middle and upper socioeconomic class population. We find that maternal weight gain is linear in early pregnancy, but there is a distinct tailoff after 32 weeks in well nourished women with a better than average overall weight gain.

We have also been doing body compositional measurements on the newborns at birth and find that 65% of the variance in birthweight at term is due to variance in body fat. We find a linear relationship between lean body mass and birthweight over the last four to six weeks of gestation. I wondered whether you had done any body compositional studies in your newborns in Sweden?

PERSSON: No.

MILNER: May I ask how you get those lean body mass and body fat estimates?

CLAPP: By treating the body as a group of cylinders.

ALBERMAN: I am uncomfortable about correcting gestational age. Has anyone followed the longitudinal growth of a twin that has survived while its co-twin has not?

CAMPBELL: I was trying to work out the effect of wrongly correcting gestational age. I think that the corrections were made around 18–20 weeks. If, for example, a fetus that was going to be large was corrected, and similarly a small fetus was also corrected, by mistake, what effect would that have?

PERSSON: That would turn the curve clockwise. It will give an S-curve.

CAMPBELL: Do you think that could be a factor?

PERSSON: Yes, in the cross-sectional curve it is definitely a factor.

CAMPBELL: Could it be in your ultrasound?

PERSSON: Yes, but a week is too much. The difference between those who are small compared with those who are large for gestational age is three days in average date of delivery, when you compare based on ultrasound.

MILNER: So, in other words you would overestimate by three days. The mother says that she is 18 weeks, but you would correct it to 17 weeks 4 days.

PERSSON: Yes; it means that the small for gestational age fetuses in our study are delivered at 278 days. Those who are large are delivered at 282 or 283 days.

CAMPBELL: I do not totally agree. Some small babies are out by more than that and there is the possibility of that artificially influencing the end part of your graph. My feeling is that there is a genuine falloff between 38 and 42 weeks, especially between 40 and 42 weeks, and that this may be masked by early correcting.

PERSSON: It is exaggerated by correcting.

MILNER: May we clarify that point because it is fundamental to the interpretation of body weight versus gestation curve.

EIK NES: I have just finished a series of 2500 consecutive women who were dated on ultrasound. Since we introduced routine screening in Norway, there is a great deal of interest in what date should be used. We want to use the ultrasound date, so we have made a statistical analysis of factors affecting dating by ultrasound. In that group of 2500 there was a sub-group that had a birthweight of more than 4.2 kg. We looked at how they delivered related to when they were predicted to deliver. We could show the three-day difference too.

MILNER: Are you saying that the babies weighing 4.2 kg delivered three days later than would otherwise have been expected? Which starting date are we using for the gestational clock? Is it based on maternal history, or is it determined on the basis of the 18 week ultrasound?

EIK NES: The problem that we face is that we have our normal populations from which the tables are made. When we date the pregnancy in the 18th week we have to assume that it is a 50 percentile pregnancy. There is no other way. Obviously there are fetuses on the 17th percentile and on the 21st percentile at 18 weeks, but we cannot know that. The error we are making in our dating is three days. It certainly does not influence the question of weight for dates.

PERSSON: There is one other experiment that can be done. One can measure other parameters. You can measure the head circumference, the distance between the eyes, the feet and whatever else you wish. You can date the pregnancy based on these parameters. It is mainly the fetal head that is affected in early pregnancy, so if you include other parameters then you would arrive at a more correct estimate of gestational age.

CLAPP: There are two issues that bother me about the conclusions being drawn based on one of the fundamental precepts of biology. The first is that in very early pregnancy you can detect the overgrown and the undergrown fetus, and that there is a restraining factor that early on. I am not familiar with rodent experimentation, but I am with the pig. With the pig at 30 days gestation there is great variation in placental size depending on where the fetus is in the horn. There is no variation in fetal size. To me it would be extremely unusual if prior to the end of definitive placentation at 18 weeks in the human one was able to see a restraint on embryonic and early fetal growth. The second issue is the idea that a cell stops growing before functional maturation occurs. I would expect to see some tailoff in growth towards term to allow that explosion of functional maturation in preparation for extrauterine existence. That is why we have definite growth curves, and that is why we express them in lean body mass. We also see a linear relationship right up through the 42nd week, but I find it disturbing from a fundamental point of view. Can anyone shed light on this issue?

RUSH: It seems to me that your data is consistent with variability at 18 weeks. You are saying that a larger fetus at 18 weeks delivers "three days later". It is probably not three days later; it is probably a larger fetus at 18 weeks.

MILNER: The point that I picked up from Professor Persson is that if you use centiles the pathobiological interpretation of being below the 10th centile at 30 weeks is dramatically different from being below the 10th centile at 40 weeks. Might we not consider using standard deviations for birthweight curves, and this concept as a clinical tool for obstetric/paediatric practice in the UK?

STEER: I think that the question of whether we ought to be using standard deviations or centiles is probably not appropriate. The only validity of centiles or standard deviations is in relation to the distribution. The mistake is that we keep equating points below 2 SDs or points below a certain centile with growth retardation, whereas it is simply a measurement of size. If we dissociate in our minds the question of the distribution from whether or not a baby is growth retarded then the whole of the argument you mentioned disappears.

STEWART: I want to ask Professor Persson how often he corrected the gestational age. How much does this reflect a purely ultrasound measurement, and how often are you agreeing with the mother?

MILNER: This is a piece of information that is often missing from the published literature.

PERSSON: We correct more that 14 days in 14 to 15% of the population, and there is no way of preselecting those who are more likely to be corrected — those who have used contraceptive pills for example. You have to examine the whole population to catch the women you must correct. The Swedish registers show gestational age at delivery of the entire population to be 280 days with one standard deviation of 13 days. If you look at those from Malmö one standard deviation is seven days. If you look at those women who do not know their gestational age one standard deviation is also seven days after dating by ultrasound. If you had a woman who has safe data, regular menstrual periods, it is back to 13 days again. This means that if you do an ultrasound examination and do not correct gestational age because the woman thinks that she knows better, you are back to the 13 days standard deviation. Looking at Swedish figures it means that ultrasound is good where you do not know the last menstrual period, and it is no use when you know it.

WIGGLESWORTH: In human pregnancies, where you do not have observed, timed matings there is only one way of determining gestational age and that is by the dates. Any other method whether it is before or after birth ends with having some population from which you construct your ultrasound charts.

SNOW: In the longitudinal studies if you make a correction for gestational age the first time you see the woman, is there information which then would say if you made the same corrections for subsequent examinations that the calculations would be different? Is there any evidence that the actual growth curve of a fetus that is small early or large early is a "wobble" towards a notional target size?

PERSON: We did longitudinal curves for each individual and then we studied the variation between the curves. Fifty percent of the variation was small and came from differences in gestational age. Fifty percent could be related to measuring error and to individual differences. In the longitudinal study gestational age was not corrected at all.

CAMPBELL: I am a passionate believer in routine ultrasound to re-date all pregnancies because it makes major contributions to good perinatal care. But I accept that when you are doing precise studies on the trend of growth perhaps it could have an influence.

MILNER: Having made that statement it is very interesting for us to hear your views on the concepts of a positively skewed or a negatively skewed birthweight versus gestational age graph at the 28 to 32 week period. If you go back to the results on which the gestational age graphs used in the UK are based there is a positive skew at 28-32 weeks. But we have heard that there is a linear relationship between lean body mass and gestational age in the last trimester. If we use ultrasonically dated age how will the clinician be informed about the fetus that causes concern?

GILLMER: To assume that all ultrasound as done by Professor Campbell is going to give you the same information as that done by a newcomer who does not see the relevance of some of the observations would be wrong. The question is what control is there over the information that is being used to re-date the pregnancies? Secondly it is not clear to me whether you are re-dating all pregnancies even where there is perhaps a day or two's difference between the estimated date on the basis of the woman's information compared to the ultrasound dating? If so, how can you justify it?

PERSSON: It is mainly statistics showing that if you correct one day then in 60% of cases you are more correct than if you rely on other dating. So when it increases to perhaps seven days, then you are correct in 80% of cases. In 14 days it is 87%

GILLMER: Surely this is akin to regression to the mean. The more correction you make the more you are going to reduce the variation with the net result that the biological variation will be wiped out.

REFERENCES

1. McKeown T, Record RG. Observations on foetal growth in multiple pregnancy in man. *J Endocrinol* 1952; **8:** 386-401.

Placental control of fetal metabolism

Professor W. W. Hay, Jr.

INTRODUCTION

The placenta is an organ that exchanges heat and matter between the fetal and maternal circulations. This exchange is the principal means by which the placenta controls fetal metabolism. This review will focus on the placental exchanges of nutrient substrates and how these affect fetal energy and protein metabolism. Other interesting aspects of placental exchange and control of fetal metabolism such as exchange of vitamins, macro-minerals, trace elements and "essential growth factors" (e.g. inositol, choline), as well as placental blood flow and the processing of various hormones (e.g. progesterone, oestrogen, placental lactogen) are equally important but beyond the scope of this review. Most of the information and concepts presented reflect animal experimentation given the paucity of data from human studies for obvious technical and ethical reasons.

Placental nutrient exchange involves three major mechanisms: (a) the direct transfer of intact nutrients, (b) the metabolism and consumption of nutrients and (c) the metabolism and processing of nutrients. These principal mechanisms are altered qualitatively and quantitatively by changes in the overall size of the placenta, the architecture of the placental tissues and developmental and pathological changes in placental transport capacity. Finally, various aspects of placental exchange can be affected by interaction with the fetus demonstrating a unity of function of the conceptus.

PLACENTAL GLUCOSE TRANSFER

Fetal metabolism

The rate of fetal glucose utilisation (including the rate of glucose oxidation) depends on the simultaneous interaction of fetal plasma glucose and insulin concentrations (Figure I) which co-vary and are directly dependent on maternal glucose concentration and the net rate of placental glucose transfer.[1-4] Thus, the placenta controls fetal glucose metabolism by regulating the rate of transfer of glucose from the maternal to the fetal circulation.

Placental glucose transfer

Placental glucose transfer has been quantified by the Fick principle (umbilical blood flow × the umbilical venous-arterial blood glucose concentration difference) and is directly related to uterine glucose uptake and the concentration of glucose in the maternal plasma (Figure II). A number of studies have demonstrated, using glucose, tracer glucose and similarly transported analogues of glucose, that placental glucose transfer follows Michaelis–Menton kinetics, demonstrating concentration gradient-dependent, saturable carrier-mediated transport. The carriers or transporters occur on both maternal and fetal sides of the trophoblast, allowing bi-directional transport and contribution to placental glucose metabolism from glucose

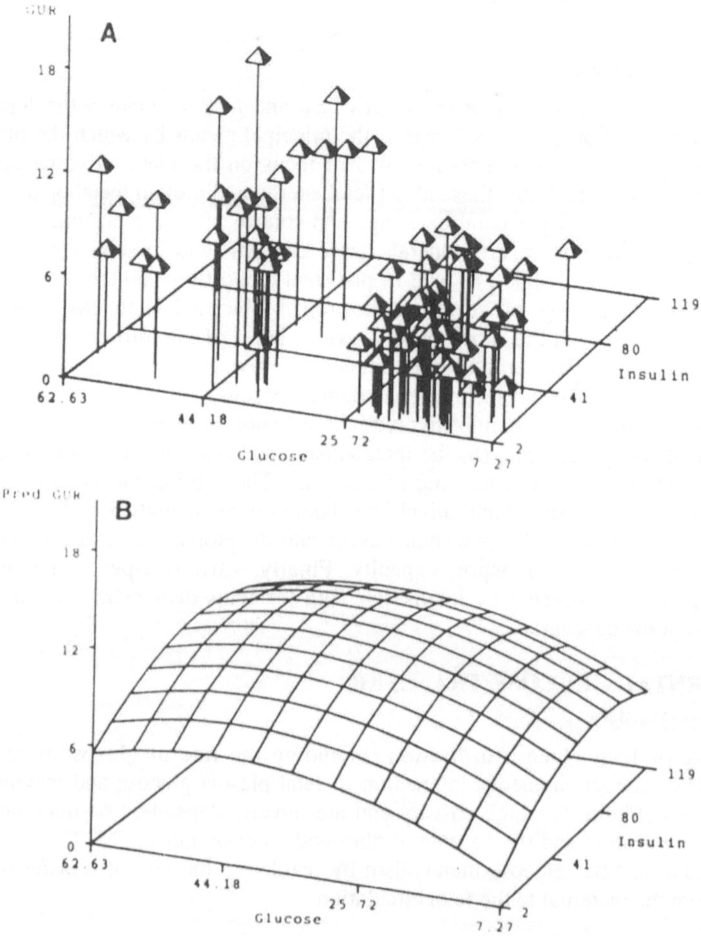

Figure I
Data from fetal sheep showing the additive effects of plasma glucose and insulin concentrations on fetal glucose utilisation rate.[1]
(a) Three-dimensional plot of individual values of glucose utilisation rate at different concentrations of glucose and insulin.
(b) Predicted three-dimensional glucose x insulin surface from the data in (a) according to the equation: GUR = –0.322 + [0.289 (glucose)] + [0.018 (insulin)] – [0.00319 (glucose)^2] - [0.000673 (insulin)^2].
GUR = glucose utilisation rate

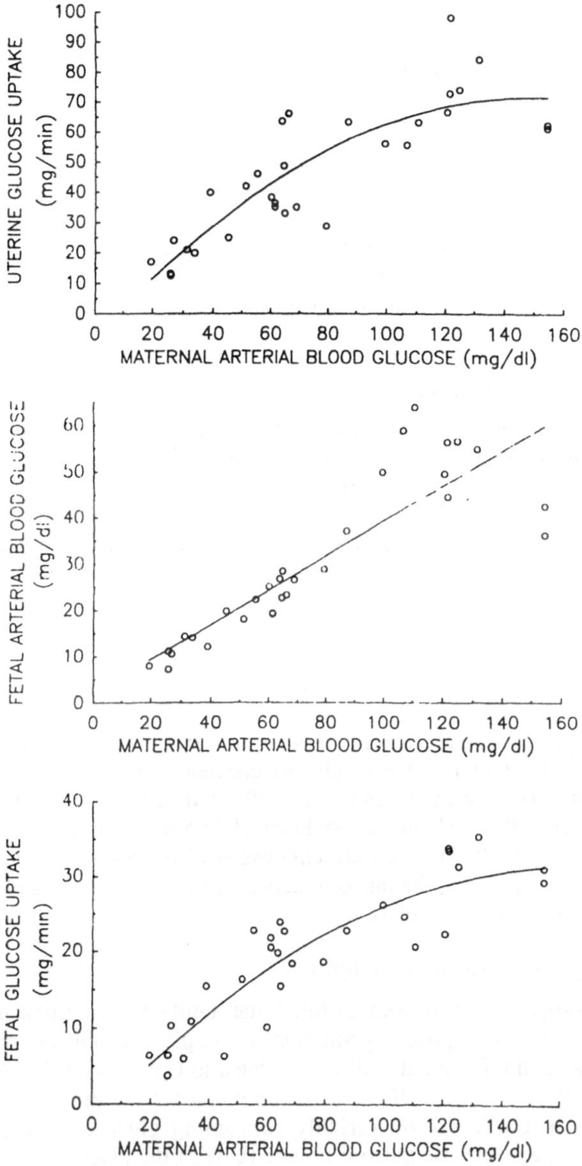

Figure II.
Data from pregnant sheep showing the relationships between: (a) fetal glucose concentration and maternal glucose concentration; (b) uterine glucose uptake and maternal glucose concentration; and (c) fetal glucose uptake (equal to placental glucose transfer) and maternal glucose concentration.[4]

molecules in the fetal as well as the maternal plasma glucose pools.[5]

Transplacental glucose gradient

Widdas first proposed that maternal-to-fetal placental glucose transfer was carrier mediated according to a Michaelis–Menton model:[6]

$$\acute{Q}_f = Vmax\ \{[G_A / (G_A + Km)] - [G_a / (G_a + Km)]\}$$

where Vmax represents the maximal flux of glucose, Km is the concentration of glucose at which the carriers are 50% saturated and $\acute{Q}_f$ = Vmax/2, and G_A and G_a represent the glucose concentrations in maternal and fetal arterial plasmas, respectively.

Placental glucose consumption

The Widdas model assumes that the placenta functions only as an exchange membrane and consumes no glucose. However according to Fick principle and *in vitro* measurements, a large portion of glucose molecules taken up by the placenta are consumed within the placental tissues (for example, this portion may be as large as two-thirds of net uterine glucose uptake in late gestation sheep) and a plot of experimental values of $\acute{Q}_f$ G_A, and G_a demonstrates a negative y-intercept. As a result, Simmons *et al.* proposed that Widdas' model must include an expression to account for net placental glucose consumption:[7]

$$\acute{Q}_f = Vmax\ \{[G_A / (G_A + Km)] - [G_a / (G_a + Km)]\} - \acute{q}_p$$

where $\acute{q}_P$ equals net placental glucose consumption from the fetal glucose pool when maternal and fetal arterial plasma glucose concentrations are equal. At actual experimental values of $\acute{Q}_f$ = 20 mg/min, G_A = 70 mg/dl, Km = 70 mg/dl, $\acute{q}_P$ = 30 mg/min, and Vmax = 209 mg/min, G_a would equal 24.5 mg/dl. If $\acute{q}_P$ were zero, G_a would equal 47.5 mg/dl.[7] Thus, the placenta exerts direct control over fetal glucose metabolism by regulating the rate of glucose transfer to the fetus and the concentration of glucose in the fetal plasma.

Placental glucose consumption variability

More recent investigations have demonstrated that, unlike the modified model of placental glucose transfer proposed by Simmons *et al.*, placental glucose consumption ($\acute{q}_P$ or UPGC) is not fixed but is directly related to G_A and G_a (Figure III).[4,8] G_A and G_a exert their effect on UPGC by determining the intratrophoblastic glucose concentration, G_P. Thus, by variably consuming glucose in response to changes in G_A, G_a, and uterine glucose uptake (UtGU) the placenta exerts additional control over fetal glucose supply and metabolism. The independent effect of G_a is important. Its slope is approximately twice that of the effect of G_A on UPGC, allowing a stronger control of G_a on UPGC than G_A. This becomes important when G_A and UtGC are very low, as during fasting hypoglycaemia. Under these circumstances, relatively small changes in G_a produced by the development of fetal

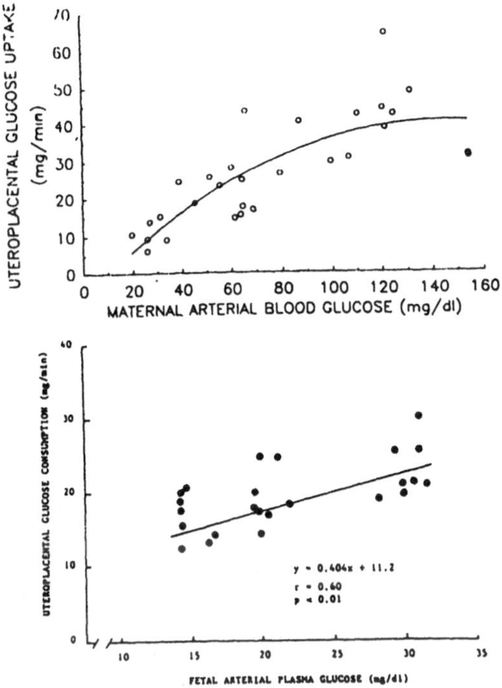

Figure III
Data from pregnant sheep showing the relationship between: (a) uteroplacental glucose consumption and maternal glucose concentration;[4] (b) uteroplacental glucose consumption and fetal glucose concentration at constant maternal arterial plasma glucose concentration of 70 mg/dl.[8]

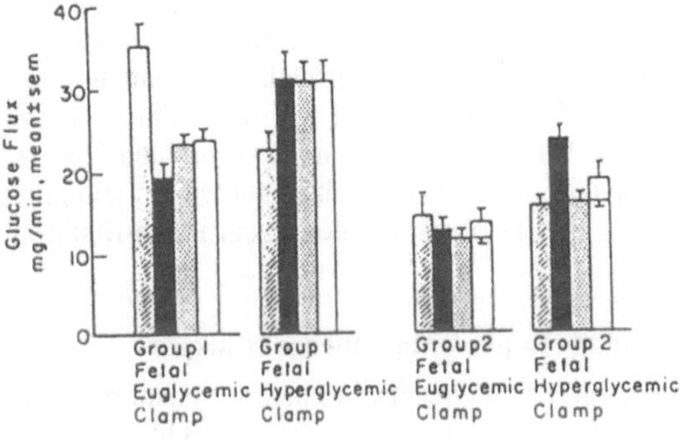

Figure IV
Glucose flux rates across the placenta in normoglycaemic sheep (left) and chronically hypoglycaemic sheep (middle and right). With chronic maternal hypoglycaemia, fetal endogenous glucose production sustains uteroplacental glucose consumption by limiting placental glucose transfer (equal to net fetal glucose entry in the control studies). A fetal glucose infusion producing an increase in fetal glucose concentration (right) exaggerated this effect, increasing uteroplacental glucose consumption without altering uterine glucose uptake.(8)

endogenous glucose production would be expected to have a significant effect on uteroplacental glucose transfer (UPGT) and UPGC. Experimental data (Figure IV) have confirmed this, providing a unique example of how the fetus and placenta cooperatively function as a metabolic unit and in the case of reduced glucose supply from the mother, can effectively secure their own autonomy without further jeopardising maternal glucose homeostasis. Since the fraction of uterine glucose uptake that is consumed by the placenta increases towards term (e.g. from ~ 10% to ~ 30% over the last half of gestation in sheep) this phenomenon becomes even more important near term as fetal viability becomes more probable.[9]

Placental size

Placental size also exerts important control over the fetus. In general, placental size and fetal size are directly related. Furthermore, experimental reduction in placental size has produced smaller fetuses. For example, Owens and colleagues performed uterine carunculectomies in sheep which reduced the endometrial implantation area resulting in a fewer number of placental cotyledons and an overall reduced placental mass and surface area.[10,11] These experiments demonstrated reduced fetal weight [3,720 ± 807 (sem) grams, control: 2,198 ± 653 (sem) grams, carunculectomy] and placental glucose transfer to the fetus [18.4 ± 2.7 (sem) mg/min, control: 11.1 ± (sem) mg/min, carunculectomy], nearly proportionate to the reduction in placental cotyledon number and weight. Of interest also was the observation that the fetal weight specific glucose transfer did not change [4.9 ± 0.7 (sem) mg/min/kg, control: 5.1 ± 2.0 (sem) mg/min/kg, carunculectomy] indicating that placental glucose transport capacity was not altered *per se*. However the fetal weight/placental weight ratio was greater in the experimental carunculectomy animals (12.6 ± 3.9) than in a normal control group (7.8 ± 1.3); thus, it is possible that the remaining placental tissues underwent further modification that allowed or promoted alternate nutrient transport. For example, amino acids could be used as alternative fuels as well as providing for a more moderate rate of growth since amino acids are taken up in excess of growth requirements under normal circumstances. A 25% reduction in the normal rate of amino acid carbon utilisation for growth (from 3.9 to 2.9 g/kg/day) and thus, an estimated 25% reduction in growth rate compared with a 50% reduction in placental weight and glucose transfer could provide about 55% of the normal glucose carbon utilisation rate (1.0 of 1.8 g/kg/day).[12]

Developmental change in placental glucose transport

Gestational or developmental changes in glucose transport capacity also have been observed. At 50% gestation in sheep placental weight is greater than at term and placental glucose transport capacity is quite low. Over the remaining half of gestation placental weight declines by about 20%, but placental glucose transport capacity increases over 8-fold. About 40% of this increased glucose transport capacity is due to a progressive decrease in G_a (perhaps due to an increased insulin-responsive tissue mass) and thus, an increase in the transplacental glucose concentration gradient, but the remaining 60% is due to increased transport capacity *per se* (Figure

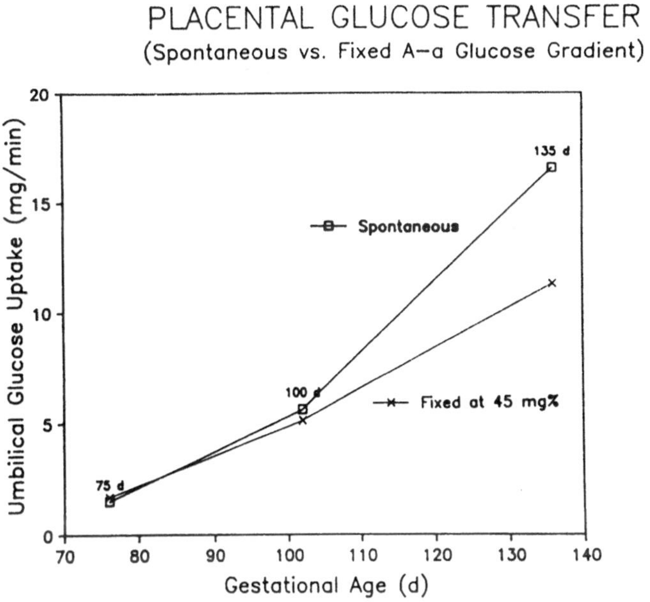

Figure V

Placental glucose transfer (measured and shown as umbilical glucose uptake) increased over gestation, even with elimination of the gestational increase in the maternal–fetal (A-a) arterial plasma glucose concentration gradient.[9]

V).[9] Experiments at different glucose concentrations at early and late gestation demonstrate no marked difference in Km; thus, the gestational increase in transport capacity most probably represents an increase in placental glucose transporter concentration rather than transporter affinity. [13]

Placental glucose processing

Placental processing of glucose also contributes to control of fetal metabolism, changing glucose into lactate and fructose. Placental lactate production in the sheep accounts for about 2 mg/min/kg that enter the fetus and an additional 6 mg/min that enter the maternal circulation (Figure VI).[14] The fetal lactate uptake is about half the rate of glucose uptake but only a third of fetal lactate utilisation.[15] Placental lactate production with net lactate supply to the fetus at normal levels of lactate and oxygen has been observed in all species studied to date including the human.[16] There is little evidence that placental lactate production is related to placental glucose uptake, but increased fetal glucose concentration that occurs at the same time is directly correlated with an increased fetal lactate concentration. Herrera *et al.* also have shown in pregnant rats a small but significant production of lactate from alanine by the placenta, indicating that glucose may not be the only

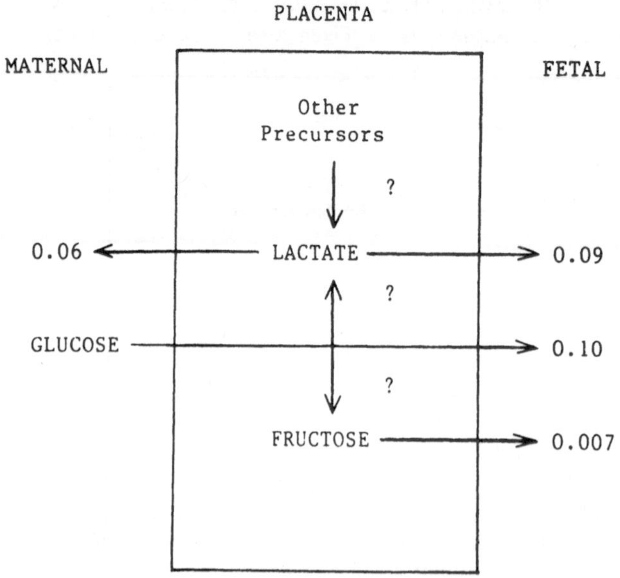

Figure VI

Placental processing of glucose with net production of lactate and fructose. Flux rates are in mmol/min at ~ 140 days gestation (term ≃ 150 days).

source of placental lactate production.[17] Fetal lactate is readily oxidised and the sum of fetal lactate and glucose uptake is directly related to fetal oxygen consumption.[18] Fetal lactate oxidation rate is directly related to fetal lactate concentration[19] but there is no measurement of the effect of lactate concentration on other pathways of lactate utilisation, such as glycogen synthesis. Gleason *et al.* have shown net ovine fetal hepatic lactate uptake[20] and Levitsky *et al.* have observed gluconeogenesis from lactate in the baboon fetus[21] and conversion to alanine with entry into protein metabolism.

Fructose is produced in the placenta from glucose via aldose reductase. Significant placental fructose production is unique to ruminants and provides a high concentration of fructose in the fetal plasma, about 80–100 mg/dl or about 4–5 times the concentration of glucose. Recent isotopic tracer studies in sheep demonstrated that net uptake of fructose by the umbilical circulation is quite low (1.27 ± 0.7 SEM mg/min/kg or about 1/5 that of glucose) but is not different from fetal fructose utilisation (0.97 ± 0.09 SEM mg/min/kg) indicating that there is no significant fructose production in the fetus (Figure VI).[22] Fructose production and utilisation vary directly with glucose supply and concentration. Fructose is metabolised in the fetus to CO_2 (about 50% is oxidised), lactate and glycogen; overall utilisation rate is directly related to fetal plasma fructose concentration.

PLACENTAL AMINO ACID TRANSFER

Active transport

For most but not all the amino acids, transport from mother to fetus occurs against a concentration gradient and involves energy dependent transport mechanisms (Table 1).[23] Even for amino acids with a fetal/maternal ratio less than 1.0 overall transport may be energy dependent because of placental concentration above

Table 1 Factors affecting placental amino acid transfer

1. Uterine/umbilical blood flow
   Δ rate → Δ distribution, under (no) perfusion versus re-perfusion
2. Hormone receptors (e.g. cAMP → ↑, i.e. Ca^{++} → activation of metabolism ± transport processes)
3. Carriers
   a. Altered carrier Vmax (no. carrier sites active, no. carriers)
   b. Altered carrier affinity
   c. Competition for carriers among substrates
   d. Altered turnover of carriers
4. Altered diffusional leaks: (a) into or out of cells; (b) via paracellular pathways
5. Altered intracellular free amino acid concentrations, altered maternal amino acid concentrations, altered fetal amino acid concentrations
6. Altered placental amino acid metabolism
7. Permissive effect of acetylcholine
8. Energy supply (substrate plus oxygen)
9. Na^+/K^+ – ATPase (inward Na^+ gradient with System A co-transport)
10. H^+ gradients (± electrochemical)

maternal levels (e.g. citrulline). Placental amino acid transport is energy dependent and thus it is not surprising that inhibition of glycolysis and aerobic metabolism can suppress placental amino acid transport. These conclusions are largely based on *in vitro* techniques and primarily using AIB rather than natural amino acids.[24] Similar energy dependency has been demonstrated *in vitro* for amino acid incorporation into placental proteins. There is practically no work looking at *in vivo* placental amino acid uptake, transport, or metabolism under conditions of energy substrate or oxygen deficiency or by selected inhibition of glycolysis or aerobic metabolism.

Uterine uptake and placental consumption

Net uptakes of amino acids by the uterus have been difficult to measure because of small arteriovenous (AV) differences and inaccuracies in the determination of uterine blood flow. In the pregnant sheep, Holzman *et al.* showed positive uterine AV differences for all amino acids tested except glutamate.[25] Because the ratio of umbilical to uterine AV differences (1.9) was about equal to the uterine to umbilical blood flow ratio, it appears that most of the uterine amino acid uptake is transported to the fetus and that placental requirements for amino acids are small relative to those of the fetus. These results were obtained at term when placental growth had ceased; earlier in gestation placental/fetal weight is several-fold higher than at term, and placental growth may still be significant relative to that of the fetus. Quantitative aspects of placental amino acid requirements have yet to be worked out. Based on placental nitrogen content at term in the human placenta, placental growth over gestation would require about 10.6 g N (or 66 g protein).[26]

The placenta near term contains a large variety of enzymes that are capable of metabolising amino acids through pathways such as gluconeogenesis, glycogen synthesis, protein synthesis, amino acid oxidation, ammoniagenesis, etc. Amino acid flux through these pathways has been demonstrated *in vitro*. Ammoniagenesis occurs *in vivo*, at least in the sheep placenta. Other pathways may operate only under select conditions. Other protein requirements include at least a small amount for oxidation and an undertermined amount for synthesis of secreted protein products (e.g. hormones such as hCG, LH and placental lactogen).

Carrier systems

Six carrier systems for amino acid uptake by animal tissues have been identified but only three of these have been found definitely in the placenta.[27] There is considerable overlap among the systems for different amino acids, but the ASC system is particularly important for transporting the bulk of the essential amino acids, with the exception of lysine, which is a basic amino acid. Competition for a carrier system exists among the amino acids transported by that carrier system; thus one can expect quantitative changes in the balance of amino acid transport produced by significant alterations in plasma amino acid concentrations. The mechanisms by which the amino acids are actively transported by placental tissues are not well understood. At least for system A, co-transport occurs with inwardly directed Na^+ transport that is energised by Na^+/K^+ – ATPase producing an outside/inside Na^+ electrochemical gradient.[28] Recently Ganapathy and colleagues have observed H^+ – amino acid co-transport that involves H^+ out/Na^+ + amino acid in, energised by Na^+/K^+ – ATPase; this mechanisms appears to apply to system L.[29] These transport mechanisms are certainly active at the maternal brush-border but may also be responsible for transport on the fetal or basal side. Studies of dual-maternal and fetal-perfused placentas with paired tracers of amino acids indicate bi-directional transport for many amino acids but with different transport kinetics such that transplacental transfer is greater in the maternal–fetal direction for all the amino acids which are taken up.[30]

Developmental and adaptive changes

Several other aspects of placental amino acid transport are worth mentioning. Both *in vitro* and *in vivo* studies indicate that reduced amino acid concentrations lead to enhanced amino acid transport (increased Vmax, reduced Km);[31,32] this can be blocked by inhibition of protein synthesis, indicating that new carriers are produced. The *in vivo* studies were conducted in pregnant rats made hypoaminoacidaemic by glucagon infusion. In these studies fetal weight was not compromised until the mother was fasted producing hypoglycaemia.[32] Thus the placenta maintained fetal amino acid levels but had no compensation for the hypoglycaemia. These results take on added importance relative to the observations by Cetin *et al.* who showed from cordocentesis data in humans that concentrations of alpha-aminonitrogen were lower in maternal and fetal plasmas of growth retarded infants. Placentas from these growth retarded infants showed reduced transport of many amino acids, particularly the essential amino acids, with a reduced transport of total alpha-aminonitrogen.[33]

The reverse process, reduction of amino acid transport, occurs with high amino acid concentration; this may be caused by *trans*-inhibition, i.e. substrate binding on the *trans*-side, limiting carrier mobility.[34] These changes appear unique to the A system. In other tissues, A-system carrier number appears to be adaptively regulated by hormones as well as substrate concentrations, but such hormonal regulation has not been found in placental tissue. Other evidence linking placental amino acid transport to placental protein synthesis is ambiguous. Similarly the placenta contains many hormone receptors (insulin, gonadotrophin, growth factors, somatomedin, beta-adrenergics, cholinergics, opiates, etc.) For the most part there is no convincing data that placental amino acid transport is regulated by these hormones, although ACh, perhaps by mediating changes in membrane potential, has been suggested as a potential regulator.[35]

Ethanol has been shown *in vitro* and *in vivo* to inhibit placental amino acid transport (primarily the L system), but at concentrations of ethanol much greater than found in chronically alcoholic pregnant women.[36] Whether acute toxic ethanol ingestion impairs amino acid transport remains to be determined. Nicotine also inhibits system A amino acid transport in the placenta; one might expect double jeopardy to the fetus from ethanol and nicotine, a common drug combination in pregnant women who produce growth-retarded infants.[37] Other drugs and toxins of many types have been implicated as inhibiting amino acid transport; mechanisms and clinical changes are not known for most. Many types of placental pathology also exist (hypertrophy, hypoplasia, infection, oedema, vascular malformations, calcium deposition, etc.), but there is no certain knowledge of their effect on amino acid transport.

Umbilical amino acid uptake

The net uptake of amino acids by the umbilical circulation represents the dietary supply of amino acids for fetal growth and protein metabolism. Although peptide uptake has been observed, this additional amount of protein probably represents little nutritional value in that total alpha-aminonitrogen uptake, at least in the fetal lamb, is not different from the alpha-aminonitrogen uptake in the form of amino acids. The uptake of amino acids by the umbilical circulation has been studied in only one experimental animal, the fetal lamb. The coefficients of extraction across the umbilical circulation show the limitation of this methodology in that for several of the amino acids the coefficient of extraction (v-a/a) is close to zero, demonstrating the high degree of accuracy needed to measure the arteriovenous concentration differences to estimate net uptakes of these amino acids by the Fick principle.[12,25]

The product of umbilical blood flow multiplied by the umbilical venous-arterial blood concentration difference for each amino acid yields the *net* uptake of each amino acid by the fetus. Figure VII shows the net uptake for each amino acid studied in the last 20% of gestation in the fetal lamb.(38) Together, the net amino acid uptakes provide 5.3 g/day/kg fetal weight of carbon and 1.6 g/day/kg of nitrogen. The net carbon uptake provides 60–70% of fetal carbon requirements (net accretion in carcass protein, glycogen and fat, and utilisation for oxidation yielding CO_2 excretion). The nitrogen uptake in this study is about 160% of the nitrogen requirement (net nitrogen accretion plus urea nitrogen excretion). Thus either there are other excretory forms of nitrogen or the accuracy of estimating nitrogen excretion, accretion or uptake in this study was quite limited. Recently using improved analytical methods for quantifying blood flow and amino concentrations, Marconi *e t al.* measured a total fetal umbilical nitrogen uptake of 0.91 g N/kg/day in fetal sheep at term, not different from the calculated requirement of about 1.0 g N/kg/day (personal communication).

Figure VII also shows the net accretion of each amino acid in fetal carcass growth. The net uptake of most of the basic amino acids exceeds their net accretion by considerable amounts. In contrast, the net uptakes of the two basic amino acids, lysine and histidine, and the neutral amino acid glycine barely exceed net accre-

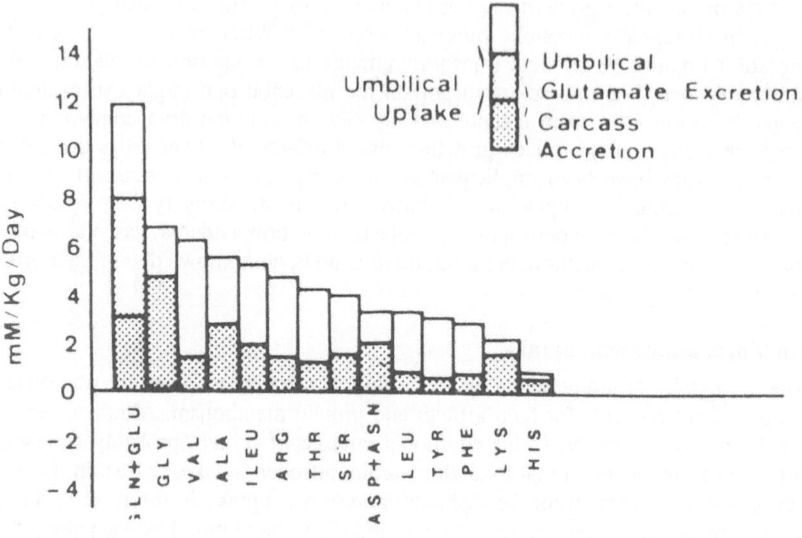

Figure VII

Net uptake of several amino acids by the late gestation fetal lamb partitioned into net carcass accretion and other fates (presumably oxidation).(38) Net uptake equals the total height of each bar.

tion. Similarly the combined accretion of asparagine and its product aspartate and the combined accretion of glutamine and its product glutamate are very close to the net uptakes of asparagine and glutamine respectively. For these amino acid pairs there is no net uptake of the acidic forms, these being derived in the fetus from deamination. Limitation of supply of these five amino acids very likely would lead to reduced protein accretion and growth.

Amino acid oxidation

The excess uptake above carcass accretion requirements for the neutral amino acids also implies that this portion of amino acid uptake is used for oxidation. Evidence for the fetal oxidation of amino acids comes from two observations, the high fetal urea production rate and the direct measurement of carbon-labelled CO_2 during fetal infusions of carbon–labelled amino acids.(39,40) Direct measurement of fetal amino acid oxidation has been made using carbon–labelled isotopic tracers of selected amino acids, quantifying net excretion of labelled CO_2, from the fetus via the umbilical circulation relative to the plasma-labelled amino acid specific activity. Central to this methodology has been the documentation that, at least in the fetal lamb, virtually 100% of fetal CO_2 production (produced, for example, by fetal infusion of NaH $^{14}CO_3$) is excreted via the umbilical circulation.(41) A limitation of this methodology is its overestimation of fetal oxidation of a specific substrate to the extent that carbon–labelled non-oxidative products derived from placental and/or maternal metabolism of the substrate re-enter and are oxidised. For example, the CO_2 production rate from tracer leucine may include CO_2 derived from the decarboxylation of ketoisocaproic acid molecules re-entering fetal plasma after the placental deamination of fetal leucine.(42) Although estimates of this additional labelled CO_2 suggest that it is a small fraction of direct amino acids oxidation, experimental verification has not been accomplished.

Several ^{14}C–labelled amino acids have been infused into fetuses *in vivo* documenting $^{14}CO_2$ production (leucine, lysine, alanine, tyrosine, glycine).(12) Oxidation rates have been calculated for leucine and lysine demonstrating that the oxidation/disposal ratio was directly related to the excess of umbilical uptake above accretion and to the plasma concentration of the amino acid.(40,43) Leucine oxidation at mid-gestation was at least as great as at term indicating that amino acids may provide carbon for fetal oxidative metabolism over a large part of gestation.

Placental-fetal amino acid cycling

In addition to net transport of amino acids to the fetus the placenta may contribute to fetal amino acid and nitrogen balance by contributing to selective interorgan cycling. For example, the placenta actively produces ammonia which is delivered into both uterine and umbilical circulations.(44,45) This process appears to be normal in mammalian metabolism, occurring in all aspects in all species studied to date.(12) A fraction of the net umbilical ammonia uptake is extracted by fetal tissues in sheep, perhaps contributing to hepatic urea formation and to other specific metabolic pathways. However the NH_3 taken up by the liver, about 6.5 µmol/min, is about 2.5 times that taken up by the umbilical circulation, demonstrating considerable fetal endogenous ammonia production, consistent with observations of net NH_3 efflux across the fetal hindlimb.[34] In a recent study in sheep Marconi *et al.* also showed that the hepatic amino acid/oxygen quotient was significantly higher than the umbilical amino acid/oxygen quotient (0.63 ± 0.87 versus 0.13 ± 0.03) implying a high amino acid utilisation by the fetal liver (personal communication). Measurements of umbilical and fetal hepatic concentrations of amino acids in the fetal sheep in these studies found reciprocal relationships between three sets of amino acids. Glutamine and glycine were taken up by the fetus from the placenta and by the liver from the umbilical vein, whereas their metabolically-related products, glutamate and serine respectively were produced by the fetal liver and taken up by the placenta. Similar but less marked relationships were found for net hepatic uptake of asparagine and release of aspartate with a reciprocal change across the umbilical circulation.

Another example of placental–fetal cycling involves the relatively high concentrations and activities of branched-chain amino acid amino transferases found in the placenta both of sheep and humans. Studies in sheep suggest that net placental uptake and transamination to the corresponding alpha-ketoacid can occur for leucine.[42] The importance of these processes to placental and fetal amino acid metabolism and growth remains to be determined, but their very existence implies a level of regulation in fetal placental metabolism far more sophisticated than originally conceived.

PLACENTAL LIPID TRANSFER

The placentas of different species have markedly different permeabilities and transport capacities for fatty acids. As a result, the fat content of fetuses varies markedly among species in direct relation to placental lipid transport.[12] However accurate measurement of placental fat transport is limited by small coefficients of extractions making precise determination of umbilical arteriovenous concentration differences difficult. Yet, the high carbon concentration of lipids (for example, palmitate has 23 carbons per mmol compared with lactate which has 3 and glucose which has 6) may make for a significant contribution of lipid carbon to fetal metabolism even though extraction ratios and actual uptakes are quite small.

Net flux of fatty acids across the placenta can occur by at least three mechanisms: (a) direct transfer by carrier-mediated transport, (b) synthesis within the placenta and subsequent release into the umbilical circulation (which may apply specifically to essential fatty acids that can be produced in the placenta by chain elongation and desaturation[46]) and (c) hydrolysis of complex triacylglycerol, lipoproteins and phospholipids derived from either maternal or fetal circulations.[47] The placenta contains lipoprotein lipase but primarily on the maternal surface; thus its role for net release of free fatty acids from maternal glycerides into the fetal circulation remains uncertain.[48] Since fetal fatty acid composition varies with maternal diet, placental selectivity in fatty acid transport probably is not of major importance.

Lipid metabolism in the fetus involves the incorporation of fatty acids into membranes as phospholipids, esterification into triacylglycerols and subsequent deposition in brown and white adipose tissue, and oxidation.(49) Considerable qualitative and quantitative variability in these processes has been observed among species and among different studies. Fetal tissues, particularly hepatic and adipose, in most species can actively synthesise fatty acids, primarily from short chain fatty acids such as acetate, lactate and amino acids, and to a lesser extent from glucose.(50) Fatty acid oxidation also is highly variable among species and among studies, reflecting quite different but generally low levels of acetyl-CoA, carnitine, palmityl-CoA synthetase, 3-hydroxyacyl-CoA dehydrogenase, carnitine acyltransferase and carnitine palmityltransferase.(51) Ketone production is generally low, probably due to relatively low levels of glucagon and thus inactive HMG-CoA synthetase, but oxidation of ketones may be quite rapid.(51)

Fetal glucose supply versus amino acid oxidation and growth

Fetal metabolic rate, as quantified by net fetal oxygen consumption, depends directly, although to only a modest extent, on energy supply. For example in fetal sheep, glucose utilisation and the sum of net fetal glucose and lactate uptakes are directly correlated with fetal VO_2.(2,16) This effect can be produced by increasing

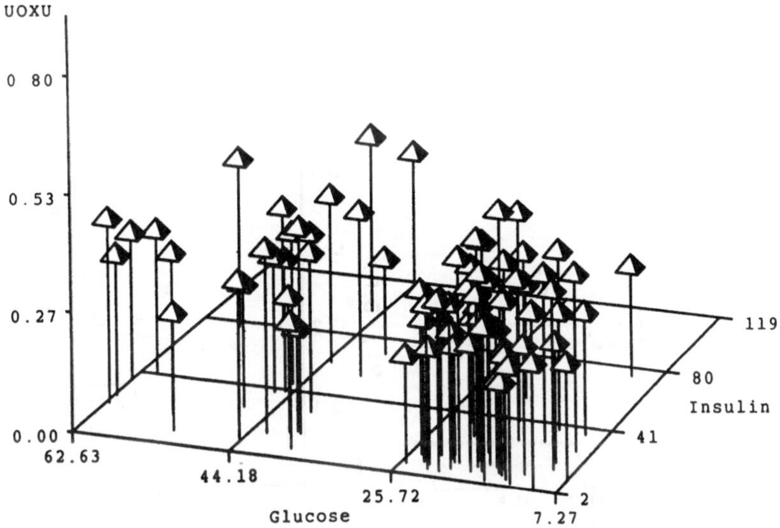

Figure VIII

Data from fetal sheep comparing net fetal oxygen consumption (measured and shown as net umbilical oxygen uptake, UOxU) with simultaneous fetal values of glucose and insulin concentrations.(2) These data are best expressed by the multiple linear correlation: UOXU = 0.303 + [0.000813 (glucose)] + [0.0000461 (insulin)].

glucose and/or insulin concentrations (Figure VIII). Thus, to the extent that the placenta determines net glucose flux to the fetus, and thereby fetal glucose and lactate concentrations, it can control to a small but significant extent (maximum of 15–25% increase in VO_2) fetal metabolic rate. However, over the physiological range of fetal glucose and insulin concentrations, fetal glucose oxidation rate changes by nearly two-fold.(1) This observation together with the simultaneous relative constancy of VO_2 indicates that a reciprocal relationship must exist between glucose oxidation and that of other energy-producing substrates. Given the limited availability and/or oxidation of other non-protein energy substrates (e.g. lipids), it appears that glucose supply can determine the relative oxidation of certain amino acids. In this regard a large amount of amino acids is taken up by the fetal sheep in excess of carcass accretion rates(38) and simultaneously, there is a high fetal urea production rate.(39) Furthermore, studies with ^{14}C-leucine have demonstrated that the fetal leucine disposal rate ratio nearly doubles with fasting-induced hypoglycaemia and reduced umbilical glucose uptake. (Figure IX).(40) There was however, no decrease in fetal protein synthesis rate in these studies. Still other studies have demonstrated fetal endogenous gluconeogenesis under these same conditions.(3) Because lactate and fructose concentrations and utilisation rates are low under these conditions amino acids are the most likely gluconeogenic precursors. These observations indicate that fetal protein catabolism is regulated by non-protein energy supply and that certain amino acids released by protein catabolism are oxidised to maintain fetal energy balance and metabolic rate or are metabolised to glucose synthesis, both at the expense of fetal growth. In these ways placental regulation of fetal energy substrate supply can control fetal protein balance and growth as well as energy balance.

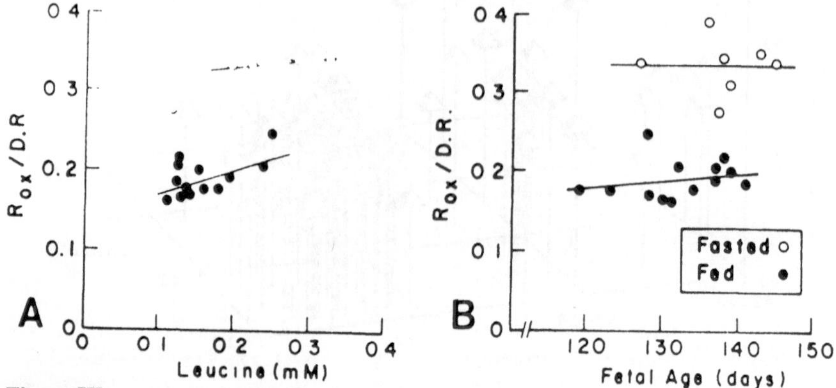

Figure IX
Demonstration in fed and fasted pregnant sheep that fetal leucine oxidation/disposal rate ratio is approximately doubled with fasting.(40) The data also show a positive correlation between leucine oxidation and plasma leucine concentration.

SUMMARY AND CONCLUSIONS

As an organ of exchange, the placenta exerts control over fetal metabolism primarily by regulating the transport of metabolic substrates to the fetus. Placental tissue contains transporters or carriers for most substrates, some of which (glucose, fatty acids) involve passive diffusion and others (amino acids) active or energy-dependent mechanisms. The quantity of placental transport of selected nutrients is affected by placental consumption of those nutrients and also by the metabolic processing of selected substrates. Developmental changes in transport capacity affect all of these substrates, but to different degrees, providing a variability in fetal diet both qualitatively and quantitatively throughout gestation that is determined by the placenta and not exclusively by fetal demand. Obviously, how much placental tissue is present determines metabolic substrate transport to a great extent. Finally, one of the most interesting aspects of placental control to emerge from recent studies is its cooperativity with fetal metabolism in processing selected substrates into different forms and in accepting fetal nutrient supply when maternal sources diminish, thereby maintaining relative autonomous viability.

ACKNOWLEDGEMENTS

Preparation of this manuscript was supported in part by NIH Project Grant No. DK-35836, NIH Program Grant No. HD-00781, and NIH P-50 Center Grant No. HD-20761.

REFERENCES

1. Hay WW Jr, Meznarich HK, DiGiacomo JE, Hirst K, Zerbe G. Effects of insulin and glucose concentrations on glucose utilization in fetal sheep. *Pediatr Res* 1988; **23**: 381-387.
2. Hay WW Jr, DiGiacomo JE, Meznarich HK, Hirst K, Zerbe G. Effects of physiologic levels of glucose and insulin on glucose oxidation and oxygen metabolism in the fetal lamb. *Am J Physiol*; In press.
3. Hay WW Jr, Sparks J W, Wilkening RB, Battaglia FC, Meschia G. Fetal glucose uptake and utilization as functions of maternal glucose concentration. *Am J Physiol* 1984; **246**: E237-E242.
4. Hay WW Jr, Meznarich HK. Effect of maternal glucose concentration on uteroplacental glucose consumption and transfer in pregnant sheep. *Proc Soc Exp Biol Med*; In press.
5. Yudilevich DL, Eaton BM, Short AH, Leichtweiss HP. Glucose carriers at maternal and fetal sides of the trophoblast in guinea pig placenta. *Am J Physiol* 1979; **237**: C205-C212.
6. Widdas WF. Inability of diffusion to account for placental glucose transfer in the sheep and consideration of the kinetics of a possible carrier transfer. *J Physiol* 1952; **118**: 23-29.
7. Simmons MA, Battaglia FC, Meschia G. Placental transfer of glucose. *J Dev Physiol* 1979; **1**: 227-243.
8. Hay WW Jr. Regulation of ovine placental glucose consumption (PGU). *Physiologist* 1987; **30**: 174. (Abstract No. 43.12).
9. Molina RD, Meschia G, Battaglia FC, Hay WW Jr. Maturation of placental glucose transfer (PGT) capacity in the ovine pregnancy. *Pediatr Res* 1988;

23: 248A. (Abstract No. 283).
10. Owens JA, Allota E, Falconer J, Robinson JS. Effect of restricted placental growth upon oxygen and glucose delivery to the fetus. In: *The Physiological Development of the Fetus and Newborn* Eds. C T Jones and P W Nathanielsz. London: Academic Press, 1985: pp.33-36.
11. Owens JA, Allota E, Falconer J, Robinson JS. Effect of restricted placental growth upon umbilical and uterus blood flows. In: *The Physiological Development of the Fetus and Newborn* Eds. C T Jones and P W Nathanielsz. London: Academic Press, 1985: pp.51-54.
12. Battaglia FC, Meschia G. *An Introduction to Fetal Physiology*. Orlando: Academic Press, Inc, 1986.
13. Molina RD, Meschia G, Battaglia FC, Hay WW Jr. Maturation of placental glucose transfer (PGT) capacity in the ovine pregnancy. *Soc Gynec Invest* 1988; **35**: 239. (Abstract No. 360)
14. Meschia G, Battaglia FC, Hay WW Jr, Sparks JW. Utilization of substrates by the ovine placenta in vivo. *Fed Proc* 1980; **39**: 245-249.
15. Sparks JW, Hay WW Jr, Bonds D, Meschia G, Battaglia FC. Simultaneous measurements of lactate turnover rate and umbilical lactate uptake in the fetal lamb. *J Clin Invest* 1982; **70**: 179-192.
16. Marconi AM, Cetin I, Ferrari MM, Pardi G, Makowski EL, Battaglia, FC. Umbilical venous-arterial lactate concentration differences in normal and growth retarded human fetuses. *Soc Gynec Invest* 1988; **35**: 68. (Abstract No. 18)
17. Herrera E, Palacin M, Martin A, Lasuncion MA. Relationship between maternal and fetal fuels and placental glucose transfer in rats with maternal diabetes of varying severity. *Diabetes* 1985; **34:(Suppl. 2)**: 42-46.
18. Sparks JW, Hay WW Jr, Meschia G, Battaglia FC. Partition of maternal nutrients to the placenta and fetus in the sheep. *Eur J Obstet Gynecol Reprod Biol* 1983; **14**: 331-340.
19. Hay WW Jr, Myers SA, Sparks JW, Wilkening RB, Meschia G, Battaglia FC. Glucose and lactate oxidation rates in the fetal lamb. *Proc Soc Exp Biol Med* 1983; **173**: 553-563.
20. Gleason CA, Roman C, Rudolph AM. Hepatic oxygen consumption, lactate uptake, and glucose production in neonatal lambs. *Pediatr Res* 1985; **12**: 1235-1239.
21. Levitsky LL, Paton JB, Fisher DE. Gluconeogenesis from lactate in the chronically catheterized baboon fetus. *Biol Neonate* 1986; **50**: 97-106.
22. Meznarich HK, Hay WW Jr, Sparks JW, Meschia G, Battaglia FC. Fructose disposal and oxidation rates in the ovine fetus. *Q J Exp Physiol* 1987; **72**: 617-625.
23. Yudilevich DL, Sweiry JH. Transport of amino acids in the placenta. *Biochim Biophys* Acta 1985; **822**: 169-201.
24. Smith CH. Incubation teçhniques and investigation of placental transport mechanisms in vitro. *Placenta* 1981; **(Suppl.2)**: 163-176.
25. Holzman IR, Lemons JA, Meschia G, Battaglia FC. Uterine uptake of amino

acids and glutamine-glutamate balance in the pregnant ewe. *J Dev Physiol* 1979; **1**: 137-149.
26. Lemons JA. Fetal-placental nitrogen metabolism. *Semin Perinatol.* 1979; **3**: 177-190.
27. Enders R H, Judd RM Donohue TM, Smith CH. Placental amino acid uptake. III. Transport systems for neutral amino acids. *Am J Physiol.* 1976; **230**: 706-710.
28. Ganapathy ME, Leibach FH, Mahesh VB, Howard JC, Devoe LD, Ganapathy V. Characterization of tryptophan transport in human placental brush-border membrane vesicles. *Biochem J.* 1986; **238**: 201-208.
29. Balkovetz DF, Leibach FH, Mahesh VB, Devoe LD, Cragoe EJ Jr, Ganapathy V. $Na^+ - H^+$ – exchanger of human placental brush-border membrane: identification and characterization. *Am J Physiol* 1986; **251**: C852-C860.
30. Eaton BM, Yudilevich DL. Uptake and asymmetric efflux of amino acids at maternal and fetal sides of placenta. *Am J Physiol* 1981; **241**: C106-C112.
31. Smith CH, Adcock EW III, Teasdale F, Meschia G, Battaglia FC. Placental amino acid uptake: Tissue preparation, kinetics, and pre-incubation effect. *Am J Physiol* 1973; **224**: 558-564.
32. Domenech M, Gruppuso PA, Nishino VT, Susa JB, Schwartz R. Preserved fetal plasma amino acid concentrations in the presence of maternal hypoammoniacidemia. *Pediatr Res* 1986; **20**: 1071-1076.
33. Cetin I, Marconi AM, Bozzetti P, Sereni LP, Corbetta CM, Pardi G, Battaglia F C. Umbilical amino acid concentrations in appropriate and small for gestational age infants: a biochemical difference present in utero. *Am J Obstet Gynecol* 1988; **158**: 120-126.
34. Smith CH, Depper R. Placental amino acid uptake. II. Tissue pre-incubation, fluid distribution and mechanisms of regulation. *Pediatr Res* 1974; **8**: 697-703.
35. Rowell PP, Sastry BVR. Human placental cholinergic system: depression of the uptake of alpha-aminoisobutyric acid in isolated human placental villi by choline acetyltransferase inhibitors. *J Pharmacol Exp Ther* 1981; **216**: 232-238.
36. Henderson GI, Turner D, Patwardhan RV, Lumeng L, Hoyumpa AM, Schenker S. Inhibition of placental valine uptake after acute and chronic maternal ethanol consumption. *J Pharmacol Exp Ther* 1981; **216**: 465-472.
37. Rowell PP, Sastry BVR. The influence of cholinergic blockade on the uptake of alpha-aminoisobutyric acid by isolated human placental villi. *Toxicol Appl Pharmacol* 1978; **45**: 79-93.
38. Lemons JA, Adcock EW III, Jones MD Jr, Naughton MA, Meschia G, Battaglia FC. Umbilical uptake of amino acids in the unstressed fetal lamb. *J Clin Invest* 1976; **58**: 1428-1434.
39. Gresham EL, James EJ, Raye JR, Battaglia FC, Makowski EL, Meschia G. Production and excretion of urea by the fetal lamb. *Pediatrics* 1972; 372-379.
40. van Veen L C, Teng C, Hay WW Jr, Meschia G, Battaglia FC. Leucine disposal and oxidation rates in the fetal lamb. *Metabolism* 1987; **36**: 48-53.

41. van Veen LC, Hay WW Jr, Battaglia FC, Meschia G. Fetal CO_2 kinetics *J Dev Physiol* 1984; **6**: 359-365.
42. Loy GL, Fennessey PV, Hay WW Jr, Meschia G, Battaglia FC. In vivo placental metabolism of leucine and alpha-ketoisocaproate in pregnant sheep demonstrated by stable isotope methodology. *Soc Gynec Invest* 1988; **35**: 240. (Abstract No. 362).
43. Meier PR, Peterson RB, Bonds DR, Meschia G, Battaglia FC. Rates of protein synthesis and turnover in fetal life. *Am J Physiol* 1981; **240**: E320-E324.
44. Holzman IR, Lemons JA, Meschia G, Battaglia FC. Ammonia production by the pregnant uterus. *Proc Soc Exp Biol Med* 1987; **156**: 27-30.
45. Holzman IR, Philipps AF, Battaglia FC. Glucose metabolism, lactate and ammonia production by the human placenta in vitro. *Pediatr Res* 1979; **13**: 117-120.
46. Noble RC, Shand JH, Christie WW. Synthesis of C20 and C22 polyunsaturated fatty acids by the placenta of the sheep. *Biol Neonate* 1985; **47**: 333-338.
47. Morriss FH Jr, Boyd RDH. Placental transport. In: *The Physiology of Reproduction*. Eds. E Knobil, J Neill. New York: Raven Press, 1988: pp.2043-2083.
48. Thomas CR, Locoy C, St. Hillaire RJ, Brunzell JD. Studies on the placental hydrolysis and transfer of lipids to the fetal guinea pig. In: *Fetal Nutrition, Metabolism and Immunology: Role of the Placenta*. Eds. RK Miller, HA Thiede. New York: Plenum Press, 1983: pp.135-148.
49. Vernon RG. Lipid metabolism in the adipose tissue of ruminant animals. *Prog Lipid Res* 1980; **19**: 23-106.
50. Vernon RG, Clegg RA, Flint DJ. Metabolism of sheep adipose tissue during pregnancy and lactation. Adaptation and regulation. *Biochem J* 1981; **200**: 307-314.
51. Jones CT, Rolph TP. Metabolism during fetal life: a functional assessment of metabolic development. *Physiol Rev* 1985; **65**: 357-430.

The placenta as an endocrine regulator

Professor T. Lind and Dr P.G. Whittaker

INTRODUCTION

The placenta once thought of as a semi-permeable membrane between the mother and her fetus is now known to have many metabolic functions amongst which is its ability to produce a wide range of hormones. Whether this capacity is regulated in any specific way is the subject of debate, though recent work has suggested some degree of autoregulation may occur for insulin-like growth factor,[1] as well as for human chorionic gonadotrophin (hCG) and human placental lactogen (hPL).[2] However few data are available and earlier investigations were designed to evaluate whether blood levels of one or more of these hormones would give some indication of placental function and fetal growth. Results have been disappointing, and if there is a relation between any of the placental hormones and either fetal growth or wellbeing it is complex and as yet imperfectly understood. The inability to "communicate" directly with the fetus *in utero* adds to the investigators' problems and studies of the maternal endocrine milieu and its possible influence upon fetal development must therefore rely upon indirect methods.

We have chosen three groups to investigate: normal healthy women who conceived spontaneously and who went on to deliver live healthy babies after uncomplicated pregnancies; mothers who underwent spontaneous abortion during the study pregnancy; and finally, mothers who were known to have insulin-dependent diabetes mellitus (IDDM). The first group offered serial data on the changes in progesterone, oestradiol, hCG and hPL occuring throughout successful pregnancies against which we could compare the endocrine findings from the other two groups. More recently we have been able to determine insulin-like growth factor (IGF-1). The second group offered serial hormone data prior to and during the time that a pregnancy was undergoing spontaneous failure. The third group was chosen because the particular metabolic disorder of IDDM is associated with babies of increased birthweight. Thus if infant birthweight is influenced by the maternal endocrine environment, such mothers might offer evidence of this effect, but bearing in mind the possible confounding influence of diabetes mellitus itself.

PATIENTS

This report contains data from three studies undertaken over several years so that the numbers of patients available has varied.

Normal group

There were data from 72 healthy women available for comparison with the mothers undergoing spontaneous abortion. Of these, 22 were in the first pregnancy and 50 were multiparous. At the time comparisons were made with the endocrinological events occurring in diabetic pregnancies there were 68 healthy mothers available.

Estimations of IGF-1 are more recent and have been undertaken on 22 of our healthy mothers.

Spontaneous abortion

There were 33 mothers studied over the time of their early pregnancy failure. Three were in their first pregnancy and 30 were multiparous. For 16 women this was their first abortion, 4 had had one previous abortion while the remaining 13 had experienced 2 or more such losses. No anatomical or other causes had been defined for the previous abortions in any of the mothers studied. Two women aborted between 6–8 weeks gestation, the remainder aborting or undergoing uterine curettage for obvious pregnancy failure between 8–16 weeks.

IDDM group

At the time our general endocrine studies were being undertaken, data were available from 27 mothers who had this metabolic disorder. For our most recent study of IGF-1 changes throughout pregnancy measurements have been made upon 38 diabetic mothers.

ASSAY METHODS

The methods used to assay progesterone, oestradiol, hCG and hPL have been published elsewhere. (3)

IGF-1

The assay used an antiserum from NIH/Chapel Hill which had a cross-reaction with IGF-2 of only 0.5%. The standard used was the MRC 86/522 derived from recombinant IGF-1 and used at concentrations from 0.3 to 20 ng/ml. Separation of IGF-1 from its carrier proteins in serum was performed with 0.1m formic acid and 80% ethanol. Spiking with standard IGF-1 showed extraction efficiency to be close to 100%. The standard curve and serum dilution curve were parallel. After overnight incubation, free IGF-1 was separated from antibody-bound by second antibody precipitation assisted by polyethylene glycol. The coefficient of variation was 4% within assay and 8% between assays (n=16).

ENDOCRINE EVENTS AND SPONTANEOUS ABORTION

Progesterone

There was a similar increase in the serum concentration of progesterone in both the normal and abortion groups until week six of pregnancy but an apparent failure to maintain levels thereafter in the latter group. By week eight the mean concentration in the abortion group was significantly lower than in the normal group ($p<0.001$) and this decline continued until week 12. Individuals within the group demonstrated a similar pattern of response, although the onset of the marked decrease in progesterone values was a function of the time that clinical symptoms occurred. For clarity the values from eight individuals only are shown in Figure I against the normal range expressed as ±2 standard deviations from the normal

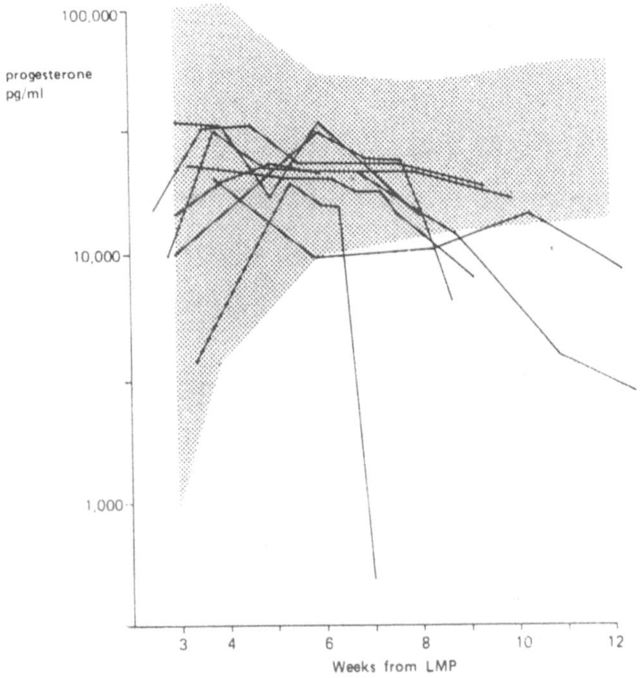

Figure I
Serum progesterone values in 8 patients undergoing early pregnancy failure plotted against the normal range expressed at ±2 standard deviations from the mean.

mean; however these individuals were representative of the group as a whole.

Oestradiol

Because of the progressive increase in the circulating levels of this hormone during normal pregnancy the changes in the abortion group were easier to determine. While a significant increase ($p<0.01$) in their serum oestradiol concentrations did occur between weeks 3–6, this was less than in the normal group ($p<0.05$). Thereafter the mean values remained static to about 10 weeks and then decreased. This became obvious when individual trends were plotted against the normal range, with the majority having values outside the lower limits before 10 weeks gestation (Figure II). Again, eight patients are used for illustration.

hCG

The trend for this placental protein hormone was different. The mean values plotted against the response of normal women were similar, though lower at each stage of gestation. The remarkable attempt of the placenta to produce this hormone, even in the absence of a fetus, is well demonstrated by the eight individuals in Figure

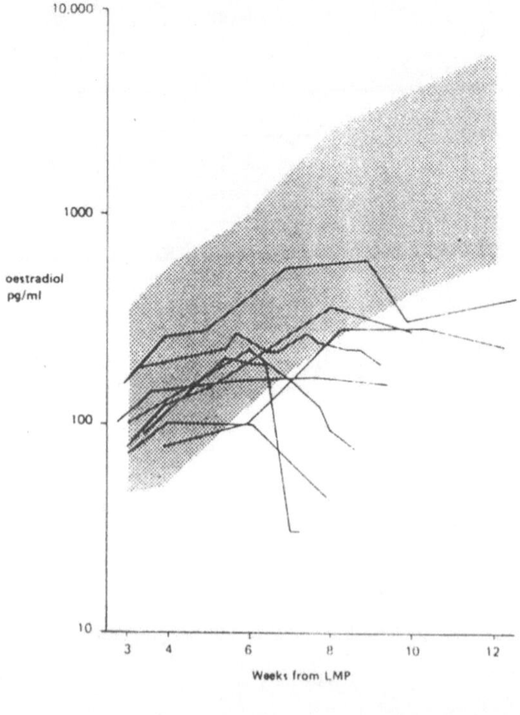

Figure II
Serum oestradiol values in 8 patients undergoing early pregnancy failure plotted against the normal range expressed at ±2 standard deviations from the mean.

III. There were sufficient data between weeks 4 and 6 for the doubling time to be calculated in 13 women who subsequently lost their pregnancies; in 12 it was not significantly different from the doubling time for the normal group (mean 2.4 versus 2.1 days). Thereafter however, the rate of increase in circulating hCG levels slowed in the abortion group to a significant extent ($p<0.001$) and the mean values at 8 weeks and beyond were all significantly less than for the normal mothers. For 13 (45%) of the 29 women reaching 8 weeks' gestation the hCG concentrations were more than two SDs below the normal mean and the decline thereafter tended to take the majority outside the normal range; interestingly, the rate of the decrease paralleled the physiological decrease occurring in normal mothers at this stage, paired analysis showing no difference.

hPL

Concentrations continued to increase though the mean concentrations achieved at 8 weeks and after were significantly lower ($p<0.001$) than for the normal group. By 8 weeks about half the women had concentrations outside the normal range but

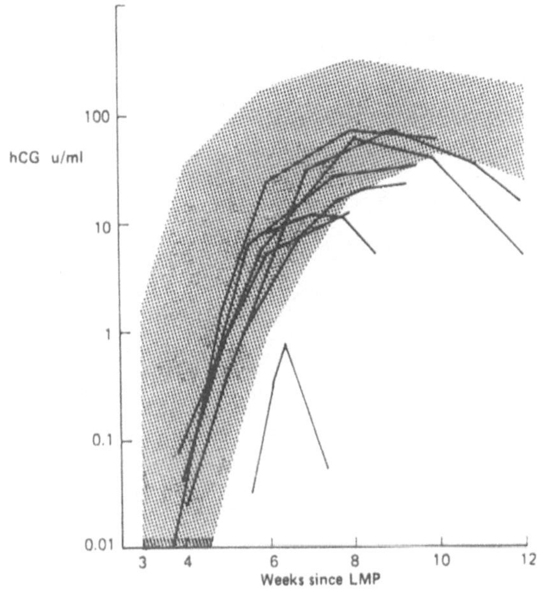

Figure III
Serum hCG values in 8 patients undergoing early pregnancy failure plotted against the normal range expressed at ±2 standard deviations from the mean.

were still showing an increase relative to previous values. Eight representative patients are shown in Figure IV.

The mean concentrations and confidence intervals for these hormones are given in Table 1. More detailed data and discussion of them are to be published elsewhere (Whittaker, Stewart and Lind; personal communication).

hPL AND GESTATIONAL AGE ASSESSMENT

During the course of our investigations into the hormonal changes occurring during the first trimester of normal viable pregnancies we observed a very close relation between the log values of maternal serum hPL and the length of pregnancy between 9–16 weeks. From work using placental explant techniques we have concluded that placental tissue is probably working maximally, and increasing hPL levels therefore reflect increasing placental mass particularly up to about 16 weeks' gestation. This has provided a valuable clinical test for the accurate assessment of gestational age over this interval. (4)

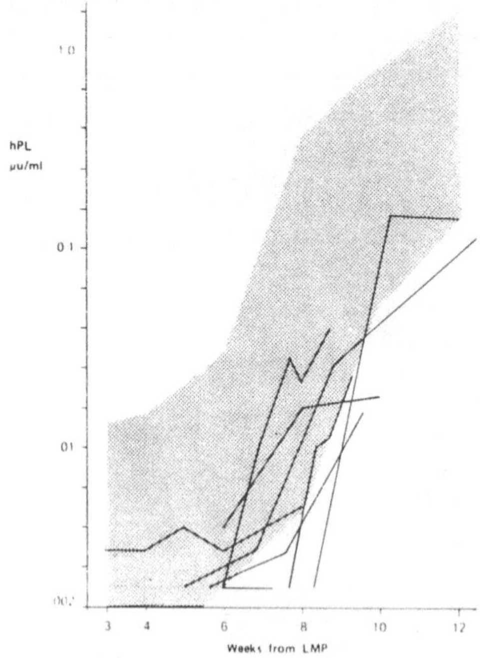

Figure IV
Serum hPL values in 8 patients undergoing early pregnancy failure plotted against the normal range and expressed at ± 2 standard deviations from the mean.

ENDOCRINE EVENTS AND IDDM

Because diabetic status might influence endocrine events this will be discussed first:

Diabetic control

A majority of patients attended during the first trimester and came regularly thereafter; each was asked to record the fasting and four preprandial blood glucose values daily for at least two days each week. We chose reasonably strict criteria for assessment: if the mean daily blood glucose level reached 10 mmol/l or if the glycosylated haemoglobin reached 10% of total haemoglobin on any two occasions during the whole of pregnancy, control was regarded as poor. On these definitions 19 women were in the well-controlled group and 8 poorly-controlled. Table 2 illustrates the mean blood glucose values in the interval between antenatal visits for both groups. Also shown are the mean glycosylated haemoglobin values; our normal pregnancy range is 5.8 – 7.3%.

Table 1. Serum hormone levels in early pregnancy. Geometric means and 95% confidence intervals in normal and women undergoing spontaneous abortion.

Gestation (weeks)	Subject group	n	Progesterone ng/ml	Oestradiol ph/ml	hCG U/ml	hPL uU/ml
3	Normal	38	10.4	128	–	–
			1.0 – 105	46 – 356		
	Abortion	14	13.2	115	–	–
			4.8 – 36.4	43 – 305	–	–
4	Normal	27	21.0	171	0.22	0.003
			3.9 – 112	51 – 568	.002 – 31.0	0.001 – 0.014
	Abortion	13	21.9	167	0.23	0.003
			12.6 – 38.1	62 – 450	.003 – 18.9	0.001 – .007
6	Normal	44	23.4	361	13.0	0.005
			9.9 – 55.7	134 – 977	1.0 – 168	0.001 – .029
	Abortion	22	18.6	207**	5.8	0.004
			7.7 – 45.0	45 – 940	0.7 – 51.3	0.001 – .012
8	Normal	63	23.9	780	72.4	0.041
			11.6 – 49.5	250 – 2547	17.0 – 309	0.005 – .369
	Abortion	29	12.8***	230***	15.4***	0.010***
			2.6 – 61.7	39 – 1352	0.55 – 430	0.001 – 0.068
10	Normal	62	27.0	1297	102.1	0.206
			12.9 – 56.8	416 – 4046	43.4 – 240	0.051 – 0.839
	Abortion	16	10.4***	244***	23.1***	0.034***
			3.2 – 34.1	64 – 923	4.4 – 122	0.005 – 0.226
12	Normal	68	29.4	1820	65.0	0.466
			13.9 – 62.4	540 – 6138	24.0 – 176	0.141 – 1.61
	Abortion	10	8.7**	203***	10.9**	0.095***
			2.0 – 38.4	29 – 1429	0.9 – 136	0.015 – 0.597

Normal versus abortion $p<.01$**
(group T test) $p<.001$ ***

The mean total daily insulin doses (Table 2) show that the requirements of both groups increased to the same proportional extent as pregnancy progressed; while the poorly-controlled mothers needed more insulin the differences between the two groups never achieved statistical significance. The incremental changes in insulin

Table 2. Mean and standard deviations (SD) of blood glucose, HbA1 and insulin requirement from 8 weeks' gestation

Gestation (weeks)		Mean daily glucose (mmol/l)	HbA1 (%)	Total daily insulin (units)
8	A	5.0(1.6)	8.6(1.9)	51.1(18.0)
	B	7.7(3.1)	10.5(1.3)	57.2(21.2)
10	A	6.6(1.1)	8.1(1.4)	51.2(13.9)
	B	6.3(1.0)	10.4(1.4)	57.2(22.3)
12	A	5.8(1.7)	8.5(1.3)	45.1(14.5)
	B	6.8(2.6)	9.7(1.1)	57.9(13.6)
16	A	5.3(2.1)	7.9(1.3)	44.4(13.2)
	B	8.0(3.8)	9.2(0.9)	54.1(15.2)
20	A	6.2(1.9)	7.6(0.9)	49.3(14.3)
	B	9.0(2.9)	9.8(1.1)	56.0(16.7)
24	A	5.9(1.5)	7.8(1.1)	57.3(17.0)
	B	7.7(1.9)	10.7(1.2)	64.6(20.6)
28	A	6.8(1.5)	7.5(1.1)	64.5(18.8)
	B	7.8(2.2)	10.2(2.5)	77.7(18.9)
32	A	5.9(1.8)	7.9(1.2)	72.3(19.3)
	B	7.0(2.7)	10.8(2.1)	84.9(19.3)
36	A	5.1(1.7)	7.9(1.2)	72.9(23.3)
	B	4.9(1.5)	8.0(0.9)	75.2(28.3)
38	A	4.6(0.7)	7.3(0.8)	75.4(28.3)
	B	–	–	–

A well-controlled
B poorly-controlled

requirements from the first trimester to term varied greatly between patients in both the well- and the poorly-controlled groups.

Birthweights and placental weights

Birthweights, expressed as the difference between actual birthweight and the expected birthweight calculated according to length of gestation, maternal parity, infant sex and maternal height and weight,[(5)] showed that the mean weights of the babies born to the diabetic mothers in both groups were significantly heavier than those of the normal mothers irrespective of the degree of metabolic control (Table 3).

Table 3. Means of the differences between the actual birthweight and the expected birthweight[5] of the babies of normal and diabetic mothers together with similar data for the placenta[6]

Patient group	Number of patients	Mean and standard deviation of birthweight differences	Mean and standard deviation of placental weight differences
Normal	69	–10 (342)	8 (117)
Well-controlled	19	613*** (655)	121* (183)
Poorly-controlled	8	746** (608)	142* (148)
All diabetic	27	652** (633)	127* (171)

Significance of difference from mean of normal group * $p<0.01$
** $p<0.001$

Well- and poorly-controlled groups not different from each other

Hormones

Figures V–VII illustrate the range for progesterone, oestradiol and hPL during normal pregnancy with the geometric mean values derived from the diabetic groups (logarithmic scale).

Progesterone: Using the diabetics as a single group the serum progesterone concentrations were significantly higher than for the normal group at 28, 32 and 36 weeks' gestation ($p<0.01$). When divided according to the degree of diabetic control it was the well–controlled mothers who achieved higher concentrations ($p<0.01$) the poorly–controlled women having values similar to the normal group.

Oestradiol: The serum levels were higher than normal at 28, 32 and 36 weeks' gestation ($p<0.001$) and even when the group was divided according to the degree of diabetes control the values remained higher than normal ($p<0.01$ for both groups).

hCG: The findings were reversed for this hormone. Taking the group as a whole the hCG values were above normal at 28 and 32 weeks' gestation ($p<0.01$) but mainly due to the poorly-controlled mothers ($p<0.001$) since the well-controlled group did not differ from the normal group.

hPL: This hormone did not differ from normal in either of the groups of diabetic mothers.

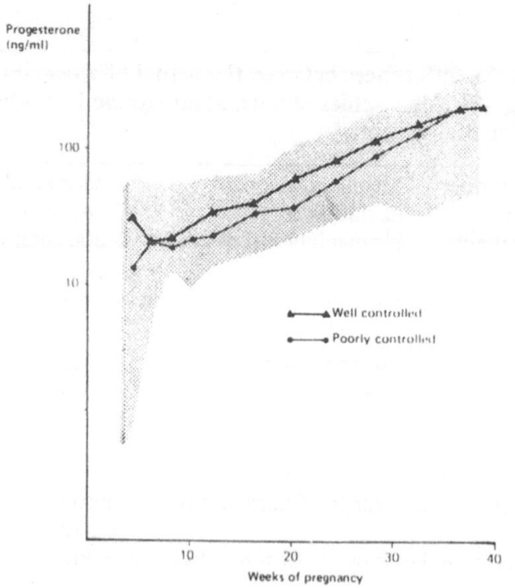

Figure V
Mean and range for serum progesterone concentrations in diabetic patients throughout pregnancy. The stippled area indicates the normal range.

Relation between hormones, birthweights and placental weights

Although the well-controlled patients had higher than normal progesterone levels in the third trimester and the poorly-controlled patients had higher than normal hCG levels during this time, it did not follow that within this diabetic group as a whole the poorly-controlled patients provided all the low progesterone concentrations or that the well-controlled patients provided the low hCG concentrations. On ranking the progesterone and hCG values at 28 and 36 weeks, the lowest progesterone values did not appear to correlate with the highest hCG concentrations (r=0.03). However in the normal group progesterone and hCG values did show a significant correlation (r=0.4, p<0.001) at 36 weeks.

Despite the lack of any change in circulating hPL concentrations in diabetic compared to normal women some interesting correlations emerged during the third trimester. Considering all the diabetic patients as one group, hPL correlated significantly with progesterone levels at 32 and 36 weeks (r=0.6, p<0.01). This persisted when they were divided into well-controlled and poorly-controlled groups (r=0.8, p<0.01; r=0.9, p<0.01 respectively). In the well-controlled group hPL also correlated with hCG at 28 and 32 weeks (r=0.6, p<0.01). Partial correlations eliminat-

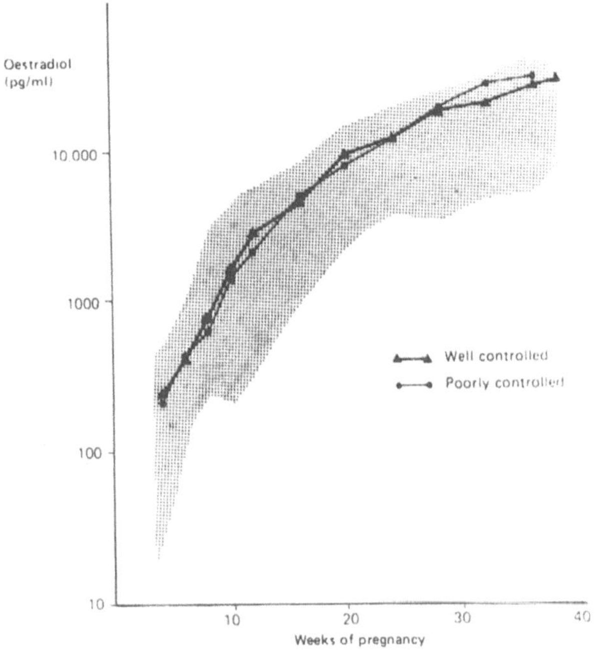

Figure VI
Mean and range for serum oestradiol concentrations in diabetic patients throughout pregnancy. The stippled area indicates the normal range.

ing the effect of time confirmed these hormonal pair correlations from 28–36 weeks for diabetic mothers but no such correlations were found in the normal pregnant women (r=0.1, r=0.3 respectively).

To determine whether the circulating levels of progesterone, oestradiol or hCG were reflecting placental mass or the birthweight of the infants the concentration of each hormone at 32 and 36 weeks' gestation was correlated with placental weight and birthweight after these had been corrected for maternal parity, stature, infant sex and length of gestation; no significant correlations were found in the diabetic group as a whole or when sub-divided according to control. However the correlation between hPL at 32 weeks (when most patients attended) and corrected birthweight was 0.48 ($p<0.02$). In our normal group of 69 women there was a correlation between serum hPL concentration and corrected placental weight (r=0.3, $p<0.01$) but not between hPL and birthweight (r=0.1).

Change in insulin requirements

No correlations ($r<0.3$) were found between hPL or any of the other hormones and the increase in insulin dosage which the majority of IDDM patients required during later pregnancy.[7]

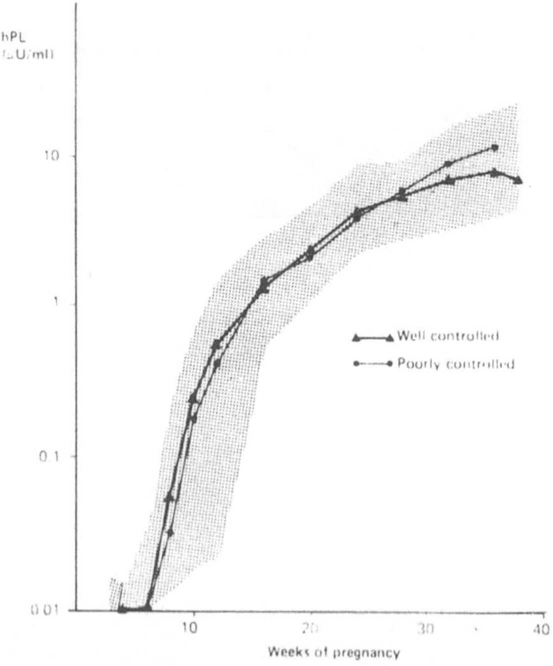

Figure VII
Mean and range for serum hPL concentrations in diabetic patients throughout pregnancy. The stippled area indicates the normal range.

IGF-1 DURING NORMAL AND DIABETIC PREGNANCY

The hormone first known as somatomedin C but now named insulin-like growth factor 1 (IGF-1) seems a likely candidate for influencing fetal growth, and several studies have tried to establish a relation with maternal circulating levels.[8] While IGF-1 does not appear to cross the placenta it has been suggested that maternal levels may influence substrate transfer across this organ thereby influencing fetal growth. To study these possibilities and the relation of IGF-1 to the other hormones we have studied serum samples from 22 normal mothers having babies of lower than average birthweight, and compared their concentrations to the data obtained from 38 mothers with IDDM in whom larger than average babies could be anticipated. At each antenatal visit sonar measurements of the fetus were undertaken so that the endocrine changes throughout pregnancy could be related to these parameters of fetal growth. Samples obtained 12 weeks post-partum were analysed whenever possible in mothers not using oral contraceptive agents.

The mean values throughout pregnancy and 12 weeks post-partum are shown in

Figure VIII for the normal and IDDM mothers and display some interesting features. Diabetic mothers have consistently lower serum levels than the normal mothers throughout pregnancy and post-partum, but the trends are similar in both groups. From early pregnancy differences in values of about 60 ng/ml, both groups show a decremental change between 6 and 12 weeks. Thereafter both groups display a steady rise in circulating concentrations, the rate of increase being the same for each. After delivery the IGF-1 levels decrease again, the 12-week concentrations being about 130 ng/ml lower than peak values for both groups.

Because of the structural similarity between hPL and human growth hormone (hGH) it has been postulated that the increase in maternal IGF-1 may be influenced by hPL. To maximise the serial nature of our data we looked at the changes within patients occurring between 24 and 36 weeks' gestation for both IGF-1 and hPL (using log values). This interval was chosen because it was the period when the circulating levels of both hormones increased rapidly. A significant correlation was found between the two hormones in both normal and diabetic mothers (0.70 and 0.54 respectively; $p<0.001$) which remained in the partial correlations allowing for the effect of time ($r=0.62$ and 0.39 respectively; $p<0.001$). We also exam-

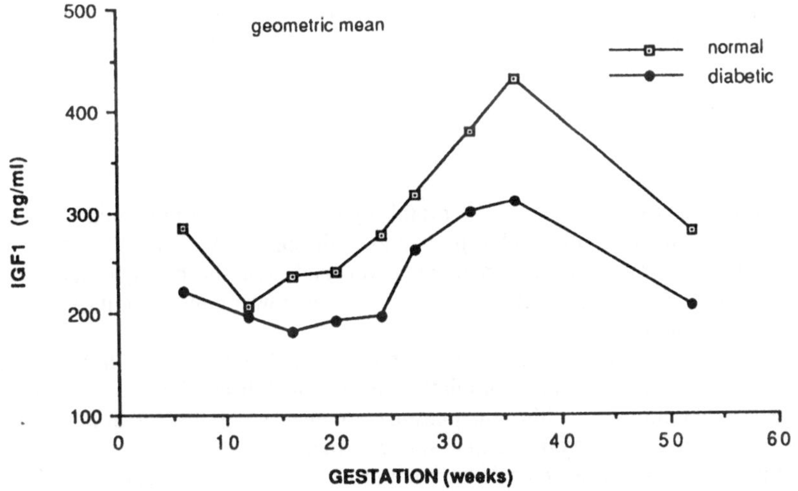

Figure VIII
Serum IGF-1 levels throughout normal pregnancies and those complicated by insulin dependent diabetes.

ined the incremental increases in both hormones over this gestational period and found that in both groups the mothers showing the biggest increases in hPL had the largest increases in IGF-1.

IGF-1, birthweight and placental weight

The increase in IGF-1 between 24–36 weeks displayed a significant correlation with birthweight ($r=0.37$; $p<0.01$). However hPL correlated with birthweight ($r=0.4$; $p<0.01$) and with IGF-1 and the latter's birthweight effect disappeared after multiple regression analysis allowed for the influence of hPL. The same was true of placental weight, the correlation between this and IGF-1 ($r=0.42$; $p<0.01$) becoming non-significant after allowing for the influence of hPL.

CONCLUSIONS

The hormonal activity of the placenta is remarkable particularly during the first trimester; over this time the maternal circulating concentrations of hPL and hCG each increase about one thousand-fold. It seems likely that these levels reflect increasing placental mass and both hormones will continue to be produced even in the absence of a fetus. For these reasons neither hormone is a useful clinical indicator of whether a pregnancy is likely to undergo spontaneous abortion or continue successfully to term. The placenta does appear to need some fetal co-operation to initiate sex–steroid production; again however they are poor clinical predictors of pregnancy outcome and sonar scanning will provide much better information concerning fetal viability.

In later pregnancy there are some relation between the hormones, but they have little obvious clinical value. While there is a relation between hPL levels and birthweight and placental weight, the correlations are of statistical significance but of minor clinical value.

Physiologically, IGF-1 seemed a promising candidate for a hormonal influence upon fetal growth but this too has proven to be disappointing. Not only is there no correlation between maternal circulating levels and infant birthweight, but IDDM mothers who on average deliver bigger babies have lower circulating IGF-1 levels than normal mothers.

As suggested at the beginning of this report, circulating levels of hormones in the maternal circulation may not relate to fetal growth because they exert a more paracrine-like influence within the placenta. Another possibility is that their influence is not direct but via effects upon substrate transfer.

While endocrine measurements have not proven to be useful for fetal assessment one valuable clinical tool has emerged from this work: the close relation between maternal hPL concentrations and the week of pregnancy has allowed a rapid and accurate estimate of length of gestation to be made between 9–16 weeks. Women attending the antenatal booking clinic during this interval can thus have pregnancy length confirmed thereby reducing the number of wasted appointments from patients attending for their 18-week scan too early; it should also help to decrease the false positive rate for interpreting maternal alpha-FP values. As more screening tests using maternal blood are described which require a knowledge of the length of gestation for their accurate interpretation the more helpful this particular endocrine test will become.

REFERENCES

1. Fant M, Munro H, Moses AC. Production of insulin-like growth factor binding protein(s) (IGF-BPs) by human placenta: variation with gestational age. *Placenta* 1988; **9**: 397-407.
2. Poisner A, Zaroff W, Richards R, Handwerger S. Partial purification from chorion and chorion-conditioned medium of a releasing factor for HPL and HCG. Presented at the 11th Rochester Trophoblast Conference, October 1988.
3. Aspillaga MO, Whittaker PG, Taylor A, Lind T. Some new aspects of the endocrinological response to pregnancy. *Br J Obstet Gynaecol* 1983; **90**: 596-603.
4. Whittaker PG, Lind T, Lawson JY. A prospective study to compare serum human placental lactogen and menstrual dates for determining gestational age. *Am J Obstet Gynecol* 1987; **156**: 178-182.
5. Altman DG, Coles EC. Assessing birth weight-for-dates on a continuous scale. *Ann Hum Biol* 1980; **7**: 35-44.
6. Thomson AM, Billewicz WZ, Hytten FE. The weight of the placenta in relation to birthweight. *J Obstet Gynaec Brit Comm* 1969; **7**: 865-872.
7. Stewart MO, Whittaker PG, Persson B, Hanson U, Lind T. *Br J Obstet Gynaecol*; In press.
8. Sara VR, Gennser G, Persson PH. Radiorecepter-assayable somatomedins during pregnancy and their relationship to fetal growth. *J Dev Physiol* 1982; **4**:187-193.

Discussion

Chairman: Professor R. D. G. Milner

CHARD: I detected a slight conflict in some of your earlier observations on various endocrine parameters in relationship to satisfactory and unsatisfactory outcome of pregnancy. Your conclusion was that all these changes were secondary to the underlying pathology, not the primary cause. Earlier it seemed that you had been trying to persuade us that there was a substantial divergence between the trophoblast proteins and the trophoblast steroids. If there is divergence could these endocrine changes have some primary effect as opposed to a secondary effect?

LIND: All I can say is that they are relationships, and if you look at the steroids, they do not seem to go on much beyond the *corpus luteum* time. If you look at the proteins, they do go well beyond the *corpus luteum* time. So you do appear to need a fetal trigger to start steroid production by the placenta.

NICOLAIDES: Is there any difference in the first trimester biochemical parameters in the group that had a blighted ovum as opposed to those who subsequently had cardio-uterine problems which resulted in spontaneous abortion? Is it cause or effect?

LIND: We only had eight who had a fetal heart detectable on sonar and did not find any differences, so we kept all 33 as a single group.

WHITTLE: I was fascinated by Dr Hay's concept that the placenta and the liver may be talking to one another metabolically. That is a very interesting idea, and I wonder whether he has observed any difference with gestational age. Maybe some of the observations that we make in growth retardation actually reflect alterations in liver function as much as placental function.

HAY: There might be changes but we do not have the answer. The studies being done at early gestation in our fetal lamb model are underway right now.

MILNER: At what gestational age is the amino acid – placental transfer data that you showed?

HAY: The data I showed you is on term fetuses. Comparable data are being obtained at around 70 to 90 days.

MILNER: The earlier information that you presented about the interaction between the fetus and the placenta with respect to glucose consumption was fascinating. From what gestational age were the results obtained?

HAY: Those data are shown from about 120 days and there appears to be no further change in those processes after 120 days. I showed you differences in transport capacity that appear to develop at least over the last half of pregnancy.

MILNER: How does that interact with the ontogeny of insulin secretion in the fetal lamb? I am interested to know if placental glucose uptake takes place in the presence of or independent of glucose-stimulated fetal insulin secretion.

HAY: We have done studies of glucose infusion, a square wave hyperglycaemic clamp, as early as 70 days and see an insulin response. This is consistent with *in vitro* data in a number of species and with other *in vivo* data from Dr Foden and her colleagues at the Physiological Laboratory in Cambridge. But the insulin response and the insulin effectiveness at 70 days is less than that at term. The decrease in fetal glucose concentration relative to that of the mother is probably less a reflection of secretion than of a change in the amount of insulin responsive fetal tissue in relationship to total fetal weight.

COCKBURN: Dr Hay, nowhere in your considerations did you refer to glycogen deposition, either in the placenta or the fetus. Glycogen deposition might explain how you got an oxygen consumption which was less than expected. Is it simply that the glucose is stored as glycogen in the placenta or in the fetus? And the same applies to amino acids. Are your amino acids measured in deproteinised plasma?

HAY: The uptake data were dependent on concentrations in whole blood, so that multiplied by blood flow gives you the net uptake.

COCKBURN: It is just that the rate of disappearance of amino acids into proteins is so rapid in the fetus. In a simple model there is a concentration gradient from maternal plasma water to placental tissue and that goes down a gradient to the fetus which is still higher than the maternal plasma water concentration. The placental amino acid concentration is extraordinarily high. One of the comments you made was that in the hypoglycaemic fasting state amino acids did not disappear so quickly—the flux was not so great. That might simply be due to the deficiency of insulin in the fetus. In the presence of glucose fetal insulin levels are high and the transfer of amino acids into fetal protein is speeded up by insulin directly. The siphoning of amino acids from maternal plasma water into the fetal tissues depends to a certain extent upon fetal insulin.

HAY: In trying to discuss placental metabolism in relation to fetal metabolism I left out a lot about the fetus and focussed on the placenta. We measure glucose utilisation with a tracer, so it represents total disappearance. We measure simultaneously but independently glucose oxidation rate, which accounts for about 50–60% of the utilisation rate. Obviously, the balance has to go somewhere, and we assume that most goes into glycogen because there is very little fat in the fetal lamb. There could also be a very large carbon exchange with carbon from glucose going into amino acids.

The amino acids are a very complex story. We know that *in vitro* and in some experimental *in vivo* conditions there is an independent effect of insulin on the transport of amino acids intracellularly. There is little evidence of how these amino acids are then metabolised. Recent studies using tracers and glucose clamp techniques suggest that if you raise the insulin concentration, everything else being the same, you can increase the oxidation of leucine which was counter to the idea that you would grow a bigger cell. These experiments were done in nongrowing organisms, namely adult humans. Comparable data have not been produced in the fetus *in utero* so we do not know what the independent effect of insulin would be on cellular amino acid uptake nor what happens to that amino acid once it is in the cell. It may be oxidised or shunted, and not contribute to synthesis unless there is an independent growth factor other than insulin present. I think that the concept of insulin as a fetal growth factor has been well discussed over many years, but it appears that it may be more a permissive growth factor allowing delivery to continue as opposed to altering the intracellular flux. The plasma leucine concentration can be raised *in vitro* or *in vivo* with an independent increase in the protein turnover rate and the oxidation rate. These studies have not been done in growing tissues so we do not know whether there is an independent effect on synthesis separate from oxidation that would alter turnover. You are quite right that the transport across the placenta is energy-dependent; I did not go into it because it affects different amino acids differently. Changing one amino acid concentration may affect its own transport, but in changing the concentration of that amino acid you may limit or exagerrate the transport of another one. The overall net balance of amino acid transport thus becomes extremely difficult to study.

HILL: I have a question for Dr Lind. There is evidence coming out of Liège and Atlanta that the placenta is secreting growth hormones and products of the growth hormone variant gene, and that most of the growth hormone in the maternal circulation in the third trimester is placental. Do you know of any information that has attempted to correlate that growth hormone with either placental or fetal growth?

LIND: None at all. You are quite right; a lot of information is coming out of America now and I think it will be postulated that changes in the small binding protein for IGF-1 may act as a feedback mechanism. I do not think that any of that work has got to the *in vivo* stage. What does concern me is that cross-sectional data are probably going to be a waste of time. We may find increases or decrements within an individual may relate better to birthweight than a given value at any given time in cross-sectional studies.

HAN: I would like to ask Professor Lind a question with regard to his maternal IGF-1 levels in normal and diabetic mothers. They are very interesting values correlating quite well with the sort of levels that you would find in the fetus. Obviously these levels are not coming in from the fetus or the placenta simply because the IGFs are bound to the binding proteins which originate in the mother. Has Professor Lind comparable data on insulin levels as well as on the weights of the infants of the normal and the diabetic mothers?

LIND: I should make it clear that these are total IGF-1 levels that were stripped from the binding protein. The weight relationships came from 22 mothers who had low birthweight babies and the diabetic mothers who had very high birthweight babies. That did establish a high correlation between birthweight and maternal IGF-1 values. Unfortunately though, when we did partial correlations with hPL we found that the association was actually due to hPL and not to IGF-1. We did not establish correlations with insulin levels because the heavy babies were of insulin-dependent diabetics.

CHARD: The earlier literature on hPL levels in diabetes was almost unanimous that overall they were elevated. More recent studies have shown no effect. Do you attribute this to some kind of treatment paradox? Perhaps by controlling pregnant diabetic women better metabolically we are eliminating a biological phenomenon of hyperplacentosis including a biochemical hyperplacentosis?

LIND: I think that the difficulty always is in defining good control. Many physicians are very convinced that the better the control the better the outcome. In principle that is probably true, but it hinges on what is good control and what is bad control. At the same time as we are getting better control of diabetes we are getting better women. They are better housed, better nourished, better educated. Statistically, progesterone, hPL, hCG and oestradiol are all higher in well-controlled diabetics. But it is only a statistical phenomenon; in practical terms they are hardly different. It is hPL which is closest to the norm.

GILLMER: In the data which you show with regard to pregnancy your observation was that the hormonal changes seemed to decline slowly, and the pregnancies you felt were failing as a result of some inherent problem rather than as a result of endocrine failure. Having had this unique opportunity to follow pregnancies can you make any observations as to the real cause of pregnancy failure?

LIND: At the 64-cell stage there are four cells which are destined to become fetus and 60 destined to become placenta. On the assumption that this sort of ratio continues for a few days I think it is understandable that the placenta can continue to produce its contribution, whereas, if the four cells which were destined to become the fetus perish then there is never going to be a pregnancy. As far as we can tell blighted ova do seem to be the commonest cause of early pregnancy failure. In other words, it must happen so early that no fetal material in the acceptable sense of the word is ever produced.

CHARD: Recent studies on quite substantial numbers of blighted ova have shown that they had very significantly elevated levels of alphafetoprotein. Perhaps the current view might incline to the thought that most blighted ova are missed abortions.

LIND: That is the point. You cannot see it on ultrasound, but histology reveals some kind of yolk sac or little "nubbins" of fetal material about 3 mm across. However, apart from the alphafetoprotein I know of no other data to suggest that fetal development ever gets off the ground.

CLAPP: In the monkey there is very good evidence for a so-called luteal rescue phenomenon if you look at progesterone levels. Do you see that in the human?

LIND: In the sense that the progesterone values are really very good between week three and week six, you could argue that hCG is promoting luteal production of progesterone and oestradiol. But after that time, unless there is a threshold phenomenon, even though hPL and hCG continue to be produced, the corpus luteum appears to fade away. Some of the women did not actually clinically abort until about week 10 or 12. So we had quite a lot of evidence on women who were still containing the products of conception.

CLAPP: So you would feel that progesterone production is primarily a luteal function until week eight?

LIND: Yes.

ALBERMAN: Most blighted fetuses are probably chromosomally abnormal, and until we look at the different chromosome abnormalities separately I think that we will confuse the matter.

LIND: The difficulty is that sufficient fetal tissue to do a karyotype is only available from a highly selected group. You would have great difficulty karyotyping a blighted ovum unless you got down to the placental level.

ALBERMAN: You could karyotype the membranes.

LIND: As long as it is still alive. We did not do this because we could rarely get a good yield.

SNOW: I have a comment on animal models as regards reduced blastocyst or embryo viability. It is true that if you reduce the cell numbers at those stages then you reduce the efficiency with which a fetus can develop. But by and large you do not interfere with the initial implantation or the initial placentation. You would expect some placental functions to continue for quite a while even in the absence of embryonic development.

SECTION 2

NORMAL FETAL GROWTH (Continued)

Genetic mechanisms of regulation of fetal growth

Dr V.K.M. Han

Growth and development of the mammalian embryo and fetus is a highly complicated sequence of events whereby a single cell zygote develops into a complex yet organized, multicellular, multisystem, fully developed animal. In mammals as in many other species, the major part of the process occurs during intrauterine life. In some organs and tissues it continues even after birth. Embryonic growth and development is controlled by two major factors, namely: (i) the genetic factors as determined by the embryonic or fetal genome, and (ii) the epigenetic or environmental factors — maternal or fetal factors that alter the expression of the embryonic or fetal genome. The relative importance of these two for the size and maturity of the infant at birth is still debated.(1) Recent studies into the control of fetal growth appear to suggest that the genome regulates the growth and development of the embryo and fetus in a predetermined pathway in which specific genes are turned on and off at specific stages of embryonic and fetal development, and that the epigenetic factors influence growth by their effect on this normal pattern of genetic expression.

Measurements of size of the newborn (weight, length, and other anthropometric data) have been used widely as endpoints of intrauterine growth both clinically and experimentally. Even though these measurements are helpful they do not determine the growth of a specific organ or tissue. In addition, anthropometric measurements at birth do not reflect the "growth potential" of the fetus which is determined to a great extent by the fetal genome, and to a lesser extent by epigenetic factors. At present, no measurement is available to determine the "growth potential" of a developing embryo. It is hoped that studies into the expression of genes encoding growth factors and related macromolecules (cell adhesion molecules, receptors, binding proteins) and the regulatory elements of the embryonic genome that control expression of these genes will lead to insights of this growth potential.

Tissue or organ development involves three different processes (i) replication or proliferation, otherwise known as "hyperplasia", (ii) migration, which involves the orderly and programmed migration of cells into definable tissues and organ rudiments, and (iii) differentiation, otherwise known as "hypertrophy", in which the cells increase in size and acquire both housekeeping and specialised functions. In this stage, a sub-population of cells acquires the capacity to synthesise macromolecules for the benefit of the entire embryo. A good example of this is the development of the endocrine tissues.

The mammalian genome contains the vital information and blueprint for these sequences of events to occur in an organised and orderly manner. How the genome, that is identical in all cells of the embryo, is differentially expressed in different somatic cells is not completely known. Studies in prokaryotes and simple eukaryotes suggest that it occurs by DNA or gene rearrangement. Rearrangements of DNA generate diversity that is required for different somatic phenotypes. Sometimes rearrangement creates new genes needed for expression in particular circumstances, e.g. immunoglobulins. In other cases, rearrangements are responsible for switching expression from one pre-existing gene to another. This latter mechanism is the predominant method by which growth and development is regulated. Any embryonic or maternal influences that alter the rearrangement mechanism will lead to growth abnormalities.

Presently, our knowledge of the mechanism and regulation of DNA rearrangement in eukaryotes is limited, but increasing rapidly. More is known about how the genome influences the phenotype and functions of cells. This is true also for cellular growth and differentiation. We believe that cellular growth and differentiation is mediated by macromolecules (e.g. cell adhesion molecules and growth factors) which are expressed at critical periods of development and coordinate the process. A good example is the coordinated regulation of cell cycle events in Balb-3T3 cells by several growth factors.(2) With some modification, this sequence of events is probably applicable for the growth of mammalian cells *i·n vivo*.

One additional concept that has emerged recently is that normal growth is a balance of expression of growth promoting factors and growth inhibitory factors. As the nomenclature implies, these have opposite effects on cell growth and differentiation. Most growth factors possess either function, but some (e.g. transforming growth factor-beta) may either promote or inhibit mitogenesis depending on the type of cell and conditions under which the biological actions occur. Any disruption of this delicate balance may lead either to undergrowth or overgrowth of the developing fetus.

Abnormalities of fetal growth that are associated with major defects of the genetic structure, e.g. chromosomal aberrations such as trisomy 18, are well known. However, it is now evident that structural defects of the chromosome, such as deletions or trisomy, need not be present for the occurrence of growth abnormalities. Products of one gene control the expression of other genes. This leads to a cascade of genetic events whereby one gene may either be turned on or off at one stage of development and this will control the expression of another gene at the next stage of development. For example, most eukaryotic genes require a promoter to determine if the gene will be transcribed or not. An active eukaryotic promoter may have an altered chromatin structure, consisting of a nucleosome-free hypersensitive site requiring *cis*-activation by an enhancer. The presence of certain factors that recognize promoter sequences and alter their structure or regulate the activity of an enhancer contributes to the regulation of gene expression. It is believed that this mechanism is active during eukaryotic development. One of these gene sequences which has been suggested to be crucial in regulation of genetic expression during development is called a homeo-box. Identification of homeo-boxes in drosophila, frog, mouse and human DNA, with similar sequences and the appearance of transcripts of these regions early in embryogenesis, suggest that these sequences are important. Even though the exact function of homeo-boxes is unknown, they may represent binding sites for proteins commonly needed for gene promoter or enhancer activation or they may encode DNA binding proteins.

Transcription of RNA does not necessarily result in the equivalent expression of the gene products. In eukaryotes, regulation of gene expression may occur at the subsequent levels of RNA stability, translation, post-translational processing, and transport. Two genetic mechanisms by which growth abnormalities may occur are as follows:

1) Firstly, minor sequence mutations in the embryonic genome involved in regulation of the expression of genes encoding growth factors and macromolecules (cell adhesion molecules, growth factor receptors) that participate in the control of tissue growth and differentiation may lead to growth impairment.

2) Secondly, epigenetic influence (alterations in maternal environment) impair growth and differentiation by altering the process of genetic rearrangement or expression of genes encoding growth promoters and inhibitors.

Very little evidence exists for these concepts which will be clarified by the increase in knowledge of the expression of the mammalian genes and their regulatory mechanisms.

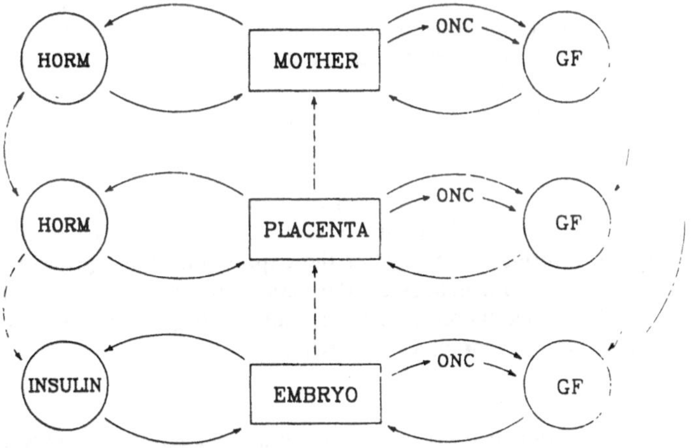

Figure I.
Genetic information transfer.

Even though the genetic regulation of growth via macromolecules is important, adequate nutrient and substrate supply to the developing cells is also of primary importance. Nutrition is an important regulator of the expression of certain growth factors, for example insulin-like growth factor 1 (IGF-1).[3] Impairment of nutrient supply due to defective placental transport is still the major cause of intrauterine growth retardation. However the molecular mechanisms underlying the process may involve alterations in the expression of growth regulating macromolecules.

We believe that the regulation of growth and development involves a series of events as illustrated in Figure I. There is substantial evidence that maternal hormones have no direct role in regulation of fetal growth, except by making the maternal environment favourable for normal embryonic development. In addition, classic fetal endocrine hormones, except insulin, play no part in fetal growth. It is likely therefore, that organ and tissue growth is regulated by growth factor macromolecules that are synthesized locally and act as autocrine or paracrine factors.

Transformation of a cell from a normal to malignant phenotype can be brought about by a variety of agents including tumour viruses. The transforming activity of a tumour virus may reside in a particular gene or genes in the viral genome. It is now believed that the tumour viruses alter the genetic regulatory switch that changes the growth properties of the target cells. Genes that confer the ability to convert cells to a tumorigenic state are called oncogenes. Viral oncogenes are closely homologous to normal cellular gene sequences (proto-oncogenes). It is believed that during evolution of retroviruses, normal cellular gene sequences have become integrated into the viral genome, and following retroviral infection of cells these genes are expressed in aberrant forms leading to neoplastic growth. One intriguing relationship between oncogenes and growth factors is that a number of oncogene products are similar to portions of growth factors or growth factor receptors, and some of the proteins that are associated with cellular proliferation.(4) As in tumorigenesis where oncogenes are aberrantly expressed, these oncogenes may be expressed in a regulated manner during normal growth and development. Expression of growth factor receptor mRNAs and/or oncogenes has been described in embryonic tissues,(5-7) placenta(8,9) and maternal tissues,(10) and they form an important element of normal growth and development.

In summary, the size and maturity of the newborn infant at birth be it term or preterm, will be determined by both the function of the embryonic genome as well as by epigenetic influences that alter the expression of the genome. Aberrent genetic or epigenetic influences on the expression of genes encoding growth factors and related macromolecules in the embryo, placenta and maternal tissues can therefore lead to abnormalities of growth.

REFERENCES

1. Robson EB. Human birth weight: natural selection and genetics. In: *The Biology of Normal Human Growth.* Eds. M Ritzen, A Aperia, K Hall, A Larsson, A Zetterberg, R Zetterstrom. New York: Raven Press, 1981· pp.183-192.
2. Stiles CD, Capone GT, Scher CD, Antoniades HN, Van Wyk JJ, Pledger WJ. Dual control of cell growth by somatomedin and platelet derived growth factor. *Proc Natl Acad Sci USA* 1979; **76**:1279-1284.
3. Underwood LE, Clemmons DR, Maes M, D'Ercole AJ, Ketelslegers J-M. Regulation of somatomedin-C/insulin–like growth factor I by nutrients. *Hormone Res* 1986; **24**:166-176.
4. Hill DJ, Strain AJ, Milner RDG. Growth factors in embryogenesis. *Oxford Rev Rep Biol* 1987; **9**:398-455.
5. Pfieffer-Ohlsson S, Goustin AS, Rydnert J, Wahlstrom T, Bjersing L, Stehelin D, Ohlsson R. Spatial and temporal pattern of cellular *myc* oncogene

expression in developing human placenta: Implications for embryonic cell proliferation. *Cell* 1985; **38**:585-596.

6. Rappolee DA, Brenner CA, Schultz R, Mark D, Werb Z. Developmental expression of PDGF, TGF-α, and TGF-ß genes in preimplantation mouse embryos. *Science* 1988; **241**:1823-1825.
7. Han VKM, Lund PK, Lee DC, D'Ercole AJ. Expression of somatomedin/insulin-like growth factor messenger ribonucleic acids in the human fetus: Identification, characterization, and tissue distribution. *J Clin Endocrinol Metabol* 1988; **66**:422-429.
8. Pfieffer-Ohlsson S, Rydnert J, Goustin AS, Larsson E, Betscholtz C, Ohlsson R. Cell-type-specific pattern of *myc* proto-oncogene expression in developing human embryos. *Proc Natl Acad Sci USA* 1985; **82**:5050-5054.
9. Goustin AS, Betscholtz C, Pfieffer-Ohlsson S, Persson H, Rydnert J, Bywater M, Holmgren G, Heldin C-H, Westermark B, Ohlsson R. Coexpression of the *sis* and *myc* proto-oncogenes in developing human placenta suggests autocrine control of trophoblast growth. *Cell* 1985; **41**:301-312.
10. Han VKM, Hunter ES III, Pratt RM, Zendegui JG, Lee DC. Expression of rat transforming growth factor alpha mRNA during development occurs predominantly in the maternal decidua. *Mol Cell Biol* 1987; **7**:2335-2343

Control of cellular multiplication and differentiation

Professor D.J. Hill and Dr V.K.M. Han

INTRODUCTION

Cell multiplication and differentiation are two aspects of a complex physiological process by which the conceptus increases in size, but they are not the only processes that constitute ordered growth. Considerable cell migration must occur in the early embryo bringing differing cell types into intimate contact with resulting inductive effects. Following blastulation epithelial-mesenchymal interactions become particularly important in shaping tissue morphology. At least three types of control govern early tissue interactions and responses: the deposition and subsequent modification of extracellular matrix molecules, the temporal expression of cellular recognition molecules and the appropriate expression of intercellular messengers such as the peptide growth factors.

Extracellular matrix components govern cell shape and proliferation rate *in vitro*, while evidence is accumulating that they can determine cell migration and the onset of differentiation *in vivo*. During the migration of neural crest cells from around the neural tube to form the peripheral nervous system, dermal pigment cells and connective tissues of the head, temporal interactions occur in the expression of fibronectin and tenascin along the migration tracts.[(1)] Tenascin appears immediately before the onset of migration and is removed immediately afterwards. This molecule, which is structurally related to fibronectin, may have a widespread role in tissue pattern formation. In addition to its potential role in cell migration tenascin has been implicated in epithelial–mesenchymal interactions which precede the induction of certain tissues, and in the differentiation of mesenchymal cells. During palate formation in the embryonic mouse tenascin fibrils appear between the mesenchyme of the two palatal shelves during shelf fusion as the intermediate epithelia make contact and degenerate. It has been suggested that tenascin may facilitate the breakdown of the mid-line epithelium and contribute to regional differentiation of the remaining palatal epithelium.[(2)] Tenascin is also expressed during condensation of mesenchyme in the wing bud of the chick embryo.[(3)] Wing bud cultures grown on tenascin showed a greater tendency to yield cartilage nodules than those grown on a plastic surface, suggesting a facilitative action in connective tissue differentiation.

A second category of developmental control involves the expression of intercellular recognition molecules by which cells recognise their anatomical position within developing structures. This system is so well developed that dispersed embryonic cells can assemble autonomously and reform tissue-like structures, and in some cases complete embryos.[(4)] Recognition molecules have been categorised into those which do not require calcium for their biological action, the cell adhesion molecules or CAMs, and those that are calcium dependent, the cadherins. Several subclasses exist within each group according to their principal or first-observed anatomical sites of expression; for instance epithelial cadherin, neural cadherin and placental cadherin. Despite this diversity their action appears to be uniform. Identical recognition molecules are expressed upon the membranes of homotypic cells during tissue condensation, or between heterotypic cells during mesenchymal-epithelial or other tissue interactions. Communication of cadherins with actin filament bundles within the cytoskeleton suggests that cells can respond directly to these molecular interactions, or lack of them, with movement. For instance, as mesoderm cells migrate through the primitive streak into the space between ectoderm and endoderm they lose epithelial–cadherin expression. When uterine decidual cells become associated with the extra-embryonic cells of the embryo to form the primordial placenta both layers express placental cadherin. This is immediately followed by invasive trophoblastic growth.

A third system of inter-cellular control during embryonic and fetal growth involves the release of hormonal messengers, of which the best characterised are the peptide growth factors.

PEPTIDE GROWTH FACTOR FORM AND FUNCTION

Those peptide growth factors that are best characterised are shown in Table 1. They are typically proteins < 30 kDa molecular weight which are synthesised and act within the local tissue environment as paracrine or autocrine hormones. Unlike classical endocrine hormones each growth factor may be synthesised by many anatomically diffuse tissues. They are generally not stored intracellularly and release is largely dependent on *de novo* synthesis. Peptide growth factors interact with receptors located on the cell membrane which are usually glycoproteins and which communicate with secondary messenger systems by conformational changes. This often involves the autophosphorylation of tyrosine residues located on the intracellular domain of the receptor. The second messenger systems utilised are diverse, and include changes to intracellular calcium levels, cyclic AMP, cellular alkalisation, and phosphoinositol metabolites. The net biological events induced by growth factors are, however, remarkably consistent and include a rapid stimulation of amino acid transport, glucose uptake and utilisation, and RNA and protein synthesis. For many, but not all growth factors, this is followed by DNA synthesis and cell replication. However, some growth factors, such as transforming growth factor ß and tumour necrosis factor, act predominantly as growth inhibitors.

The somatomedins or insulin-like growth factors (IGFs) are single chain polypeptides of ~ 7.5 kDa which share structural and functional similarities with insulin. Two peptide species exist: IGF-1 which has 70 amino acids and is encoded by a gene on human chromosome 12, and IGF-2 which has 67 amino acids and derives from a gene on the short arm of chromosome 11.[5] The IGFs are potent mitogens for cells derived from all primitive germ layers. In postnatal life the IGF-1 gene is under tight transcriptional control by growth hormone, circulating levels being severely reduced in hypopituitarism and elevated during acromegaly. While the major source of IGFs was originally thought to be liver it is now recognised that they are synthesised by most body tissues both before and after birth.[6,7]

Epidermal growth factor (EGF) is a single chain polypeptide of 53 amino acids with molecular weight 6 kDa. Mouse EGF was first isolated from male

Table 1. Peptide growth factors

Insulin-like growth factors somatomedins	IGF-1 & -2	Mitogen and differentiating agent for cells derived for all primitive germ layers.
Epidermal growth factor Transforming growth factor α	EGF TGF α	Mitogens for epithelial and mesodermal tissues. Inhibit differentiated function in ovary. Enhance maturation of skin and teeth. Promote release of HCG and HPL from placenta.
Fibroblast growth factor	Acidic FGF Basic FGF	Mitogen for mesodermal and endodermal cell types. Induce mesoderm formation in *Xenopus* embryo. Inhibit differentiation in muscle but potentiate hormone release in pituitary. Cause angiogenesis.
Platelet–derived growth factor	PDGF	Mitogen for mesodermal cell types. Chemotactic for fibroblasts, smooth muscle cells, monocytes and neutrophils.
Transforming growth factor β	TGF β	Inhibitor of epithelial cell proliferation but biphasic action on mesodermal cell types. Induce mesoderm formation on *Xenopus* embryo. Inhibit differentiation in muscle. Chemotactic for monocytes, and fibroblasts. Promote fibronectin and collagen synthesis.

submaxillary glands and the equivalent human peptide, urogastrone, from urine.(8,9) A structural analogue of EGF is transforming growth factor α (TGF α). This has a molecular weight of 7.5 kDa and shows a 30–40% amino acid homology with EGF.(10) TGFα reproduces all the biological actions of EGF and interacts with the receptor. EGF is a potent mitogen for epithelial and mesodermal cell types *in vitro* including connective tissues, glial cells and ovarian granulosa cells.

Fibroblast growth factor (FGF) has been isolated from bovine pituitary and brain in both an acidic (pI 4.5) and basic (pI 9.6) form, each being approximately 16–17 kDa.[11,12] FGFs are potent mitogens for tissues derived from mesenchyme or neuroectoderm such as chondrocytes, fibroblasts, myoblasts, glial cells, adrenal cortex and ovarian granulosa cells.[13] They are the most effective mitogens so far identified for vascular endothelial cells and additionally promote cell migration, invasion and the production of plasminogen activator, all necessary features of angiogenesis *in vivo*. Platelet-derived growth factor (PDGF) was first identified within the α storage granules of platelets. Human PDGF is a highly basic glycoprotein (pI 10.2) with two biologically equipotent variants, PDGF1 which contains 7% carbohydrate and has a molecular weight of 31kDa, and PDGF2 with 4% carbohydrate and molecular weight 28 kDa. In platelets both forms contain an A-chain of 15–17 kDa and a B-chain of 14 kDa linked by disulphide bridges. the B-chain of PDGF shows extensive sequence homology with the viral p28 protein encoded by the v-*sis* oncogene,[14] and the cellular *sis* gene was subsequently shown to encode the precursor protein for PDGF B-chain.[15] In tissues other than platelets PDGF usually consists of a homodimer of two B-chains. PDGF stimulates proliferation in many cell types derived from mesoderm including fibroblasts, smooth muscle cells, glial cells and ovarian granulosa cells.[16]

Transforming growth factor β (TGFβ) differs from the other growth factors outlined in that it predominantly acts as an inhibitor of cell proliferation. It is a homodimer of 25 kDa found in abundance in, and purified from, platelets. TGFβ is a potent inhibitor of epithelial cell replication *in vitro* at pM concentrations.[17] For mesodermal cells it can act as a bifunctional growth regulator either enhancing the actions of other growth factors on cell replication or serving as a growth inhibitor depending on the cellular substratum, the age of development of the tissue, and whether the cells are virally transformed.[18] TGFβ stimulates fibronectin and collagen release, major constituents of extracellular matrix, by some fibroblast types; increases the release of plasminogen activator from other fibroblasts leading to a degradation of extracellular matrix glycoproteins; and modulates cell adhesion molecule receptors. These properties suggest a potential role in tissue modelling.

Mitogenesis

The overlapping biological properties of growth factors such as IGFs, EGF, PDGF, and FGF as cell mitogens may represent, at first sight, gross evolutionary overcapacity. However, some selectivity exists since differing cell types may recognise each growth factor with a different relative sensitivity. Additionally, each growth factor appears to fulfil a particular role within the cycle of cell replication.

Many fundamental studies on cell cycle control have been performed using Balb/c-3T3 fibroblasts which were originally derived from an embryonic mouse. It was found that PDGF alone and at concentrations similar to those found in tissues was unable to initiate proliferation in quiescent, density-arrested Balb/c-3T3 cells and that an addition of plasma was needed for cells to enter S phase and DNA synthesis.[19] Similarly, platelet-poor plasma alone could not stimulate cell replication although it maintained cell survival. A sequential addition of PDGF followed by platelet-poor plasma enabled cells to progress to S phase with a lag period of 12 hours following exposure to PDGF. The percentage of nuclei stimulated to initiate DNA synthesis depended on the concentrations of PDGF and plasma. Only a transient exposure to PDGF was necessary and the sensitising effect lasted for 3–5 hours. In contrast, plasma was required for the whole of the remaining period of G_1. It was concluded that PDGF induced a state of "competence" which rendered quiescent cells capable of traversing the cell cycle from G_0 to G_1 in response to other plasma factors. FGF fulfilled a similar role for this cell type.

The need for plasma to enable synchronised Balb/c-3T3 cells to progress through G_1 could be replaced by a mixture of EGF and IGF-1, although the latter could be substituted by pharmacological concentrations of insulin.[20] The temporal order of exposure to these "progression" factors is important for subsequent entry into DNA synthesis, EGF being necessary for the first six hours of G_1 and IGF-1 for the remaining period until approximately 2.5 hours before the G_1/S boundary when cell replication becomes growth factor independent. The ability of cells to traverse the final part of G_1 without growth factor stimulation is probably due to the transcription of DNA-synthesising enzymes such as thymidine kinase and thymidylate synthase having been completed by this time. Their transcription earlier in G_1 is stimulated by IGF-1.[21] Growth arrested Balb/c-3T3 cells could therefore be induced to traverse the full cell cycle in defined culture medium containing only PDGF, EGF and IGF-1 in sequential order. Each growth factor may render the cells responsive to the next since exposure of cells to PDGF caused a change in affinity of the EGF receptor for EGF,[22] while plasma caused a doubling of IGF-1 receptor number approximately 3 hours into G_1 and prior to the onset of IGF sensitivity.[20]

The ability of Balb/c-3T3 cells to traverse the cell cycle in growth factor-supplemented medium was dependent on the availability of amino acids, especially those in group β such as cysteine, isoleucine, lysine, phenylalanine and tyrosine.[23] In medium deficient in amino acids cells become arrested at a point midway through G_1 coincident with the time from which IGF-1 is necessary. An additional amino acid-dependent restriction point was found in human fibroblasts 2–3 hours before the G_1/S boundary, coincident with the completion of DNA-synthesising enzyme transcription. This suggests that two periods within G_1 in particular require protein synthesis and that both may be dependent on IGF-1.

This model of growth factor action during Balb/c-3T3 cell proliferation does not hold true for all cell types although the concept of "competence" and "progression" factors appears to be universal. Human fibroblasts have a greater endogenous ability to release IGFs *in vitro* than do embryonic mouse fibroblasts.[24] Additionally, PDGF is necessary throughout G_1 as well as at the G_0/G_1 interface for optimal proliferation to occur.[25] Other cell types differ more radically; for instance EGF appears to act as a competence factor for isolated hepatocytes while IGF-1 fulfils this role for chondrocytes.

The mitogenic actions of some growth factors are influenced by associations with specific binding proteins or extracellular matrix components. An IGF binding protein of 26 kDa is released by multiple cell types *in vitro* and is found throughout extracellular fluids and the circulation.[26] It greatly extends the biological half-life of the IGF peptides. One form of this binding protein, purified from human amniotic fluid, avidly attaches to some cell membranes *in vitro* including those of fibroblasts.[27] Exogenous binding protein enhanced the mitogenic capacity of IGF-1 on adult human fibroblasts, while other closely related species, also isolated from amniotic fluid, did not associate with cell membranes and antagonised IGF-1 biological activity.[28] This may represent an additional level of growth control in which cells can up- or down-regulate IGF action by the synthesis of specific binding proteins.

A different mechanism may be responsible for prolonging the biological half-life of FGF within tissues. FGF avidly associates with heparin sulphate, a glycosaminoglycan produced in large amounts by vascular and corneal endothelium and a structural component of their extracellular matrix. The FGF gene does not encode a conventional signal peptide sequence which is necessary for vesicle-associated exocytosis.[13] The peptide may therefore leave the cell associated with extracellular matrix molecules and either interact immediately with FGF receptors as an autocrine stimulus or remain stored within the matrix. FGF bound to matrix components retains full biological activity. Since organogenesis involves an interaction of cells with newly-synthesised extracellular matrix in order to promote stem cell growth and stabilise their specialised phenotype, it is possible that FGF could exert both mitogenic and differentiating effects from a matrix store.

Tissue induction

Two peptide growth factors, FGF and TGFß, have been shown to promote the induction of mesoderm from primitive ectoderm in the early embryo. Such induction in the amphibian embryo depends on diffusable morphogens from the vegetal pole ectoderm causing mesodermal development from the animal pole ectoderm. FGF is a mesoderm-inducing factor for cultured animal pole ectoderm from *Xenopus* embryos; the structures which develop being primarily derived from ventral mesoderm and consisting of concentric patterns of loose mesenchyme, mesothelium and blood cells enclosed by ectoderm. Some dorsal mesodermal structures, such as muscle cells, were also identified.[29] TGFß also induced mesoderm formation in *Xenopus* ectoderm, especially muscle which was identified by the presence of α actin mRNA.[30] A synergism existed between FGF and TGFß in this respect.[31] The most potent natural source of mesoderm-inducing activity is conditioned medium from *Xenopus* XTC cell cultures, a known source of TGFß. The ability of TGFß antiserum to block the mesoderm-inductive capacity of XTC conditioned medium suggests that an amphibian TGFß may be the major bioactive moiety.[30]

Tissue differentiation

Growth factors can augment or antagonise the onset of differentiated cell function. A potentiation of differentiation need not exclude a mitogenic role since an immediate action on proliferation may be followed by a later tendency to promote terminal differentiation. Separate growth factors can co-operate or compete during the induction of differentiated function, while some show synergistic interaction with endocrine hormones. While growth factor action is most obvious during the progressive differentiation of the fetus and neonate, considerable interest has been shown in tissues which retain a high degree of anatomical and functional rearrangement in adult life, such as the ovarian follicles.

A well-studied model of tissue differentiation *in vitro* is the fusion of myoblasts into polynuclear, post-mitotic myotubes. This process can be quantitated by measuring the rise in myotube–associated enzymes such as myokinase and creatine phosphokinase, or the aquisition of acetyl choline receptors. Muscle differentiation largely occurs *in utero* in man but can still be observed in the first week post-partum in the rat. Physiological concentrations of IGF-1 or pharmacological concentrations of insulin promoted the proliferation of newly-isolated myoblasts and of established myoblast cell lines.(32,33) However, after one or two replicative cycles myoblasts ceased to proliferate in response to IGF-1 and were instead stimulated to differentiate terminally.(34) This action of IGF-1 on myoblast differentiation was still apparent when proliferation was abolished by exposure of cells to cytosine arabinoside. Primary and established myoblast cultures also proliferated in response to FGF. However, FGF inhibited myoblast differentiation to maintain an expanding population of cells.(35) TGFß exerted rapid anabolic actions on isolated myoblasts, such as an increase in amino acid transport, but had little effect on myoblast proliferation and inhibited myoblast differentiation.(36) When myoblasts differentiated spontaneously at high cell density the number of cellular receptors for TGFß was greatly reduced, a process also noted for EGF and FGF receptors.(37) Thus differentiation of tissues may be associated with gross changes in growth factor responsiveness.

The myoblast model demonstrates that separate growth factors, which in the short term have similar mitogenic actions, can have opposite effects on long-term tissue phenotype; FGF blocking and IGF-1 stimulating differentiation. Two observations suggest that IGFs are also involved in the differentiation of brain cell types. Firstly, when isolated cells from day old rat cerebellum were exposed to IGF-1 glial cell differentiation was directed towards the production of oligodendrocytes rather than astrocytes.(38) Secondly, IGF-2 synergised with nerve growth factor to promote neurite outgrowth from rat sensory and sympathetic ganglia.(39) IGF-1 has also been reported to potentiate the differentiation of fetal rat calvaria, chondrocytes, and erythroid precursor cells.

EGF modulates the differentiation of epithelial structures in the fetus and neonate. When administered to the fetal lamb for two weeks in the third trimester EGF caused hypertrophy of skin epithelium and the growth of the adrenal, thyroid, liver and kidney.(40) In the fetal rabbit and lamb exogenous EGF induced lung epithelial maturation and surfactant production,(41,42) while in cultures of embryonic chick skin EGF inhibited glucocorticoid-induced epidermal keratinisation.(43) Receptors for EGF are abundant in human placenta, especially on the microvillus plasma membranes in contact with the maternal circulation, and on the basolateral membranes adjacent to the fetal circulation.(44) This distribution implies an interaction between EGF and the syncytiotrophoblast, and studies with isolated trophoblasts and placental cultures have shown that EGF modulates trophoblast differentiation and function. In homogeneous cultures of term trophoblasts EGF caused a dose–related release of human placental lactogen (hPL) and human chorionic gonadotropin (hCG).(45) There was no change in trophoblast cell number within these experiments but EGF induced a differentiation of cytotrophoblasts to form a syncytium. Parallel experiments with early and late placental explants yielded similar results for hormone release.(46) It is not known whether the EGF that interacts with placenta *in vivo* is fetal, maternal or placental in origin. However, infusion of EGF into the fetal lamb caused an increased release of hPL into the maternal circulation. EGF is abundant in milk, especially colostrum, and may contribute to the proliferation and maturation of the neonatal gut.

GROWTH FACTORS IN EMBRYOGENESIS

Peptide growth factors appear very early in development. Indeed mRNA for TGF α and PDGF A chain are present in the fertilised mouse egg, being of maternal origin.(47) As the embryonic genome is activated at about the 4-cell stage so mRNAs for TGFß, IGF-2 and the type-1 IGF receptor become detectable when amplified by a polymerase chain reaction prior to hybridisation with specific cDNA probes. IGF-1 mRNA does not appear until around 8 to 9 days consequent when placentation begins. This suggests that IGF-1 expression may be driven by placental factors. Messenger RNA for IGF-2 was identified in embryonic chick eye, heart and wing bud mesenchyme.(48) Using immunocytochemistry we have investigated the presence of IGF-like peptides in the chick embryo from 2–10 days incubation (Hamberger and Hamilton stages 16–36).(49) In the developing wing bud IGF peptides were demonstrated throughout the undifferentiated mesenchyme of the wing bud. By stage 24 cartilage had begun to differentiate in the proximal limb bud and staining for IGFs disappeared in the region of chondrogenesis. This was coincident with a switch from type I to type II collagen production within this tissue and an increase in tenascin deposition. At stage 28 the cartilaginous rudiments of the long bones are clearly defined, and by stage 36 the epiphyseal growth plates are seen. At this time strong staining for IGF peptides became apparent within the maturing and hypertrophic chondrocytes. Myogenic regions of the chick stained strongly for IGFs from as early as stage 20 while the central and peripheral nervous system stained strongly throughout development. Parallel studies have demonstrated that the chick limb contains substantial amounts of FGF, particularly in the early stages when the structure is undifferentiated mesenchyme. The picture that emerges from studies with chick embryos is one of peptide growth factors appearing and disappearing in particular tissue structures coincident with major events of morphogenesis and differentiation. It is interesting that no growth factor has been shown to fulfil the role of morphogen in dictating the three dimensional structure of the limb.

In the rat embryo mRNA for IGF-2 was localised by cDNA/mRNA *in situ* hybridisation to yolk sac, hepatic bud, branchial arch mesoderm, and dermatomyotome between 10.5 and 14.5 days' gestation, and was additionally present in differentiated muscle, perichondrium, chondrocytes and gut epithelium in later gestation.[50] In the mouse embryo EGF receptors appear with the first differentiated cell type, trophoectoderm.[51] It is unclear whether the peptide that might activate these receptors is EGF or TGFα. Although TGFα was detected in the mouse embryo with the highest levels on day seven of gestation, *in situ* hybridisation studies in rat suggested that the embryo does not express TGFα at this time.[52] However, abundant TGFα mRNA was present in maternal decidua, especially adjacent to the embryo. Decidual expression appeared following implantation, peaked at day eight and slowly declined to day 15 in parallel with decidual resorption. Peak levels of TGFα may therefore be available to the embryo from a maternal source during gastrulation and neurulation. FGF mRNA is detectable in the *Xenopus* blastula[31] while the peptides are present in chick embryo brain, retina and vitreous from day 11 of gestation.

Goustin *et al.* [53] found expression of PDGF in human placenta from as early as 21 days post-conception. By *in situ* hybridisation the expression of the c-*sis* gene was localised to trophoblasts. Explants of first trimester placenta released radioreceptor-assayable PDGF, while cultured trophoblast cell lines were rich in high affinity PDGF receptors, and responded to exogenous PDGF with an increased expression of the proto-oncogene c-*myc* accompanied by DNA synthesis. Since the expression of c-*myc*, which encodes a DNA binding protein and is one of the first intracellular events to take place following interaction of PDGF with its receptor, was also localised to trophoblasts this may represent an autocrine action of PDGF on trophoblast proliferation during the early invasive growth of the placenta. TGFß mRNA was found in the vegetal pole ectoderm of *Xenopus* embryos and is transcribed by a maternally-derived gene Vgl.[54] An ectodermal cell line, XTC, obtained from a metamorphosing tadpole releases a TGFß–like peptide *in vitro*.[30] In the 11–18 day mouse embryo TGFß has been localised immunohistochemically to differentiated and undifferentiated mesenchyme, including bone and connective tissues, particularly that derived from neural crest such as palate, larynx, facial mesenchyme and teeth.[55] Staining was most intense around sites of tissue morphogenesis involving mesodermal interaction with adjacent epithelia, including hair follicles, teeth and secondary palate. In late fetal rat development TGFß bioactivity was identified in multiple tissues, levels being greatest in muscle, lung, liver and kidney,[56] while TGFß was released by isolated fetal rat calvaria and by myoblasts.[56,57] Following birth, TGFß concentrations in rat tissues decline rapidly to barely detectable levels,[56] although in the human TGFß remains widely distributed amongst cells of the immune system including monocytes and T-lymphocytes. Its presence in the latter has been hypothesised to constitute an autocrine negative feedback system on interleukin 2-dependent lymphocyte clonal expansion.[58]

PEPTIDE GROWTH FACTORS IN THE HUMAN FETUS

While it is not possible to study early events of embryogenesis in the human, fetal tissues are available from late first trimester until approximately 18 weeks from abortuses. In the early second trimester human fetus IGFs were localised by immunohistochemistry to epithelia within the gut, kidney and lung; hepatocytes, adrenal cortical cells from the fetal zone, differentiated skeletal and cardiac muscle fibres, haemopoietic tissue and dermal skin.(59) This distribution may depend on an association with specific IGF binding proteins which share a similar cellular distribution.(60) The binding proteins may contribute to a sequestration of IGF peptides within certain cell populations, since analysis of IGF-1 and 2 mRNA distribution in human fetal tissues by *in situ* hybridisation suggested that the majority was present in fibrous mesenchymal tissues adjacent to the cell types positive for IGF peptides.(61)

By early second trimester EGF is present in the human fetus within cells at the base of the gastric and pyloric glands in the stomach, the Brunner's glands in the duodenum, the epithelium of the distal convoluted kidney tubules, anterior pituitary, pseudostratified columnar epithelium of the trachea and the placenta.(62) In later fetal development mRNA for PDGF was identified in the human kidney.(63) Recently it was reported that TGFß was expressed by osteoblasts and osteoclasts within the human fetal epiphyseal growth plate.(64) This is of interest since TGFß has been reported to favour a switch from a chondoblast phenotype, typified by type II collagen production, to an osteoblast phenotype characterised by type I collagen synthesis.(65)

CONTROL OF GROWTH FACTOR EXPRESSION

Since the genomic drive to growth is balanced by the constraints of maternal size, placental function, and nutritional sufficiency, the expression of peptide growth factors is likely to depend on nutritional availability and oxygenation. However, there is evidence that a fetal hormone, insulin, may also influence growth factor expression. Almost all available evidence concerns IGF expression. Insulin is clearly essential to optimal fetal development since clinical or experimental fetal hypoinsulinaemia is associated with severe growth retardation, poor muscle mass and a failure of tissue IGF release.(66) Even when euglycaemia is maintained, as in the pancreatectomised fetal lamb, a lack of insulin impairs growth and causes a sharp reduction in circulating IGF-1.(67) Paradoxically, circulating IGF-2 levels were elevated. Fetal hyperinsulinaemia, either induced in animals or occurring in the human infant of the diabetic mother, is not accompanied by sizeable somatic tissue overgrowth or oversecretion of IGF peptides, although in the human and monkey adiposity is greatly increased. This suggests that insulin is largely permissive to fetal growth and to IGF-1 expression. The available evidence suggests that this is too simplistic a concept and that a variety of mechanisms may operate in different tissues and at different stages of development.

In the chick embryo insulin at physiological concentrations of 1–10 nM/l increased parameters of tissue growth, metabolism and muscle differentiation.(68) In mammalian fetal development insulin has not been shown to exert any direct mitogenic actions on isolated connective tissues at physiological concentrations. However, we have recently found that insulin will promote DNA synthesis by isolated newborn rat astroglial cells with a half-maximal concentration of 1–2 nM/l (Han, unpublished observation). This may be related to the release from these cells of a carrier protein which binds insulin and may increase the biological half-time.[69] Some previous observations on the growth-promoting ability of insulin *in utero* may have been compromised by inappropriate culture conditions. We recently found that insulin enhanced the release of IGF-1, IGF-2 and IGF binding protein from human fetal fibroblasts, although no effects were seen below a concentration of 17 nM/l.[70] However, insulin was only effective on sparse, rapidly growing cultures and was without action on confluent cells. Thus, there is no evidence that insulin at physiological concentrations will modulate IGF expression, and the permissive action of insulin on connective tissue growth may be mediated by a stimulation of nutrient uptake and utilisation. The creation of such an anabolic environment would favour growth factor synthesis.

COMMENTS

Peptide growth factors provide an infinitely variable, fundamental level of intercellular communication influencing all aspects of cell behaviour throughout life and anteceding the appearance of the endocrine system. Their sphere of influence is predominantly within each local tissue environment and this level of control, coupled with interactions between cells and extracellular matrix components, provides the fundamental drive to embryonic development. Each tissue has the potential to release a cocktail of peptide growth factors, some growth stimulatory and some inhibitory, some which potentiate differentiation and some which block it. The balance of this paracrine environment is likely to vary between tissues and with development. The paracrine system may be modulated by external variables which enhance or retard overall body growth or differentiation. Such influences are likely to include the nutritional–insulin axis.

A paracrine system is difficult to sample in a representative manner for diagnostic purposes during the pathogenesis of abnormal human fetal growth. Circulating levels of IGF-1 or 2, for instance, may tell the clinician nothing of the degree of differentiation of the lungs or liver. However, one tissue that is amenable to biopsy is the placenta. We have recently found that the placentae from infants severely growth retarded for gestational age are deficient in mRNA for IGF-1 (Han, unpublished observation). While it is not possible to extrapolate the efficiency of the paracrine growth system in placenta to the tissues of the fetus, the growth of the placenta is directly related to fetal growth potential by its ability to transport nutritional metabolites and undertake gaseous exchange from the maternal circulation. The quantitation of mRNA for key growth factors from needle biopsies offers a potential diagnostic tool for the early confirmation of abnormal growth or maturation *in utero*.

REFERENCES

1. Epperling H-H, Halfter W, Tucker RP. The distribution of fibronectin and tenascin along migratory pathways of the neural crest in the trunk of the amphibian embryo. *Development* 1988; **103**: 743-756.

2. Fyfe D, Ferguson MWJ, Chiquet-Ehrisman R. Tenascin immunolocation during palate development in mouse and chicken embryo. *J Anat Embryol;* In press.
3. Mackie EJ, Thesleff I, Chiquet-Ehrismann R. Tenascin is associated with chondrogenic and osteogenic differentiation in vivo and promotes chondrogenesis in vitro. *J Cell Biol* 1987; **105**: 2569-2579.
4. Dan-Sohkawa M, Yamanaka H, Watanebe K. Reconstruction of bipinnaria larvae from dissociated embryonic cells of the starfish, Asterina pectinifera. *J Embryol Exp Morphol* 1986; **94**: 47-60.
5. Tricoli JV, Rall LB, Scott J, Bell GI, Shows TB. Localization of insulin–like growth factor genes to human chromosomes 11 and 12. *Nature* 1984; **310**: 784-786.
6. D'Ercole AJ, Stiles AD, Underwood LE. Tissue concentrations of somatomedin-C: further evidence for multiple sites of synthesis and paracrine or autocrine mechanisms of action. *Proc Natl Acad Sci USA* 1984; **81**: 935-939.
7. Rotwein P, Pollock KM, Watson M, Millbrandt JD. Insulin-like growth factor gene expression during rat embryonic development. *Endocrinology* 1987; **121**: 2141-2144.
8. Cohen S. Isolation of a submaxillary gland protein accelerating incisor eruption and eyelid opening in the newborn animal. *J Biol Chem* 1962; **237**: 1555-1562.
9. Gregory H. Isolation and structure of urogastrone and its relationship to epidermal growth factor. *Nature* 1975; **257**: 325-327.
10. Marquardt H, Hunkapiller MW, Hood LE, Todaro GJ. Rat transforming growth factor type 1: structure and relation to epidermal growth factor. *Science* 1984; **223**: 1079-1082.
11. Gospodarowicz D, Cheng J, Lui GM, Baird A, Böhlen P. Isolation of brain fibroblast growth factor by heparin-Sepharose affinity chromatography: identity with pituitary fibroblast growth factor. *Proc Natl Acad Sci USA* 1984; **81**: 6963-6967.
12. Esch F, Baird A, Ling N, Ueno N, Hill F, Denoroy L, Klepper R, Gospodarowicz D, Böhlen P, Guillemin R. Primary structure of bovine pituitary basic fibroblast growth factor (FGF) and comparison with the amino-terminal sequence of bovine brain acidic FGF. *Proc Natl Acad Sci USA* 1985; **82**: 6507-6511.
13. Gospodarowicz D, Neufeld G, Schweigerer L. Fibroblast growth factor: structural and biological properties. *J Cell Physiol.* 1987; **Suppl 5**: 15-26.
14. Waterfield MD, Scrace GT, Whittle N, Stroobant P, Johnsson A, Wasteson A, Westermark B, Heldin CH, Huang JS, Deuel TF. Platelet-derived growth factor is structurally related to the putative transforming protein of p28sis of simian sarcoma virus. *Nature* 1983; **304**: 35-39.
15. Johnsson A, Heldin CH, Wasteson A, Westermark B, Deuel TF, Huang JS, Seeburg PH, Gray A, Ullrich A, Scrace G, Stroobant P, Waterfield MD. The c-sis gene encodes a precursor of the B chain of platelet-derived growth factor.

Embo J 1984; **3**: 921-928.

16. Deuel TF, Huang JS. Platelet-derived growth factor. Structure, function and roles in normal and transformed cells. *J Clin Invest* 1984; **74**: 669-676.
17. Strain AJ, Hill DJ, Milner RDG. Divergent action of transforming growth factor beta on DNA synthesis in human foetal liver cells. *Cell Biol Int Rep* 1986; **10**: 855-860.
18. Roberts AB, Anzano MA, Wakefield LM, Roche NS, Stern DF, Sporn MB. Type beta transforming growth factor: a bifunctional regulator of cellular growth. *Proc Natl Acad Sci USA* 1985; **82**: 119-123.
19. O'Keefe EJ, Pledger WJ. A model of cell cycle control: sequential events regulated by growth factors. *Mol Cell Endocrinol* 1983; **31**: 167-186.
20. Van Wyk JJ, Underwood LE, D'Ercole AJ, Clemmons DR, Pledger WJ, Wharton WR, Loef EB. Role of somatomedin in cellular proliferation. In: *Biology of Normal Human Growth*. Eds. M Ritzen, A Aperia, K Hall A Larsson, A Zetterburg, R Zellerstrom. New York: Raven Press, 1981: pp.223-239.
21. Yang HC, Pardee AB. Insulin-like growth factor I regulation of transcription and replicating enzyme induction necessary for DNA synthesis. *Cell Physiol* 1986; **127**: 410-416.
22. Sinnett-Smith JW, Rozengurt E. Diacylglycerol treatment rapidly decreases the affinity of the epidermal growth factor receptors of swiss 3T3 cells. *J Cell Physiol* 1985; **124**: 81-86.
23. Cooper JL, Wharton W. Late G1 amino acid restriction point in human dermal fibroblasts. *J Cell Physiol* 1985; **124**: 433-438.
24. Clemmons DR, Underwood LE, Van Wyk JJ. Hormonal control of immunoreactive somatomedin production by cultured human fibroblasts. *J Clin Invest* 1981; **67**: 10-19.
25. Westermark B, Heldin CH. Similar action of platelet-derived growth factor and epidermal growth factor in the prereplicative phase of human fibroblasts suggests a common intracellular pathway. *J Cell Physiol* 1985; **124**: 43-48.
26. Ooi GT, Herington AC. The biological and structural characterization of specific serum binding proteins for the insulin-like growth factors. *J Endocrinol* 1988; **118**: 7-18.
27. Clemmons DR, Elgin RG, Han VKM, Casella SJ, D'Ercole AJ, Van Wyk JJ. Cultured fibroblast monolayers secrete a protein that alters the cellular binding of somatomedin-C/insulin-like growth factor I. *J Clin Invest* 1986; **77**: 1548-1556.
28. Elgin RG, Busby WH, Clemmons DR. An insulin-like growth factor (IGF) binding protein enhances the biological response to IGF-1. *Proc Natl Acad Sci USA* 1987; **84**: 3254-3258.
29. Slack JMW, Darlington BG, Heath JK, Godsave SF. Mesoderm induction in early Xenopus embryos by heparin-binding growth factors. *Nature* 1987; **326**: 197-201.
30. Rosa F, Roberts AB, Danielpour D, Dart LL. Spron MB, Dawid IB. Mesoderm induction in amphibians: the role of TGF B2-like molecules.

Science 1988; **239**: 783-785.
31. Kimelman D, Kirschner M. Synergistic induction of mesoderm by FGF and TGF-beta and the identification of an mRNA coding for FGF in the early *Xenopus* embryo. *Cell* 1987; **51**: 869-871.
32. Ewton DZ, Florini JR. Relative effects of somatomedins, multiplication-stimulating activity, and growth hormone on myoblasts and myotubes in culture. *Endocrinology* 1980; **106**: 577-583.
33. Hill DJ, Crace CJ, Nissley SP, Morrell D, Holder AT, Milner RDG. Fetal rat myoblasts release both somatomedin-C (SM-C)/insulin–like growth factor I (IGF I) and multiplication stimulating activity: partial characterization of myoblast-derived SM-C/IGF I. *Endocrinology* 1985; **117**: 2061-2072.
34. Ewton DZ, Florini JR. Effects of the somatomedins and insulin on myoblast differentiation in vitro. *Dev Biol* 1981; **56**: 31-39.
35. Linkhardt TA, Clegg CH, Hauscha SD. Myogenic differentiation in permanent clonal mouse myoblast cell lines: regulation by macromolecular growth factors in the culture medium. *Dev Biol* 1981; **86**: 19-30.
36. Massagué J, Chiefetz S, Endo T, Nadal-Ginard B. Type beta transforming growth factor is an inhibitor of myogenic differentiation. *Proc Natl Acad Sci USA* 1986; **83**: 8206-8210.
37. Ewton DZ, Spizz G, Olson EN, Florini JR. Decrease in transforming growth factor β binding and action during differentiation in muscle cells. *J Biol Chem* 1988; **263**:4029-4032
38. McMorris FA, Smith TM, De Salvo S, Furlanetto RW. Insulin-like growth factor I/somatomedin-C: a potent inducer of oligodendrocyte development. *Proc Natl Acad Sci USA* 1986; **83**: 822-826.
39. Recio-Pinto E, Ishii DN. Effects of insulin, insulin-like growth factor-II and nerve growth factor on neurite outgrowth in cultured human neuroblastoma cells. *Brain Res* 1984; **302**: 323-334.
40. Thorburn GC, Waters MJ, Young IR, Dolling M, Buntine D, Hopkins PS. Epidermal growth factor: a critical factor in fetal maturation? In: *The Fetus and Independent Life* (Ciba Found Symp 86). Ed. J Whelan. London: Pitman, 1981: pp.172–191.
41. Catterton WZ, Escobedo MB, Sexson WR, Gray ME, Sundell HW, Stahlman MT. Effect of epidermal growth factor on lung maturation in fetal rabbits. *Pediatr Res* 1979; **13**: 104-108.
42. Sundell HW, Gray ME, Serenius FS, Escobedo MB, Stahlman MT. Effects of epidermal growth factor on lung maturation in fetal lambs. *Am J Pathol* 1980; **100**: 707-725.
43. Obinata A, Akimoto Y, Hoshino A, Hirano H, Endo H. Inhibition by epidermal growth factor of glucocorticoid-induced epidermal alpha-type keratinization of chick embryonic skin cultured in the presence of delipidized fetal calf serum. *Dev Biol* 1987; **124**: 153-162.
44. Roa CV, Carman FR, Ghegini N, Schultz GS. Binding sites for epidermal growth factor in human fetal development. *J Clin Endocrinol Metab* 1984; **58**: 1034-1042.

45. Morrish DW, Bhardwaj D, Dabbagh LK, Marusyk H, Siy O. Epidermal growth factor induced differentiation and secretion of human chorionic gonadotropin and placental lactogen in normal human placenta. *J Clin Endocrinol Metab* 1987; **65**: 1282-1290.
46. Maruo T, Matsuo H, Oishi T, Hayashi M, Nishino R, Mochizuchi M. Induction of differentiated trophoblast function by epidermal growth factor: relation of immunohistochemically detected cellular epidermal growth factor receptor levels. *J Clin Endocrinol Metab* 1987; **64**: 744-750.
47. Rappolee DA, Brenner CA, Schultz R, Mark D, Webb Z. Developmental expression of PDGF, TGF alpha, TGF beta genes in preimplantation mouse embryos. *Science* 1988; **241**: 1823-1825.
48. Engstrom W, Bell KM, Schofield PN. Expression of the insulin-like growth factor II gene in the developing chick limb. *Cell Biol Int Rep* 1987; **11**: 415-421.
49. Ralphs JR, Wylie L, Hill DJ. Distribution of insulin-like growth factor peptides in the developing chick embryo. *Development* 1989: In press.
50. Beck F, Samani NJ, Penschow JD, Thorley B, Tregear GW, Cochlan JP. Histochemical localization of IGF I and II mRNA in the developing rat embryo. *Development* 1987; **101**: 175-184.
51. Adamson ED. Meek J. The ontogeny of epidermal growth factor receptor during mouse development. *Dev Biol* 1984; **103**: 62-70.
52. Han VKM, Hunter ES, Pratt RM, Zendegui JG, Lee DC. Expression of rat transforming growth factor alpha mRNA during development occurs predominantly in the maternal decidua. *Mol Cell Biol* 1987; **7**: 2335-2343.
53. Goustin AS, Betscholtz C, Pfeiffer-Ohlsson S, Persson H, Rydnert J, Bywater M, Holmgren G, Heldin C-H, Westermark B, Ohlsson R. Coexpression of the *sis* and *myc* proto-oncogenes in developing human placenta suggests autocrine control of trophoblast growth. *Cell* 1985; **41**: 301-312.
54. Weeks DL, Melton DA. A maternal mRNA localized to the vegetal hemisphere in Xenopus eggs codes for a growth factor related to TGF-beta. *Cell* 1987; **51**: 861-868.
55. Heine VI Munoz EF, Flanders KC, Ellingsworth LR, Lam H-Y-P, Thompson NL, Roberts AB, Sporn MB. Role of transforming growth factor beta in the development of the mouse embryo. *J Cell Biol* 1987; **105**: 2861-2876.
56. Hill DJ, Strain AJ, Milner RDG. Presence of transforming growth factor beta-like activity in multiple fetal rat tissues. *Cell Biol Int Rep* 1986; **10**: 915-922.
57. Centrella M, Canalis E. Transforming and non-transforming growth factors are present in medium conditioned by fetal rat calvariae. *Proc Natl Acad Sci USA* 1985; **82**: 7335-7339.
58. Kehrl JH, Wakefield LM, Roberts AB, Jakowlew S, Alvarezmon M, Derynck R, Sporn MB, Fauci AS. Production of transforming growth factor beta by human T lymphocytes and its potential role in the regulation of T cell growth. *J Exp Med* 1986; **163**: 1037-1050.
59. Han VKM, Hill DJ, Strain AJ, Towle AC, Lauder JM, Underwood LE, D'Ercole AJ. Identification of somatomedin/insulin-like growth factor

immunoreactive cells in the human fetus. *Pediatr Res* 1987; **22**: 245-249.
60. Hill DJ, Clemmons DR, Wilson S. Han VKM, Strain AJ, Milner RDG. Immunological distribution of one form of insulin-like growth factor (IGF)-binding protein and IGF peptides in human fetal tissues. *J Molec Endocr* 1989; In press.
61. Han VKM, D'Ercole AJ, Lund PK. Cellular localisation of somatomedin (insulin-like growth factor) messenger RNA in the human fetus. *Science* 1987; **236**: 193-197.
62. Kasselberg AG, Orth DN, Gray ME, Stahlman MT. Immunocytochemical localization of human epidermal growth factor/urogastrone in several human tissues. *J Histochem Cytochem* 1985; **33**: 315-322.
63. Fraizer GE, Bowen-Pope DF, Vogel AM. Production of platelet-derived growth factor by cultured Wilm's tumour cells and fetal kidney cells. *J Cell Physiol* 1987; **133**: 169-174.
64. Sandberg M, Vuorio T, Hirvonen H, Alitalo K, Vuorio E. Enhanced expression of TGF–beta and c-fos mRNAs in the growth plates of developing human long bones. *Development* 1988; **102**: 461-470.
65. Rosen DM, Stempien SA, Thompsom AY, Seyedin SM. Transforming growth factor–beta modulates the expression of osteoblast and chondroblast phenotypes *in vitro*. *J Cell Physiol* 1988; **134**: 337-346.
66. Hill DJ, Milner RDG. Insulin as a growth factor. *Pediatr Res* 1985; **19**: 879-886.
67. Gluckman PD, Butler JH, Comline R, Fowden A. The effects of pancreatectomy on the plasma concentrations of insulin-like growth factors 1 and 2 in the sheep fetus. *J Dev Physiol* 1987; **9**: 79-88.
68. Girbau M, Gomez JA, Lesniak A, DePablo F. Insulin and insulin-like growth factor I both stimulate metabolism, growth and differentiation in the post-neurula chick embryo. *Endocrinology* 1987; **121**: 1477-1482.
69. Han VKM, Lauder JM, D'Ercole AJ. Rat astroglial somatomedin/insulin-like growth factor binding proteins: characterization and evidence of biological function. *J Neurosci* 1988; **8**: 3135-3143.
70. Hill DJ, Hubner C, Rashid P, Strain AJ, Clemmons DR. Insulin-like growth factor (IGF) binding protein release by human fetal fibroblasts: dependency on cell density and IGF peptides. *J Endocrinol* 1989; In press.

Discussion

Chairman: Mr R.B. Fraser

FRASER: There is a prevailing feeling that there might be a fairly simple relationship between several of the peptide growth factors and size at birth.

HILL: There is a loose statistical correlation between cord blood levels of IGF-1 and birthweight. There is much less convincing evidence that IGF-2 in the fetal circulation is related to birth size. The problem is to determine what circulating IGF-1 or IGF-2 tells you. Is it simply a representation of total anabolic status of the fetus, or is it, as the biology would imply, mainly a product of hepatic function because most circulating IGF seems to come from the liver? So it might tell you about the liver, but not about any other tissue.

SNOW: Can you distinguish between IGF which is produced because the fetus is a particular size rather than IGF which has caused it to become that size? Are these longitudinal data, and are there any data on conditions that would distinguish cause and effect?

HAN: Whether the reproduction of the expression of these growth factors is as a result of the cause or whether it is a cause of the reduction in growth is a very valid question, but we do not have data to support it. In experimental growth retardation models created by carunculectomy Robinson's group looked at IGF-1 and IGF-2 expression or IGF-1 and IGF-2 blood levels. IGF-2 blood levels appeared to go up while the IGF-1 levels appeared to go down. I think that we still need to do longitudinal studies to find out the cause and the result.

BRUDENELL: Would you expect there to be a relationship between insulin growth factors in the cord blood *in utero* obtained by cordocentesis and the birthweight?

HAN: A group in the US last year looking at cordocentesis blood longitudinally *in utero* found a correlation between the IGF-1 level in the cord and the ultrasound diagnosed fetal size but not with the IGF-2 levels.

BRUDENELL: And with birthweights rather than ultrasound estimations?

HAN: Ultimately with birthweight as well.

CAMPBELL: We know in hypoxic intrauterine growth retardation there is poor growth of the liver because of redistribution of the fetal circulation; blood is diverted to the brain and the visceral circulation is reduced. So it may just be a manifestation of this redistribution. Could that be the case?

HILL: Yes, the circulation levels are mainly a reflection of hepatic production.

DRIFE: It was mentioned this morning that an insulin-like growth factor binding protein is the main protein product of the decidua. The production is maximal around about the beginning of the second trimester. At the moment we are still puzzling over whether this is a protective measure or a regulatory mechanism. I wonder whether you have any ideas whether the decidua might be a controller of fetal growth for at least part of the pregnancy.

HILL: At present there is no known function for the binding protein which is present in massive amounts in amniotic fluid — in the region of 140 μg/ml. You must consider though that the decidua is a massively active endocrine tissue; it is producing enormous amounts of prolactin and other hormones as well as the IGF binding proteins.

CHARD: An inverse correlation between PP12, IGF binding protein levels and fetal weight has been clearly demonstrated. So as a phenomenon there is a very powerful inverse relationship.

HILL: But that is probably a product of the fact that there is a good inverse correlation between IGF-1 and the binding proteins, at least in postnatal life, so that is maybe what you are picking up.

CLAPP: With regard to the flow redistribution, I think that is a very late phenomenon in growth retardation. I would doubt that the flow interrelationships over time would be related to IGF production from the liver.

CAMPBELL: I would disagree. Whenever hypoxia occurs there will be flow redistribution. We could demonstrate it at 24 weeks' gestation.

CLAPP: I think that the responses have been clearly shown experimentally in response to acute hypoxia, but the response to a gradual onset hypoxia is not that of early flow redistribution. If you go acutely hypoxic below a certain level you will kill the fetus very abruptly. Until you get to that level the fetus adapts to the change in its oxygen environment quite nicely and flow redistribution does not occur until long after the initial event occurs.

CAMPBELL: It depends what you mean by late, but chronic hypoxia can exist in a fetus of 24 – 26 weeks and that hypoxia will cause a flow redistribution.

CLAPP: But if you look at the continuum between perfect health and death, flow redistribution is one of the last of the adaptive mechanisms that the fetus uses to survive.

CAMPBELL: I disagree, but I hope to convince you tomorrow.

CLAPP: I will try to convince you tomorrow.

Maternal diet and fetal substrate provision

Mr R.B. Fraser and Mrs F.A. Ford

It seems logical that pregnancy has an energy cost greater than the non-pregnant state. Energy is required for deposition as the products of conception, the energy cost of maintenance of the new tissues and energy deposited in maternal fat stores during pregnancy. Energy consumption in pregnancy may be reduced by alterations in patterns of exercise but national and international authorities have advised pregnant and lactating women to increase their energy intakes to meet the demands of reproduction.[1,2] For pregnancy these recommendations derive from the theoretical calculations of Hytten and Leitch,[3] which were that an additional 80 000 Kcal are required on average. Advice on the qualitative aspects of diet in pregnancy is usually limited to general comments on proportions of carbohydrate and protein to be selected.

QUANTITATIVE REQUIREMENTS OF DIET IN PREGNANCY

Durnin recently published the results of longitudinal studies of energy balance in healthy pregnant women in Glasgow[4] in which the food intake of 67 women was recorded longitudinally in pregnancy. This study showed a gradual rise in intakes over the duration of pregnancy, but the calculated extra energy intake of pregnancy was less than 20 000 Kcal. Basal Metabolic Rate (BMR) calculated by indirect calorimetry showed a fall in early pregnancy followed by a rise during the last 10 weeks. There was no excess requirement in the first 30 weeks of pregnancy, and the increase in the last quarter might have been met by a small increase in energy intake or a reduction in physical activity.

Durnin's study was expanded by further recruitment to become part of a collaborative international project in which longitudinal studies of maternal fat deposition and BMR were performed in Scotland,[5] the Netherlands,[6] the Gambia,[7] Thailand,[8] and the Phillipines.[9] Similar studies have been reported from Sweden[10] and England.[11]

The changes in BMR relative to the non-pregnant state are shown in Figure I. There is good agreement between the pattern observed in Scotland, England and The Netherlands, with a larger increase in Sweden. The Gambian women in contrast show a decreased metabolic rate followed by a shallow rise. This energy saving can only be achieved by a suppression of metabolism in the mother. When energy supplements were provided the BMR showed a significant increase suggesting that the energy cost of pregnancy can vary in response to caloric supply. This obviously represents a major adaptive benefit for times when food is in short supply. Indeed calculations of the cumulative maintenance costs of pregnancy in these women reveals a value of 1 000 Kcal for the supplemented women and an actual saving of 10 700 Kcal in the unsupplemented group!

In addition to the fall in BMR other energy sparing mechanisms include a

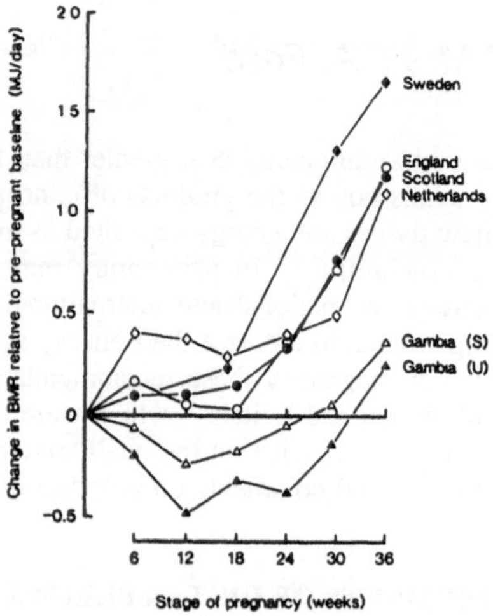

Figure I
Recent longitudinal studies of basal metabolic rate in pregnancy (S) supplemented (U) unsupplemented. (see text for references).

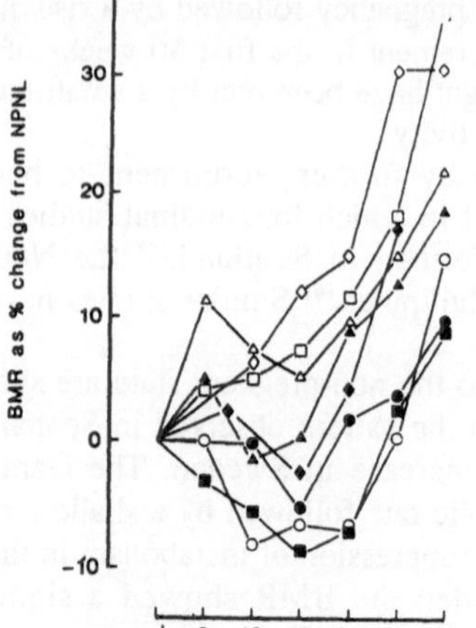

Figure II
Effect of pregnancy on BMR in individual women in Cambridge. NPNL = non-pregnant non-lactating. Average NPNL BMR was 6.1 MJ/day (Reference 2, with permission).

possible reduction in diet-induced thermogenesis[12] and highly significant reductions in energy expenditure on standardised activities when expressed per kg bodyweight, representing an increased work efficiency in pregnancy.[11] Thus, international studies reveal healthy women reproducing with net energy costs which vary from minus 10 700 Kcal in the Gambia to plus 120 000 Kcal in Sweden.

Prentice has suggested that studies based on group mean values of BMR may obscure considerable individual variation, and indeed whole body calorimetry studies performed in Cambridge reveal that some women respond like the Gambian mean and others like the Swedish mean.[11] Changes in BMR up to 24 weeks were significantly correlated with maternal fatness prior to pregnancy, with thin mothers tending to be energy sparing (Figure II). The doubly-labelled water technique measures total energy expenditure (TEE) in free-living subjects by a stable isotope method depending on calculations of CO_2 production derived from the differential elimination of ^2H and ^{18}O from the body water pool. With this technique applied to pregnant women, Davies *et al.*[13] reported similar individual variation in TEE confirming the existence of 'energy sparing' and 'energy profligate', normal women.

ENERGY LACK OR ENERGY EXCESS?

There must be speculation about what represents a physiological energy intake in pregnancy. Women are apparently reproducing successfully within a very wide range of energy intakes, and powerful adaptive mechanisms exist. Is the energy sparing thin woman responding normally to pregnancy or is she adapting at

Table 1. Changes in body weight and total body fat studied longitudinally in 22 healthy Swedish women.[10]

	Maternal body weight (Kg)	Total body fat (Kg)
prepregnancy	61.0 ± 9.9	17.2 ± 6.9
16 weeks	63.7 ± 9.7	20.7 ± 6.0
30 weeks	70.2 ± 9.9	22.6 ± 6.9
36 weeks	72.7 ± 10.3	22.3 ± 7.1
5–10 days post partum	67.6 ± 10.8	22.9 ± 7.8
6 months post partum	61.9 ± 10.9	20.4 ± 7.9

considerable personal cost to inadequate energy intake and poor pre-pregnancy stores? Do the unsupplemented Gambian women represent the limit of that adaptation and verge into a pathological state marked by retarded fetal growth? The supplementation studies suggest that a mean birthweight increase of 200 g can be achieved by supplements of as little as 400 Kcal. On the other hand are the well nourished energy profligate Swedes consuming excess energy at a time of a physiological switch to 'energy conservation' which leaves them with a net fat gain which they are unable to clear from their stores, and which may predispose to obesity in later life? Forsum's figures (Table 1) show two most interesting features on which to base speculation: firstly, that the first trimester of pregnancy is intensely anabolic, and secondly, that six months after delivery and despite lactation, a significant net maternal fat gain persists.[10] She also reported a significant positive correlation between resting metabolic rate and birthweight.

QUALITATIVE ASPECTS OF DIET IN PREGNANCY

The wide range of anabolic and catabolic pathways modified by insulin are shown in Figure III, modified from the work of Fritz.[14] Freinkel stated that "the disposition of most maternal fuels is intimately linked to the adequacy of insulin secretion in the mother. This means that maternal insulinisation might be the pre-potent arbiter of the incubation medium in which the conceptus develops".[15] Both prevailing insulin concentrations and tissue sensitivity to its actions must be considered. For instance, the dynamics of the maternal fat stores referred to above seem to alter with pregnancy, lipogenesis being a feature of the first two trimesters

Enhanced Insulin Activity	Anabolic Processes Lipid synthesis Protein synthesis Glycogen synthesis Catabolic Lipolysis Fatty acid oxidation Ketogenesis Glycogenolysis Proteolysis Gluconeogenesis	Reduced Insulin Activity

(Modified from Fritz – Ref 14)

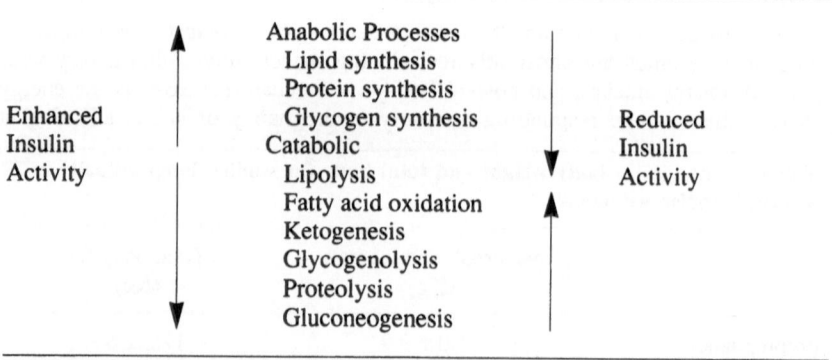

Figure III.
Metabolic processes influenced by alterations in insulin concentration and/or sensitivity to its action.

and lipolysis a feature of the third.[16] Since plasma insulin levels are higher in the third trimester this implies a loss of sensitivity to its actions.

The components of the substrate mix present in the placental blood supply are reviewed, with observations on the effects that qualitative changes in maternal diet may have on that mix by alterations in insulin sensitivity. From the model of maternal diabetes mellitus, there is evidence that the fetus may be unable to prevent excessive transfer of substrates, producing fetal hypertrophy. In chronic maternal malnutrition birthweight falls. These abnormal states are considered later in this volume.

GLUCOSE HOMEOSTASIS IN PREGNANCY

Glucose is the principal substrate for fetal growth and metabolism and its homeostasis is altered by pregnancy.

Fasting state

In normal pregnancy fasting plasma glucose levels fall progressively from about eight weeks amenorrhoea until term.[17] The level at 12 weeks' gestation is significantly lower than the non-pregnant level but there is no significant change as pregnancy progresses thereafter. The level of plasma insulin shows a small but significant rise during the last 10 weeks of pregnancy, i.e. the change is not contemporaneous with the fall in plasma glucose.[18] The fall in fasting glucose levels occurs too early in pregnancy to be simply explained by the demands of the conceptus, and is probably a resetting of the maternal internal environment designed to favour the fetus. How it might exert this benefit is not clear. The physiological nature of this reduction in plasma glucose appears to be confirmed by the fact that it is not accompanied by hypoinsulinaemia.[19,20] Hypoinsulinaemia only appears when the period of fasting exceeds 14 h,[21] a relatively rare occurrence in normal pregnant women.

Response to glucose loading in pregnancy

The observations of Lind *et al'*. are typical of studies performed in developed countries (Figure IV).[18] In early pregnancy the curve of maternal plasma glucose response shows a slightly smaller 'area under the curve' than in the non-pregnant state. This phenomenon is accompanied by similar plasma insulin levels. In late pregnancy, in contrast, there is a progressively greater area under the glucose curve because of a rise in the peak value and a delay in the time to reach the peak. These supposedly physiological changes have been considered to reveal a 'diabetogenic' influence of pregnancy.

Possible explanations of this state of relative insulin resistance (or loss of insulin sensitivity) include an increased secretion of hormones with an anti-insulin effect (such as glucagon, human placental lactogen (HPL), oestrogens, progesterone and cortisol).[22] This insulin resistance might be effected through alterations in tissue insulin receptor numbers or binding activity, or post-receptor phenomena within the insulin responsive cell. Ryan's group reported reduced glucose disposal rates

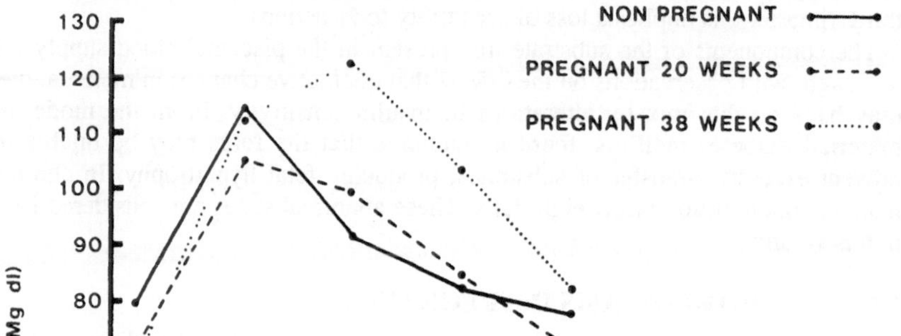

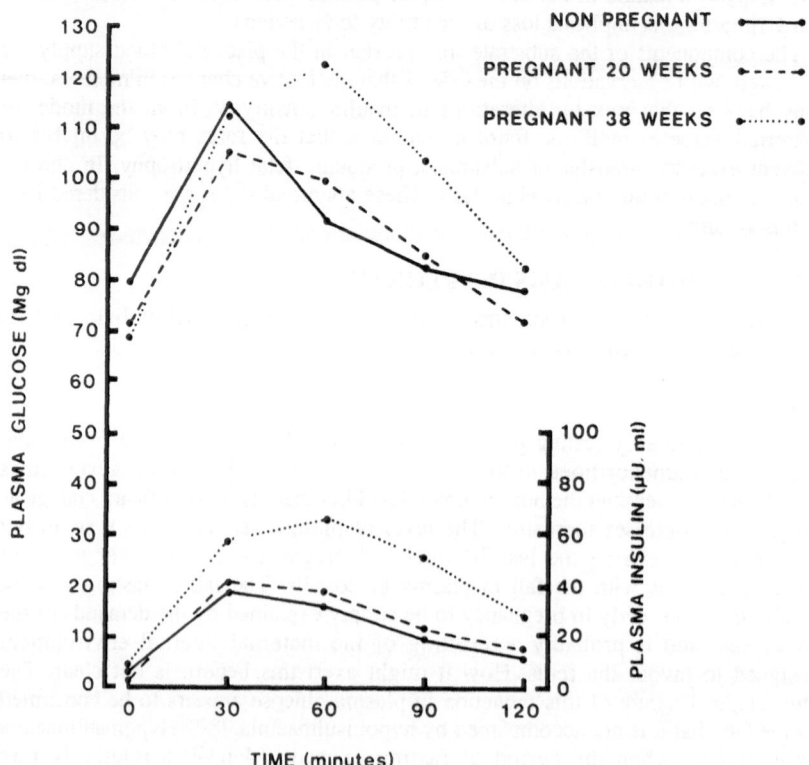

Figure IV
Longitudinal study of Oral Glucose Tolerance Test response in 19 healthy primigravids studied at 20 weeks, 38 weeks and as their own non-pregnant controls (Reference 18)

which were accompanied by normal erythrocyte insulin binding and they suggested a post-receptor defect in insulin activity in pregnancy.[23]

Glucose homeostasis and mixed meal feeding in pregnancy

Gillmer *et al.* studied plasma glucose and insulin levels during 24 h feeding experiments with normal diets containing 180 g of carbohydrate.[24] Nine normal women were studied in early pregnancy (12–22 weeks' gestation) and again in the third trimester. The mean diurnal plasma glucose was 4.5 mmol/l in early pregnancy and 4.8 mmol/l in late pregnancy. The level only exceeded 5.6 mmol in the hour after meals. These levels were comparable with profiles obtained in men and non-pregnant women, but the preprandial glucose levels were lower and the postprandial levels higher in pregnancy. An increased insulin response was required to maintain this normoglycaemia, a finding which was thought to confirm increased peripheral resistance to insulin activity in late pregnancy. In a study of obese non-diabetic pregnant women the insulin resistance of obesity was superimposed on that of pregnancy.[25]

Our own studies confirmed the increased insulin resistance in normal women habituated to low dietary fibre (DF) diets with advancing pregnancy, but in women habituated to high DF diets there appeared to be enhanced insulin sensitivity associated with a lower diurnal plasma glucose in the third trimester of pregnancy, compared to late second trimester.[26,27] We speculated that qualitative changes in diet might have an important effect on the substrate mix by altering the rate and proportions of nutrient absorption, but also have a more general effect by enhancement of insulin sensitivity.

Cousin's group studied 24 hour excursions of glucose, insulin and C-peptide in a longitudinal design in which six non-obese, non-diabetic women had profiles performed during the second and third trimesters and 6–11 weeks post-partum.[19] They ate to appetite from normal diets. Mean plasma glucose levels were significantly lower during pregnancy than post-partum — a difference entirely accounted for by reduced levels during overnight fasting. The 2 h postprandial glucose was significantly higher in the third trimester compared to the second trimester and post-partum studies. Mean plasma insulin levels over the 2 h were significantly higher in the third trimester, but all the differences occurred during the day and evening. During overnight fasting the insulin levels were similar in all three profiles.

Freinkel's group have compared the diurnal profiles of plasma glucose, insulin, free fatty acids (FFA), triglycerides, cholesterol and individual amino acids in late normal pregnancy and in age and weight matched non-pregnant women.[20] There were eight women in each arm of the study and the pregnant subjects were between 33 and 39 weeks gestation. They were given three equal portions of a standardised liquid formula diet at 0800 h, 1300 h and 1800 h and sampling was continued over a 24 h period. The diet contained 2100 Kcal/24 h with 275 g carbohydrate and 75 g protein. Preprandial glucose levels were lower and postprandial peaks were higher in the pregnant subjects. Their glucose levels were lower throughout the overnight fast. Preprandial insulin levels were similar, but postprandial insulin levels were three times higher in the pregnant subjects. Insulin levels during overnight fasting were similar.

Preprandial mobilisation of FFA was greater in the pregnant than the non-pregnant subjects.

Two hypotheses were generated to explain the observed changes in glucose homeostasis. The first, 'Facilitated Anabolism' suggests that the relative hyperglycaemia in the postprandial phase in pregnant women is a device to encourage fetal growth by allowing an increased transfer of maternal plasma glucose to the fetus. The second, 'Accelerated Starvation' suggests that the lower maternal plasma glucose levels in the post-absorptive phase and during overnight or more prolonged fasting, lead to enhanced lipolysis. The mother metabolises fats, thus sparing glucose for transfer across the placenta for fetal metabolism and growth.[28]

We have recently reported a similar experiment in which 15 non-pregnant and 14 pregnant women, studied in the third trimester, had diurnal profiles performed after habituation to three different diets in a crossover design.[29] Diet I contained 40% of energy from carbohydrate and 10 g DF representing typical Western intakes. Diet II contained 40% of energy as carbohydrate but 52 g of DF, and Diet III, designed to imitate typical Third World intakes contained 60% of energy as carbohydrate and 84 g of DF.

Our hypothesis was that the low DF diet would induce a similar response pattern to that described by Freinkel's group, but that the enhanced insulin sensitivity introduced by the high DF intakes would lead to improved glucose homeostasis on Diets II and III. Figure V reveals that there was no deterioration in glucose homeostasis in pregnancy on any of the three diets, and this study does not support the hypothesis of Facilitated Anabolism. Ketonaemia, as a measure of lipolysis and FFA oxidation was enhanced in pregnancy on the low DF diet, Diet I, but showed no enhancement on the two high DF diets, despite marked differences in glycaemia and insulinisation (Figure VI). This provides indirect support for the hypothesis that short-term dietary manipulation can affect post-receptor insulin sensitivity.

Other fetal substrates

Glucose is the principal energy substrate of the human fetus and as the precursor of fetal glycogen and lipid is a major source of the energy reserves of the newborn infant. It crosses the placenta by facilitated diffusion up to a saturable maximum which exceeds 17 mmol/l.[30]

Free fatty acids (FFA) cross the placenta and enter the fetal circulation, and might be a major source of nutrient supply to the fetus. Triglycerides can cross into the fetal circulation but to what extent they do so in the human is uncertain.[31]

Ketone bodies cross the placenta freely.[28] They are present in the maternal circulation when lipolysis is active. Ketonuria is very common in early pregnancy when nausea and vomiting reduce energy intakes in most women. The fetal brain has the appropriate enzyme systems from early pregnancy to oxidise ketones for energy. B-OH butyrate is a major potential alternate fuel which can replace glucose in the fetal brain in early human development.[32] The rate of ketone body oxidation by the brains of fetus, infant, child and adult depends on circulating concentrations. In addition, enzyme systems exist within the fetal brain from early gestation which are capable of incorporating carbon derived from ketone bodies into cerebral lipids and cerebral proteins.[33]

Despite this evidence of an important, if not essential, role for ketone bodies in fetal substrate provision there is a widely held view that ketonaemia should be minimised in pregnancy.[6] This view arises from the studies of Churchill and Berendes who reported that children of diabetic and non-diabetic mothers who had recorded episodes of ketonuria during pregnancy had lower motor and mental scores at eight months of age, and lower IQ values at four years of age than children of mothers who had no recorded ketonuria.[34,35]

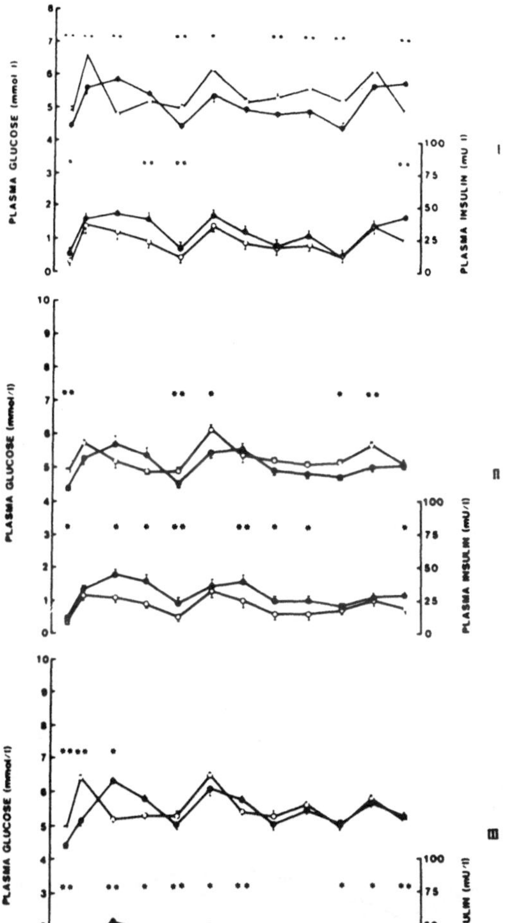

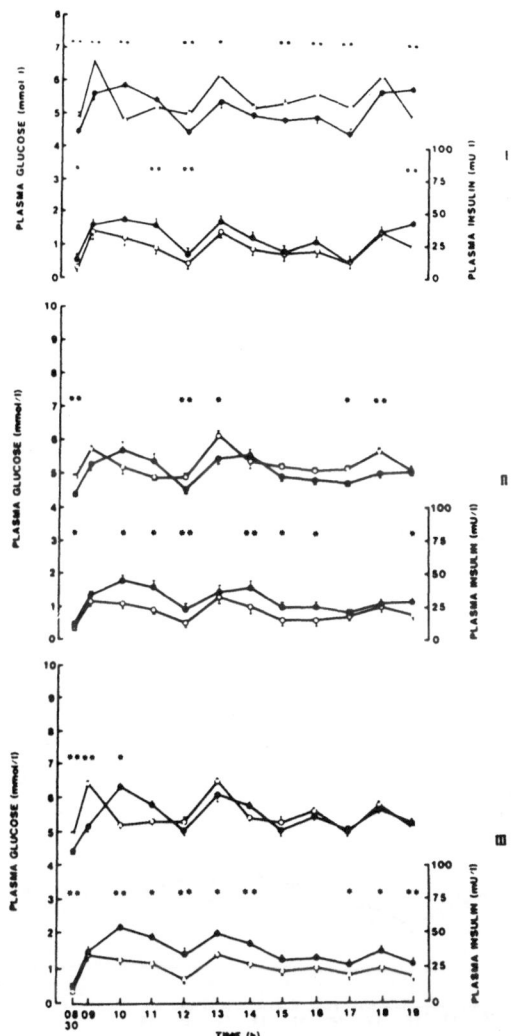

Figure V
Diurnal profiles of mean (±SE) blood BOH butyrate levels (mmol/l) on Diets I, II, and III. ●--------● pregnant subjects O--------O non-pregnant subjects. Statistical significance of difference * $p<0.05$ ** $p<0.01$ (Reference 29, by permission of the editor, *Br J Obstet Gynaecol*)

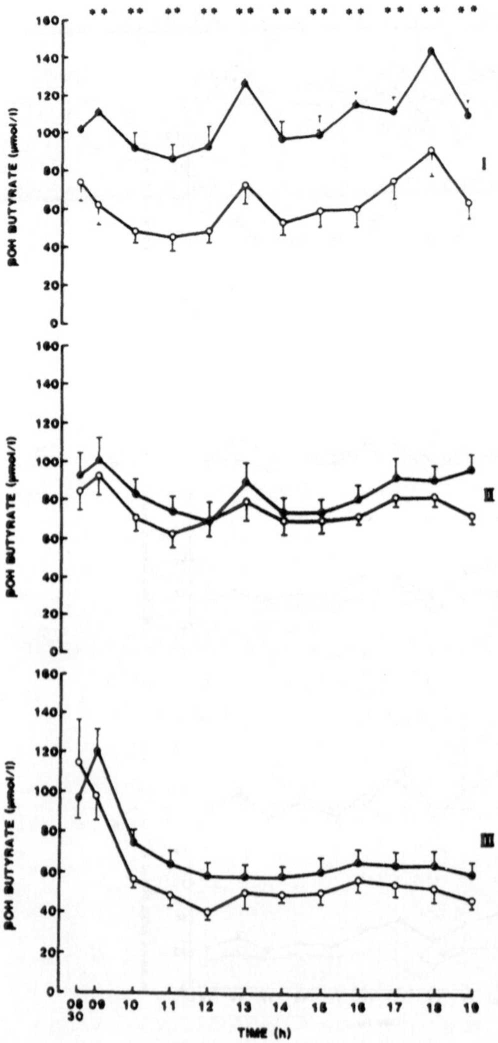

Figure VI
Diurnal profiles of mean (±SE) blood BOH butyrate levels (mmol/l) on Diets I, II, and III. ●---------● pregnant subjects ○---------○ non-pregnant subjects. Statistical significance of difference * $p<0.05$ ** $p<0.01$ (Reference 29, by permission of the editor, *Br J Obstet Gynaecol*)

In a reworking of the data of the Collaborative Perinatal Projects, Naeye and Chez corrected for non-nutritional factors which affect psychomotor performance and were unable to detect any influence of maternal IQ on the infants of non-diabetic mothers.[36]

Transplacental active transport of neutral and basic amino acids appears to be concentration dependent.[14] Their main role in the fetus is presumably related to protein synthesis. Physiological adjustments in pregnancy reduce circulating levels, and placental transfer is thought to be concentration dependent.[5] The effect of these changes on fetal growth and metabolism is speculative.

CONCLUSIONS

The principal metabolic fuel of the human fetus is glucose, but the importance of alternate fuels in both normal and adverse circumstances is not yet clear. All fetal substrate concentrations vary with meal frequency and content, both quantitative and qualitative. The volume and nature of the ingested food may have profound effects on the secretion rate of insulin and peripheral sensitivity to its action. Whether or not these substrate variations in well nourished women have any detectable effect on overall fetal growth, or more subtle effects particularly on brain growth and maturation, may await discovery.

Acknowledgement

We are grateful to Dr Andrew Prentice of the MRC Dunn Clinical Nutrition Centre in Cambridge for permission to reproduce Figures I and II, and for his helpful comments on those parts of this chapter which refer to energy intakes in pregnancy.

REFERENCES

1. FAO/WHO. Energy and Protein Requirements. *WHO Tech Rep Ser. No.* 522. Geneva: WHO, 1973.
2. DHSS. Recommended daily amounts of food energy and nutrients for groups of people in the United Kingdom. *Report on Health and Sound Subjects No.15*. London: HMSO, 1979.
3. Hytten FE, Leitch I. *The Physiology of Human Pregnancy*. Oxford: Blackwell Scientific Publications, 1971: pp.411-412.
4. Durnin JV, McKillop FM, Grant S, Fitzgerald G. Is nutritional status endangered by virtually no extra intake during pregnancy? *Lancet* 1985; **ii**: 823-825.
5. Durnin JV, McKillop FM, Grant S, Fitzgerald G. Energy requirements of pregnancy in Scotland. *Lancet* 1987; **ii**: 897-900.
6. van Raaij JMA, Vermaat-Miedema SH, Schonk CM, Peek MEM, Hautvast JGAJ. Energy requirements of pregnancy in the Netherlands. *Lancet* 1987; **ii**: 953-955.
7. Lawrence M, Lawrence F, Coward WA, Cole TJ, Whitehead RG. Energy requirements of pregnancy in The Gambia. *Lancet* 1987; **ii**: 1072-1076.

8. Throngprasert K, Tanphaichitre V, Valyasevi A, Kittigool J, Durnin JVGA. Energy requirements of pregnancy in rural Thailand. *Lancet* 1987; **ii**: 1010-1012.
9. Tuazon MAG, van Raaij JMA, Hautvast JGAJ, Barba CVC. Energy requirements of pregnancy in the Philippines. *Lancet* 1987; **ii**: 1129-1131.
10. Forsum E, Sadurskis A, Wager J. Resting metabolic rate and body composition of healthy Swedish women during pregnancy. *Am J Clin Nutr* 1988; **47**: 942-947.
11. Prentice AM, Goldberg GR, Murgatroyd PR, Davies HL, Scott W. Energy sparing adaptations in human pregnancy assessed by whole-body calorimetry. *Br J Nutr*; In press.
12. Illingworth PJ, Jung RT, Howie PW, Isles TE. Reduction in postprandial energy expenditure during pregnancy. *Br Med J* 1987; **294**: 1573-1576.
13. Davies HL, Prentice AM, Coward WA, Goldberg GR, Black AE, Murgatroyd PR, Scott W, Ashford J, Sawyer M. Individual variation in the energy cost of pregnancy. Doubly labelled water method. *Proc Nutr Soc* 1988; **47**: 47-45A.
14. Fritz IB. *Insulin Action.* New York: Academic Press, 1972.
15. Freinkel N, Metzger BE. Pregnancy as a tissue culture experience: the critical implications of maternal metabolism for fetal development. In: *Pregnancy Metabolism, Diabetes and the Fetus.* Eds. K Elliot, M O'Connor. Ciba Foundation Symposium 63 (new series). Amsterdam: Exerpta Medica, 1979.
16. McDonald-Gibson RG, Young M, Hytten FE. Changes in plasma non-esterified fatty acids and serum gycerol in pregnancy. *Br J Obstet Gynaecol* 1975; **82**: 460-466.
17. Lind T, Aspillaga M. Metabolic changes during normal and diabetic pregnancy. In: *Diabetes Mellitus in Pregnancy.* Eds. EA Reece, Dr Coustan. New York: Churchill Livingstone, 1988: pp.71-102.
18. Lind T, Billewicz WZ, Brown G. A serial study of changes occurring in the oral glucose tolerance test during pregnancy. *J Obstet Gynaecol Br Commonw* 1973; **80**: 1033-1039.
19. Cousins L, Rigg L, Hollingsworth D, Brink G, Auran J, Yen SS. The 24-hour excursion and diurnal rhythm of glucose, insulin, and C-peptide in normal pregnancy. *Am J Obstet Gynecol* 1980; **136**: 483-487.
20. Phelps RL, Metzger BE, Frienkel N. Carbohydrate metabolism in pregnancy. XVIII. Diurnal profiles of plasma glucose, insulin, free fatty acids, triglycerides, cholesterol, and individual amino acids in late normal pregnancy. *Am J Obstet Gynecol* 1981; **140**: 730-736.
21. Metzger BE, Ravnikar V, Vileisis RA, Freinkel N. 'Accelerated starvation' and the skipped breakfast in late normal pregnancy. *Lancet* 1982; **i**: 588-592.
22. Kühl C, Hornnes PJ, Andersen O. Etiology and pathophysiology of gestational diabetes mellitus. *Diabetes* 1985; **34 Suppl 2**: 66-70.
23 Ryan EA, O'Sullivan MJ, Skyler JS. Insulin action during pregnancy: Studies with the euglycaemia clamp technique. *Diabetes* 1985; **34**: 380-389.
24. Gillmer MDG, Beard RW, Brooke FM, Oakley NW. Carboydrate metabolism in pregnancy. Part 1. Diurnal plasma glucose profile in normal and diabetic

women. *Br Med J* 1975; **iii**: 399-404.
25. Gillmer MDG, Persson B. Metabolism during normal and diabetic pregnancy and its effect on neonatal outcome. In: *Pregnancy Metabolism, Diabetes and the Fetus*. Eds. K. Elliott, M O'Connor. Ciba Foundation Symposium 63 (new series). Amsterdam: Excerpta Medica, 1979: pp. 93-126.
26. Fraser RB, Ford FA, Milner RDG. A controlled trial of a high dietary fibre intake in pregnancy — effects on plasma glucose and insulin levels. *Diabetologia* 1983; **25**: 238-241.
27. Fraser RB. High fibre diets in pregnancy. In: *Nutrition in Pregnancy*. Eds. DM Campbell, MDG Gillmer. London: Royal College of Obstetricians and Gynaecologists, 1983: pp.269-277.
28. Freinkel N, Phelps RL, Metzger BE. Intermediary metabolism during normal pregnancy. In: *Carbohydrate Metabolism in Pregnancy and the Newborn 1978*. Eds. HW Sutherland, JM Stowers. Berlin: Springer-Verlag, 1979: pp.1-31.
29. Fraser RB, Ford FA, Lawrence GF. Insulin sensitivity in third trimester pregnancy. A randomized study of dietary effects. *Br J Obstet Gynaecol* 1988; **95**: 223-229.
30. Hytten FE. Placental transfer. In: *Clinical Physiology in Obstetrics*. Eds. FE Hytten, G Chamberlain. Oxford: Blackwell Scientific Publications, 1980: pp.468-492.
31. Hull D, Elphick MC. Evidence for fatty acid transfer across the human placenta. In: *Pregnancy Metabolism, Diabetes and the Fetus*. Eds. K. Elliott, M O'Connor. Ciba Foundation Symposium 63 (new series). Amsterdam: Excerpta Medica, 1979: pp.75-91.
32. Adam PAJ, Räiha N, Rahiala EL, Kemomäki M. Oxidation of glucose and D-B-OH Butyrate by the early human fetal brain. *Acta Paediatr Scand* 1975; **64**: 17-24.
33. Patel MS, Johnson CA, Rajan R, Own OE. The metabolism of ketone bodies in developing human brain: development of ketone-body-utilising enzymes and ketone bodies as precursors for lipid synthesis. *J Neurochem* 1975; **25**: 905-908.
34. Churchill JA, Berendes HW, Nemore J. Neuropsychological deficits in children of diabetic mothers. *Am J Obstet Gynecol* 1969; **105**: 257-268.
35. Churchill JA, Berendes HW. Intelligence of children whose mothers had acetonuria during pregnancy. In: *Perinatal Factors Affecting Human Development*. Washington DC: Pan American Health Organisation, 1969. Scientific Publication M185: pp.30-35.
36. Naeye RL, Chez RA. Effects of maternal acetonuria and low pregnancy weight gain on children's psychomotor development. *Am J Obstet Gynecol* 1981; **139**: 189-193.

Environmental influences on fetal growth: effects and consequences

Dr M.H.L. Snow

The evidence briefly reviewed in Section 1 of this volume indicates that for each mammalian species the growth rate of the embryo/fetus is characteristic, within a fairly narrow range. Significant departures above or below the accepted normal range are regarded as pathological and may be caused by any of several factors. Aneuploidy, gene mutation and gross abnormality (perhaps resulting from ingestion of teratogenic substances) are all associated with altered growth, generally with growth retardation. These are extreme examples but many other factors are known that influence embryonic/fetal growth in more subtle ways, e.g. maternal smoking, alcohol intake, maternal nutrition, metabolic disorders, medication and other drugs.

Brief inspection of embryological texts and tables of normal embryonic and/or fetal development generates the impression of a regular and closely controlled relationship between age, size and developmental stage. Detailed study of embryos developing normally does little to shake that belief; it reveals some variation in the size and development of embryos of a given age, but largely confirms the view that the component parts of a single embryo grow in harmony and that morphogenesis is highly co-ordinated. In the light of our knowledge that the formation of many organs requires the closely timed mutual interaction of tissues with different temporal and spatial origins, we might conclude that close co-ordination between parts is essential for embryogenesis to be successful. If the growth and development of an embryo departs from these tacit bounds then surely abnormality must result — but does it? Clinically there is an association between intrauterine growth retardation and susceptibility to developmental abnormality, both physical and physiological,(1-4) and teratologists have long been aware of the association of growth retardation with teratogenesis.(5) In this paper I will briefly review circumstances in which the mammalian embryo is confronted with the problem of being an inappropriate size for its age and developmental stage and will describe an extreme situation in which the harmony of development within the embryo is sacrificed, yet abnormality or death are not unavoidable outcomes.

There is a strong underlying presumption in this discourse – namely that the embryo has some notion of its own size, and how big it should be for its developmental age, and that homeostatic mechanisms are automatically deployed in order to seek and maintain this "target size" against any circumstance that would persuade it to depart from the normal growth curve. This viewpoint may seem extreme but is supported by observations on catch-up growth,(6,7) responses to teratogenic insult,(8) and certain other embryological data.(9)

TOO LARGE

Experimentally this condition can only be achieved by manipulation prior to implantation. Cells are added to the cleavage stage embryo, usually by the aggregation of whole embryos, or by the injection of cells into the blastocyst cavity. The latter method increases the size of the inner cell mass, from which the embryo proper will develop but probably does not increase the size of the trophectodermal lineage, whereas aggregation of earlier, 8– to 16–cell stages should contribute to all cell lineages. Normal viable chimaeric offspring are routinely produced from aggregates of two embryos in many mammalian species, including inter-species combinations, and in the mouse have been made with three or four embryos (see reference 9 for review). Normal development to fetal stages has been reported from aggregates of 16 eight-cell mouse embryos.(10) When born the chimaeric embryos are of normal size. The downward regulation in size of these embryo aggregates is made shortly after implantation, between the stage at which the pro-amniotic cavity is formed and that at which the primitive streak appears.(11-13) The mechanism of size regulation seems to involve a lengthening of the cell cycle during this approximately 24 h period, since cell death is not recorded at above normal levels and autoradiography shows no increase in the proportion of non-dividing cells. Lewis and Rossant (1982)(12) comment that pro-amniotic cavity formation occurred at different times in control and experimental double-embryos and suggest that this event may be linked to total cell number and not to the number of cell cycles undergone since fertilisation. However, Rands (1986)(13) does not find this association in the regulation of quadruple-embryos where the process seems to be age related. It is not known whether this size regulation is brought about by nutritional constraints imposed by the uterine environment or by regulatory mechanisms intrinsic to the embryo. The time of regulation coincides with the period during which the implanted embryo is furthest from a maternal blood supply but since the mouse embryo at this stage consists of only 200–400 cells (400–800 in double embryos) the nutritional demand should not be great. Size regulation in these circumstances is completed before the onset of organogenesis so tissue interactions involved in those processes are not compromised and the subsequent normal development is perhaps to be expected. There is no data to indicate when size regulation takes place in the other mammalian species in which chimaeras have been made.(9)

I am not aware of any experimental technique that will increase embryonic size during organogenesis above normal. There is a negative correlation between litter size and fetal weight at birth, and for the two days preceding birth in the mouse(14-16) so artificially reducing litter size is potentially a method for increasing fetal weight. We have attempted to exploit this by removing one fallopian tube, thus effectively halving litter size.(17) We found no significant increase in the $14^1/_2$ d or earlier stage weights of experimental over control fetuses although a highly significant difference is apparent at $17^1/_2$ d, $18^1/_2$ d and at birth (see Section 1). We are therefore of the opinion that the reduction in birthweight associated with large litter size is a function of late gestation, and probably due to crowding and/or nutritional constraints becoming acute shortly before birth. In this respect they may be similar to human multiple pregnancies.

TOO SMALL

From pre-implantation stages

A widely held view for many years has been that insults to the pre-implantation embryo which reduce cell-number or retard development will either be lethal or will be compensated for and not result in post-implantation developmental disturbance or long-term deleterious effects. At the beginning of the 1980's there was little data that questioned that view; it was known that the inner cell mass (ICM), from which the embryo proper develops, was more susceptible to damage than the extra-embryonic lineages, but the feeling was that below a certain size the ICM was inviable whereas above that size it would maintain normal embryonic development.(18-20) More recently several reports have appeared which seriously challenge that conclusion and expose threshold conditions which survive beyond implantation and impinge upon development through organogenesis. The long-term consequences of such conditions are not yet known but this subject is a matter of considerable concern with the growth in demand for *in vitro* fertilisation and human embryo transfer. Furthermore, it is essential information in assessing the applicability to man of pre-implantation diagnosis of genetic disease by molecular analysis following blastomere sampling.

Removing cells experimentally from embryos will reduce size. As with large embryos considerable autoregulation of embryonic growth can occur, for example viable newborn rabbits can be obtained from one cell taken from the 8–cell stage.(21) The experimental data on the timing of this upward regulation comes from analyses of mouse half-embryos and provides a less clear picture than has been provided for downward regulation. It has been claimed, but the data not published,(12) that regulation of half-embryos occurs at the same time as the double-embryos. The initial study of half-embryos(22) had rather few experimental embryos to analyse but found that regulation was complete by about 10 d gestation, and thought it probably occurred over the preceding day or two. This would be some 3–4 days later than the downward regulation. A more recent study(23) comes to a similar conclusion, based on a larger series of half embryos, clearly showing no regulation in late primitive-streak stages (7.5 d) but finding 10 and 11 d half-embryos to be of normal size. After regulation to normal size half embryos seem to fall behind again so that they are significantly small at 13.5 d gestation. Tsunoda and McLaren(24) reported that at 18 d gestation the average weight of fetuses in a large sample of half-embryos was significantly reduced. A similar catch-up and fall back, in the same time frame has been reported for XO female mouse embryos,(25,26) and in the recovery from cytotoxic damage caused by Mitomycin C given at late primitive-streak stages (Table 1).(17) The later time for upward regulation coincides with the development of full placental function and could therefore be related to nutritional status.

The manufacture of half-embryos by surgical manipulation of pre-implantation stages is a very laborious and different experimental system from which to obtain

Table 1. Fetal weights of control Q strain embryos, and of embryos from females treated with 100μg Mitomycin C (MMC) at 7.6 d of gestation.

Age (d)	Control No. embryos (No. litters)	Control log_{10} wt (mg)	MMC No. embryos (No. litters)	MMC log_{10} wt (mg)
9.5	15(2)	0.515±0.037	20(2)	0.309±0.037**
10.5	15(2)	1.094±0.021	29(3)	0.848±0.037**
11.5	49(4)	1.541±0.018	38(4)	1.293±0.036**
12.5	14(1)	1.774±0.028	46(4)	1.837±0.011
13.5	28(3)	2.087±0.010	37(4)	2.057±0.013
14.5	136(12)	2.324±0.007	49(6)	2.296±0.013
15.5	21(2)	2.652±0.087	29(3)	2.451±0.016**
16.5	8(1)	2.777±0.019	38(5)	2.690±0.008
17.5	–	–	–	–
18.5	32(3)	3.014±0.011	17(3)	2.918±0.051*
birth	66(6)	3.114±0.006	89(10)	3.073±0.005**

p – significantly different from control
* $p < 0.05$
** $p < 0.001$

large numbers of post-implantation embryos, so there is no detailed analysis of the impact on morphogenesis and little on the long term, post-natal effects that might result. No anatomical malformations are reported but half-embryos have been found to be retarded in development at the onset of organogenesis.[23] In another report on adult identical twins produced from 8-cell mouse embryos divided in half, behavioural studies reveal significant departures from normal with the monozygotic twins being less active, less emotional, less aggressive and less socially interested than their unmanipulated litter mates.[27] It was noted that in swimming tests the monozygotic twins seemed to prefer to float passively rather than to swim.

Reduction of cell number in pre-implantation stages by the use of cytotoxic agents is far harder to control than the surgical removal of blastomeres and in general the all-or-none effect described earlier is assumed to be the outcome, with few studies closely examining organogenesis stage embryos. A common observation is that the early post-implantation rat or mouse embryo (the egg-cylinder stage) is absent or malformed and unlikely to survive.[28-31] However, survival into late gestation of 50% or more transferred mouse blastocysts in which the ICM cell number is reduced to ~ 70% of normal has recently been reported.[32] At 10 d these embryos have 13 pairs of somites compared to 19 in controls but by

13-14 d they are essentially normal.

The consensus from these studies is that if upward regulation in size is called for it takes place during organogenesis, in a period of development noted for its high cell proliferation rate. The growth profiles are very similar, and strikingly like those found for embryos reduced in size by Mitomycin C at stages immediately preceding organogenesis (see below). It may be that our Mitomycin studies reveal the extremes to which the embryo can go in upward size regulation. They illustrate the subsequent developmental difficulties which are probably encountered irrespective of the cause of size reduction.

From post-implantation stages

Many factors, including social habits, can operate to reduce embryonic size after implantation but if the constraint is removed the embryo can make good the deficit to a greater or lesser extent by an acceleration in growth rate.(8) The success of such restorative growth is likely to decline with increasing embryonic age as the ensuing, conflicting demands of differentiation arise and restrict the freedom for tissues to act independently. Attempts to recover from being undersized in the fetal period may already be compromised by having passed the developmental stage during which an increase in organ sub-units (e.g. neurons, germ cells) is possible. In these instances fetal tissues seem similar to adult organs and may be severely restricted in the compensatory mechanisms available to them.(33)

The ability to recover from a size deficit present or induced just prior to organogenesis seems to be good but the level above which smallness no longer jeopardises normal development is not at present definable. The studies with Mitomycin C represent a case in which an extreme size reduction is produced and illustrate some of the problems that restorative growth can produce.

Mitomycin C is an alkylating agent which cross links DNA and inhibits further replication. In the mouse single intra-peritoneal injections into pregnant females when embryos are at mid-primitive-streak stages causes the immediate death of cells undergoing DNA replication. This removes up to about 50% of cells. A mitotic delay follows while surviving cells move through their division cycles. These two events can result in reduction of the late primitive-streak stage embryo to ~ $^1/_{10}$th of normal size (containing on average 1300–1400 cells rather than 13 000). Immediately thereafter cell proliferation increases, variably in different tissues and over some 6 d the embryos grow back to normal size as measured by weight and length.(34) The elevation of cell proliferation rates to different levels in different tissues rapidly produces physical distortion. The neural ectoderm, in which mitotic activity is most increased, outgrows the predominantly mesodermal components of the underlying body resulting in the neural tube being thrown into a wavy configuration. Nevertheless we realised that neural tube morphogenesis proceeded approximately according to its normal chronological timetable despite being extremely small, but that somitogenesis was initially slowed down.(35,36) The extent of the developmental mismatch is maximal in mid-organogenesis and is illustrated by the different somite stages at which otic placode/vesicle and limb-bud formation occurs (Table 2). Further developmental disharmony is observed in the timing of limb-bud formation, proliferation and migration of germ cells and gonad formation, vertebral morphogenesis and vertebral numbers, and in the early formation of gut and haemopoietic lineages.[35,37-40] Since the cytotoxic insult is extremely brief and the cellular debris rapidly cleared away many hours or even days prior to the appearance of affected organs, it can be concluded that all the developmental aberrations are the consequence of the disturbances to growth, and not the result of direct action on primordia.

Although anatomical recovery from the cytotoxic damage is satisfactory insofar as fetuses are born in normal numbers and of normal birthweight, there are severe

Table 2. Developmental asynchrony between normal Q strain embryos and those exposed to Mitomycin C (MMC) at 7.0 d gestation. The asynchrony is expressed in hours, either with reference to somite stage, a common measure of embryonic development, or with reference to the chronological age of the embryo. + means MMC embryos are advanced, - means retarded.

	Somite No. (age, d)		Asynchrony (h)	
	Control	MMC	By somite	By age
Otic placode forms	12–13 (8.9)	7–8 (9.0)	+5 to 6	0 to –2
Otic vesicle forms	14–16 (9.0)	12–13 (9.3)	+3	–7 to –8
Otic vesicle closes	25–27 (9.6)	22–23 (10.0)	+3 to 4	–9 to –10
Fore limb-bud	19–20 (9.2)	20–23 (9.9)	0 to –2	~ –15
Hind limb-bud	31–33 (10.0)	27–28 (10.4)	+5 to 6	–8 to –9

post-natal consequences. About half of the offspring fail to survive to weaning, their death usually being associated with runting and ataxia. It seems plausible to relate this problem to the neural tube/somite mismatch during neural crest migration and early spinal nerve development, resulting perhaps in abnormal ganglia and nerve distribution. However, our observations show that development seems normal, at least at the level of conventional histology.[17,39] The implication is that, if neuronal errors underlie the post-natal mortality they are subtle, perhaps involving the specificity of neuroeffector junctions, or nerve conductivity. The newborn that survive to weaning appear normal, but reduced fertility or sterility is common. This is due to the disturbance in normal germ-cell migration and proliferation in the early embryo.[37] The runting in some of the offspring may reflect undernutrition, the result of unsuccessful competition with more co-ordinated litter-mates. We have seen one or two litters in which all members showed some ataxia and in these, although post-natal growth was slow, mortality was not high. The pups in these litters were reminiscent of spastics, or sufferers from multiple sclerosis. It is clear that our observations with Mitomycin C represent an extreme effect on the potential for embryogenic repair. Further increase of Mitomycin C doses results in heavy embryonic mortality.

It is necessary to ask to what extent lesser disturbances of embryogenesis might compromise normal development. In this respect the axial skeleton seems to be a sensitive indicator in both our Mitomycin C studies and other potentially teratogenic circumstances.(38,41) In some mouse strains minor skeletal variations, such as the presence of an extra rib, a third molar or 27 presacral vertebrae instead of 26, are present at known frequency. The incidence of these variants can be altered by very small changes in growth rate, produced for example by changes in diet(42) or growth of the embryos in the uterus of a more rapidly growing strain.(43,44) In mice selected for high or low body weight(45) similar changes in incidence of these variants has been correlated with size.(46) These morphological consequences of altered growth are clearly not life threatening and should be regarded as illustrating the normal range of phenotype. However what may be a known variant in one strain may appear as a rare occurrence in another, perhaps associated with a known incident during pregnancy. In such circumstances they may be regarded as a reflection of pathological embryonic growth. In the absence of anatomical abnormality it remains possible in the light of our experience with Mitomycin C that an embryopathy might result in impaired neurological development or lowered fertility.

In considering clinical implications attention has been drawn to the similarity between the Mitomycin C–induced skeletal aberrations and those present in the Klippel-Feil, and Wildervanck Syndromes.(38) If Mitomycin C is given during early organogenesis the condition known as sacral agenesis or caudal regression may occur (unpublished observations). This condition is rare in humans generally but is found at relatively high frequency (about 1%) in infants of mothers with diabetes mellitus.(47,48) There is evidence that the embryos of diabetic mothers are significantly small in early gestation then grow faster and have a tendency to become larger than normal unless the diabetes is well controlled.(49) Experimentally induced diabetes in the rat is associated with lumbo-sacral skeletal anomalies(50,51) and with growth retardation in early organogenesis.(52-54) These developmental defects are prevented by strict control of the diabetes during organogenesis.(55)

Earlier I referred to the experimental production of monozygotic twins in the mouse, their embryonic/fetal development and the analysis of their postnatal behaviour. The spontaneously generated monozygotic twins in man experience a similar reduction in size due to the process of twinning which leads to the formation of two embryonic axes within a normal sized single implanted blastocyst. Each twin embryo can be presumed to be half normal size at this stage. Clinical data suggest that each embryo or fetus is of comparable size to a singleton fetus in the second trimester(9) but declines in size in the last 10 weeks of pregnancy. Twin fetuses thus go through a phase of accelerated growth in the period which includes organogenesis. Monozygotic twins constitute a high-risk group for susceptibility to malformation. This may be due to their small size *per se*(3) but it seems more likely that the risk is generated by the higher than normal growth rate that they experience at a critical time in their development.

REFERENCES

1. Neligan GA, Kolvin I, Scott DM, Garside RF. *Born too soon or born too small.* London: W Heinemann Medical Books Ltd, 1976.
2. Naftolin F. *Abnormal fetal growth: Biological bases and consequences.* W. Berlin: Dahlem Konferenzen, 1978.
3. Spiers PS. Does growth retardation predispose the fetus to congenital malformation? *Lancet*: 1982; **1**: 312-314.
4. Gould JB. The low-birth-weight infant. In: *Human Growth* 2nd Edition, Vol 1. Eds. F Falkner, JM Tanner. New York, London: Plenum Publishing Corporation, 1986: pp.391-413.
5. Brent RL, Jensh RP. Intra-uterine growth retardation. *Advances in Teratology* 1967; **2**: 139-227.
6. Tanner JM. The regulation of human growth. *Child Dev* 1963; **34**: 817-847.
7. Williams JPG. Catch-up growth. *J Embryol Exp Morphol* 1981; **65**:(Supplement): 89-101.
8. Snow MHL. Restorative growth in mammalian embryos. In: *Issues and Reviews in Teratology*, Vol 1. Ed. H Kalter. New York: Plenum Publishing Corporation, 1983: pp.251-284.
9. Snow MHL. Control of embryonic growth rate and fetal size in mammals. In: *Human Growth*, 2nd edition Vol 1. Ed. F Falkner, JM Tanner. New York, London: Plenum Publishing Corporation, 1986: pp.67-82.
10. Hillman N, Sherman MI, Graham C. The effect of spatial arrangement on cell determination during mouse development. *J Embryol Exp Morphol* 1972; **28**: 263-278.
11. Buehr M and McLaren A. Size regulation in chimaeric mouse embryos. *J Embryol Exp Morphol* 1974; **31**: 229-234.
12. Lewis NE, Rossant J. Mechanism of size regulation in mouse embryo aggregates. *J Embryol Exp Morphol* 1982; **72**: 169-181.
13. Rands GF. Size regulation in the mouse embryo. I. The development of quadruple aggregates. *J Embryol Exp Morphol* 1986; **94**: 139-148.
14. Healy M, McLaren A, Michie D, Foetal growth in the mouse. *Proc Royal Soc* Ser B, 1960; **153**: 367-379.
15. McCarthy JC. Genetic and environmental control of foetal and placental growth in the mouse. *Animal Production* 1965; **7**: 347-361.
16. McLaren A. Genetic and environmental effects on foetal and placental growth in mice. *J Reprod Fertil* 1965; **9**: 79-98.
17. Gregg BC. *An investigation into the relationship between pattern formation and growth in the mouse vertebral column.* Ph.D. Thesis, University College London, 1985.
18. Ansell JD, Snow MHL. The development of trophoblast *in vitro* from blastocysts containing varying amounts of inner cell mass. *J Embryol Exp Morphol* 1975; **33**: 177-185.
19. Snow MHL, Aitken J, Ansell JD. Role of the inner cell mass in controlling

implantation in the mouse. *J Reprod Fertil* 1976; **48**: 403-404.
20. Copp AJ. Interaction between inner cell mass and trophoectoderm of the mouse blastocyst. I. A study of cell proliferation. *J Embryol Exp Morphol* 1978; **48**: 109-125.
21. Moore NW, Adams CE, Rowson LEA. Developmental potential of single blastomeres of the rabbit egg, *J Reprod Fertil* 1968; **17**: 527-531.
22. Tarkowski AK. Experimental studies on regulation in the development of isolated blastomeres of mouse eggs. *Acta Theriologica* 1959; **2**: 251-175.
23. Rands GF. Size regulation in the mouse embryo II. The development of half embryos. *J Embryol Exp Morphol* 1986; **98**: 209-217.
24. Tsunoda Y and McLaren A. Effect of various procedures on the viability of mouse embryos containing half the normal number of blastomeres. *J Reprod Fertil* 1983; **69**: 315-322.
25. Burgoyne PS. Evans EP, Holland K. XO monosomy is associated with reduced birth weight and lowered weight gain in the mouse. *J Reprod Fertil* 1983; **68**: 381-385.
26. Burgoyne PS, Tam PP, Evans EP. Retarded development of XO conceptuses during early pregnancy in the mouse. *J Reprod Fertil* 1983; **68**: 387-393.
27. Baunack E, Falk U, Gärtner K. Monozygotic vs. dizygotic twin behavior in artificial mouse twins. *Genetics* 1984; **106**: 463-477.
28. Spielmann H, Eibs HG and Merker HJ. Effects of cyclophosphamide treatment before implantation on the development of rat embryos after implantation. *J Embryo Exp Morphol* 1977; **41**: 65-78.
29. Spielmann H, Jacob-Müller U. Investigations on cyclophosphamide treatment during the preimplantation period. *Teratology* 1981; **23**: 7-13.
30. Spindle AI. Inhibition of early postimplantation development of cultured mouse embryos by bromodeoxyuridine. *J Exp Zool* 1977; **202**: 17-26.
31. Yu HS, Tam PP, Chan ST. Effects of cadmium on preimplantation mouse embryos *in vitro* with special reference to their implantation capacity and subsequent development. *Teratology* 1985; **32**: 347-353.
32. Tam PP. Postimplantation development of Mitomycin C-treated mouse blastocysts. *Teratology* 1988; **37**: 205-212.
33. Goss RJ. Modes of growth and regeneration: Mechanisms, Regulations, Distribution. In: *Human Growth*, 2nd Edition, Vol 1. Eds: F Falkner, JM Tanner. New York, London: Plenum Publishing Corporation 1986: pp.3-26.
34. Snow MHL, Tam PP. Is compensatory growth a complicating factor in mouse teratology? *Nature* 1979; **279**: 555-557.
35. Snow MHL, Tam PP, McLaren A. On the control and regulation of size and morphogenesis in mammalian embryos. In: *Levels of Genetic Control in Development*. Ed. S Subtelny. New York: A R Liss Inc, 1981: pp.201-217.
36. Tam PP. The control of somitogenesis in mouse embryos. *J Embryol Exp Morphol* 1981; Supplement **65**: 103-128.
37. Tam PP, Snow MHL. Proliferation and migration of primordial germ cells during compensatory growth in mouse embryos. *J Embryol Exp Morphol* 1981; **64**: 133-147.

38. Gregg BC, Snow MHL. Axial abnormalities following disturbed growth in Mitomycin C treated mouse embryos. *J Embryol Exp Morphol* 1983; **73**: 135-149.
39. Snow MHL, Gregg BC. The programming of vertebral development. In: *Somites in Developing Embryos*. NATO ASI Series A, Vol 118. Eds: R Bellairs, DA Ede, JW Lash. New York, London: Plenum Press, 1986: pp.301-311.
40. Snow MHL. Uncoordinated development of embryonic tissues following cytotoxic damage. In: *Approaches to Elucidate Mechanisms in Teratogenesis*. Ed. F Welsch. New York, London: Hemisphere Publishing Corporation, 1987: pp.83-98.
41. Kimmel CA, Wilson JG. Skeletal deviations in rats: Malformations or variations. *Teratology* 1973; **8**: 309-316.
42. Deol MS, Truslove GM. Genetical studies on the skeleton of the mouse. XX. Maternal physiology and variation in the skeleton of C57B1 mice. *J Genet* 1957; **55**: 288-312.
43. McLaren A, Michie D. Factors affecting vertebral variation in mice. 2. Maternal effects in reciprocal crosses. *J Embryol Exp Morphol* 1956; **4**: 161-166.
44. McLaren A, Michie D. Factors affecting vertebral variation in mice. 4. Experimental proof of the uterine basis of a maternal effect. *J Embryol Exp Morphol* 1958; **6**: 645-659.
45. Falconer DS. Replicated selection for body weight in mice. *Genet Res* 1973; **22**: 291-321.
46. Truslove GM. The effect of selection for body-weight on the skeletal variation of the mouse. *Genet Res* 1976; **28**: 1-10.
47. Kucera J, Lenz W, Maier W. Malformations of the lower limbs and the caudal part of the spinal column in children of diabetic mothers. *German Medical Monthly* Vol X 1965; 393-396.
48. Grix A, Curry C, Hall BD. Patterns of multiple malformations in infants of diabetic mothers. In: *Birth Defects*, Vol 18. New York: A R Liss Inc., 1982: pp.55-77.
49. Pedersen JF, Mølsted-Pedersen L. Early growth retardation in diabetic pregnancy, *Br Med J* 1979; **1**: 18-19.
50. Deuchar EM. Effects of maternal diabetes on embryonic development in mammals. In: *Maternal Effects in Development* Eds: DR Newth, M Balls. Cambridge: Cambridge University Press, 1979: pp.375-394.
51. Eriksson UJ, Dahlström E, Hellerström C. Diabetes in pregnancy. Skeletal malformations in the offspring of diabetic rats after intermittent withdrawal of insulin in early gestation. *Diabetes* 1983; **32**: 1141-1145.
52. Eriksson UJ, Lewis NJ, Freinkel N. Growth retardation during early organogenesis in embryos of experimentally diabetic rats. *Diabetes* 1984; **33**: 281-284.
53. Rashbass P, Ellington SKL. Development of rat embryos cultured in serum prepared from rats with streptozotocin–induced diabetes. *Teratology* 1988; **37**: 51-61.

54. Sadler TW. Effects of maternal diabetes on early embryogenesis: I. The teratogenic potential of diabetic serum. *Teratology* 1980; **21**: 339-347.
55. Baker L, Egler JM, Klein SH, Goldman AS. Meticulous control of diabetes during organogenesis prevents congenital lumbosacral defects in rats. *Diabetes* 1981; **30**: 955-959.

Discussion

Chairman: Mr R.B. Fraser

NICOLAIDES: I refer to Dr Snow's work on identical twinning where there is not much evidence, certainly from ultrasound, of an early onset growth retardation. So presumably in the first trimester there must have been a catch-up in growth.

SNOW: I have looked at the human literature on twins because it does seem to be an example where you know at the onset of organogenesis that you have got something which is half size. The ultrasound data strongly suggest that catch-up growth does occur. But some of the literature does not go early enough to answer the question.

NICOLAIDES: What is your suggestion to explain the late falloff in growth? Is it environmental? Is it a blood supply problem? Is it related to insulin?

SNOW: No, I am sure that using the mouse as an experimental model you can rule out placental problems with the monozygotic twins. They are separated pre-implantation and they implant at quite different sites. They have their own membranes and their own placenta. So there is not a circulatory problem which would account for the decline in growth in that situation.

NICOLAIDES: It has also been my experience that it is not necessarily the result of a twin transfusion syndrome.

STEWART: When you say that your mice, no matter what disastrous things you may have done to them, apparently turn out as normal, how are you judging normality?

SNOW: That is a very important point. The vast majority of laboratories go on anatomical criteria and maybe on longevity and breeding performance. There are very few places that would either deliberately test or pick up any behavioural oddities by casual observation. There is one study in the mouse literature on monozygotic twins in which the birthweight is low and in which behavioural tests were carried out postnatally.(1) The monozygotic twins were significantly underemotional and underagressive; they were lethargic. It has no parallel in man that I know of. There is an argument over IQ level discordancies in twins but I do not believe that there are any behavioural oddities.

STEWART: This is the problem because the outcome for "small for gestational age" babies does not differ too much from that of normally grown babies of equivalent gestation. But as they grow older and you are able to test better there may be considerable differences.

SNOW: We are very bad with mice in recognising what might be wrong postnatally. If it has only three legs then we would notice it, but if it is clumsy I doubt if many people would pick it up.

FRASER: I wonder if these differences provide a model of any typical human malformations?

SNOW: It is a question that I have asked myself. Hunting around in the human syndromes I can drum up two: one is called Wildervanck, and the other is Klippel-Feil, which seem to be very similar to some of our size-reduced mice insofar as one can make a comparison across such a wide species gap.

LIND: There is a human model from which we can take some comfort, and that is women with renal transplants. They are on noxious drugs prior to conception and throughout their pregnancy. A review of the world literature so far has shown that they have no higher incidence of fetal anomalies than anyone else, that birthweight is not reduced relative to other people with equivalent renal disorders. I think that is quite amazing. So we come back again to joyous hope that things which ought to disrupt people do not seem to have the disastrous effects that we would anticipate.

STEWART: That is in terms of skeletal or structural abnormalities. It is the fundamental cognitive processing and things like that which concern me.

LIND: That is only part of the problem. People have assumed that drugs like folic acid antagonists would have caused skeletal or other physical disorders. The fact that they do not is encouraging.

SNOW: If we had carried out our cytotoxic drug studies in a conventional fashion with early treatment and examination of the fetal anatomy the day before birth, we would probably have discontinued the studies after a couple of months because nothing was happening. But that was not the rationale behind the study, which was undertaken to look at part of the primitive streak-stage embryo which has a very high self-proliferation rate. The notion was to block this with a cytotoxic drug and observe what developmental abnormalities we got in the next 24 hours or 48 hours. The amount of damage was absolutely horrendous. The embryos were knocked sideways by the treatment in a totally unexpected way, but because the lab had an interest in the origins of germ cells and the formation of the gonad which started within that next 24 hour period we kept some for an extra day to see if they would survive. The following day, although they were very small, the embryos were not obviously morphologically abnormal. We thought the experiment had failed. However, we repeated it several times, monitoring embryonic/fetal development at different stages of organogenesis and found that the initial cytotoxic damage was reliably uniform and severe, and that recovery from the damage took place during organogenesis with the resulting loss of developmental harmony within the embryo that I have described. Casual inspection of the fetus shortly before birth would have regarded the fetuses as normal and given no cause to suspect the trauma undergone in early embryogenesis. There would have been no apparent reason to anticipate post-natal problems, and had there not been an interest in gonadal development (and hence in reproductive performance) in another group in our unit, the offspring would probably not have been given the chance to survive beyond birth. The spasticity of the pups and associated mortality might never have been realised. Dozens of teratological studies with cytotoxic agents, including Mitomycin C, conducted over the last 30 years have not revealed the recuperative ability of the embryo.

LEVENE: Dr Stewart has referred to subsequent abnormal behaviour in your animals. I think that in the model you have described it is inappropriate to talk about apparently subtle neurological abnormalities. You caused a massive insult at the neural crest stage, and I would have expected an all-or-nothing effect because the higher cerebral function centres have not developed by that stage. By the stage they had developed the insult presumably is no longer operating, so we would not necessarily expect to see an effect. Your model is not particularly relevant in terms of looking at more subtle behavioural or even motor function disorders.

SNOW: With regard to motor function, the mismatch between the developing neural tube and the somatic elements in the limbs is such that spinal ganglia formation and the emergence of ventral nerves occur before the tissues that they would normally pass through have been formed. The possibilities for bad wiring at that level seem enormous, and you might expect motor function coordination to have been scrambled completely. But that by and large is not true; later on in fetal stages the appropriate connections seem to be there. We pick up a low frequency of missing spinal ganglia, double spinal ganglia and a few errors in nerve pathways. But it is a very low frequency in terms of what seemed possible.

LEVENE: Have you looked at DNA content?

SNOW: Unfortunately not. We have looked at other parameters which point us in that direction. We have measured tissue volume at various stages of embryonic development, at cell density within tissues and nucleus–cytoplasmic ratio. We cannot find significant changes which would lead us to suspect that they are dramatically short of cells and what we are dealing with is a hypertrophy rather than a hyperplasia problem.

FRASER: I was interested in what Professor Lind was saying about the renal transplant and the possible human model of the high risk embryo. Is there an increased rate of spontaneous abortion in this group? Perhaps the human is more efficient in recognising and eliminating the abnormal conceptus.

LIND: Not that we are aware of, but not too many women with renal transplants continue their reproductive career long enough to lose a lot of babies.

CLAPP: Mr Fraser, it seemed to me that you showed a great deal of variability in metabolic efficiency in pregnant women. You made inference that this was related to fatness. Is that right?

FRASER: They looked for all sorts of correlations for variations in basal metabolic rate, and the most significant was prepregnancy fatness related to metabolic rate at 24 weeks gestation.(2)

CLAPP: I think that there are very significant pitfalls in the doubly-labelled water technique and one should be aware of them before putting too much confidence in the data.

FRASER: Indeed, and this technique has been subject to a certain amount of criticism. What was reassuring was that they were able to demonstrate apparently similar patterns of expenditure with the two methods.

ALBERMAN: Dr Snow, the picture you describe would account very neatly for some cases of cerebral palsy which are more common in monozygotic twins and growth retarded children for no obvious reason. There is increasing interest in intergenerational studies and I wondered whether, as you have been breeding the mice that you treated, were you able to look at the birthweight of their offspring?

SNOW: We did, and they do not seem to depart from normal, but we have not done a great number of those studies. Having demonstrated that they were fertile we were more interested in going back to the embryos and identifying the low fertility.

ALBERMAN: Are the litters smaller? Is that part of the low fertility?

SNOW: No. Overall the litter size from the females is not significantly lower than normal.

REFERENCES

1. Baunack E, Falk U, Gaertner K. Monozygotic vs dizygotic twin behaviour in artificial mouse twins. *Genetics* 1984; **106**: 463-478.
2. Prentice AM, Goldberg GR, Murgatroyd PR, Davies HL, Scott W. Energy sparing adaptations in human pregnancy assessed by whole body calorimetry. *Br J Nutr*; In press.

SECTION 3

FETAL OVERGROWTH

Fetal growth: an overview

Professor F. Cockburn

"Mary, Mary, quite contrary
How does your fetus grow?"
"To tell the truth kind Sir," she said,
"I really do not know"
"Well listen Mary while I tell
The where, the why and how"

We have learned that the genetic material contained in the fertilised ovum controls cell division and tissue development, given that the environment surrounding the embryo and the fetus, provided by the mother, is satisfactory.

THE WHERE

Fetal growth takes place within the uterus and uterine size is a major determinant of fetal growth which can override genetic factors. Walton and Hammond(1) demonstrated this in elegant studies on crosses between the large Shire horse and tiny Shetland mare, and tiny Shetland pony and large Shire mare where the uterine size of the mare was the overriding determinant of the size of the newborn foal. The larger uterine size of the Shire mare promotes fetal overgrowth in the "genetically" small Shetland pony – Shire mare cross. In the human, larger women tend to have larger uteruses and larger babies, but also tend to have larger husbands. There are extreme examples of recurrence of high birthweight without obvious cause such as the family described by Penrose(2) in which a mother had seven children weighing over 13 lb (5.9 kg) with the heaviest being 17 lb 3 oz (7.8 kg). The mother was large with presumably a capacious uterus and an effective uterine blood flow.

Extrauterine pregnancies generally result in light for date infants when the pregnancy reaches viability. This small size could result from many factors, but effective placental blood supply is likely to be a major determinant of fetal growth.

THE WHY

It is difficult to understand why there should be advantage in fetal overgrowth. In situations of generalised fetal overgrowth such as in the large infant of the diabetic mother there can be positive disadvantage in terms of difficulty and/or preterm delivery. Similarly, no advantage can be envisaged to a fetus from focal overgrowth of an individual limb or organ. However, in phenylketonuria or cystic fibrosis the healthy siblings of affected individuals appear to have higher than average birthweights.(3,4) Phenylketonuria and cystic fibrosis are autosomal recessive disorders in which, in the untreated state, the affected individuals have greatly reduced reproductive fitness. This should result in a gradual reduction in gene frequency given that there are no new mutations. To explain how the gene frequency has been maintained it is necessary to postulate that carriers of the defective gene for these disorders (heterozygotes) have a slightly higher than normal reproductive fitness called heterozygote advantage. A higher than average birthweight close to the optimum for survival is one possible explanation.[5]

AND HOW

Fetal growth rate is governed by the rate of cell division in different cells and tissues, and total size reflects changes in cell number rather than changes in cell size or quantity of extracellular materials. Given a normal genetic potential, maternal health and nutrition and normal uterine size and blood supply, what other factors are there which could increase the rates of cellular division and produce fetal overgrowth?

Pedersen[6] in 1954 put forward the hypothesis that it was maternal hyperglycaemia which resulted in fetal hyperglycaemia and hyperinsulinaemia which in turn accelerated fetal growth and produced the fetal anomalies found in infants of diabetic mothers (IDMs). The classic description of these infants was given by Farquhar in Edinburgh:[7] "These infants are remarkable not only because like fetal versions of Shadrach, Meshach and Abednego they emerged at least alive from within the fiery metabolic furnace of diabetes mellitus, but because they resemble one another so closely that they might well be related. They are plump, sleek, liberally covered with vernix caseosa, full-faced and plethoric. The umbilical cord and the placenta share in the gigantism."

Insulin is a major growth promoting factor in fetal growth and its effects on growth may well be mediated in many ways.[8,9] It can increase the rates of transfer of nutrients including amino acids into cells,[10] promote protein synthesis[11] and is conducive to anabolism and tissue growth by inhibiting the effects of catabolic hormones.[12] In fetal rat brain insulin has a direct effect in the regulation of brain cell growth.[13]

THE PLACENTA

The mechanisms of control of the rate of cell division in the embryo and placenta in the first trimester are unknown. Growth of the first trimester placenta appears to be exponential, with flattening of the curve beginning in the early second trimester, and progressive slowing until delivery.[14] Syncytiotrophoblast cells produce human chorionic gonadotrophin (hCG) which probably elicits the trophic support of progesterone production.

Trophoblast receptors for insulin and peptide growth factors appear at the blastocyst stage and increase in number throughout gestation.[15,16] These receptors are on the microvillar surface where they could be stimulated by maternal insulin and insulin-like growth factors (IGF-1 and IGF-2). Placental growth also requires fetal trophic factors.[17]

Antigenic differences between mother and fetus may influence the rates of fetal and placental growth. Allogeneic mouse placentas are approximately 25% larger than those of syngeneic matings.[18] Antipaternal antibodies shield critical fetal antigens from recognition by the maternal immune system and may also be actively involved in promoting fetal growth.[19]

The most consistent feature of placentas of IDMs is their increased size compared to those of non-diabetic mothers.[20] The feto-placental weight ratios are significantly smaller in both gestational and insulin-dependent diabetic pregnancies than in normal pregnancies.[21] Specific binding of both IGF-1 and insulin to the placental membranes and lectin purified placental receptors from diabetic patients with good glycaemic control is no different from normal whilst there is an increase in receptor numbers in diabetic patients with poor glycaemic control.[22]

FETAL OVERGROWTH

Naeye[23] has reported that macrosomic IDMs demonstrate a 10–15% increase in body length. The greater size of the fetus and its viscera is due to increased cell number and the resultant organomegaly is an effect of insulin and not an effect of excess substrate.[24]

Cardiomegaly with septal and ventricular wall hypertrophy may be related to chronic fetal hyperinsulinaemia and to the numbers of myocardial insulin receptors.[25,26] Hepatomegaly is a result of hepatic cellular hyperplasia, hepatic cellular hypertrophy with up to 60% increase in cytoplasm, in part due to increased fat and glycogen content together with an excessive amount of haemopoietic tissue.[23]

LOCALISED FETAL OVERGROWTH

Vascular naevi particularly of a limb can result in gigantism of that limb, and similarly regional overgrowth may occur in association with lymphangiomas and neurofibromatosis.

Asymmetrical overgrowth of unknown aetiology may involve the whole of one side of the body or one limb, with normally functioning and structured tissues. There may be associated defects such as mental retardation, hypertrophy of internal organs on the enlarged side and rarely an association with Wilms' tumour or adrenal carcinoma.

The association of hemihypertrophy and Wilms' tumour is also seen in the Beckwith-Wiedemann syndrome in which the main features are macroglossia, abdominal wall defects, visceromegaly, gigantism, hypoglycaemia, ear creases, naevus flammeus and mid-facial hypoplasia.[27,28] Transmission of the condition is most consistent with autosomal dominant inheritance with incomplete penetrance and in some instances there is a chromosomal defect related to duplication of the short arm of chromosome 11.[29] This syndrome is discussed further elsewhere in this volume. Wilms' tumours are particularly common in children with hemihypertrophy, and it is interesting that gene mapping indicates that IGF-2, insulin and the oncogene HRAS-I are found on the short arm of chromosome 11. There is recent evidence for an association of increased expression of IGF-2 mRNA and IGF-2 protein in Wilms' tumour cells and type 1 IGF receptors which respond to IGF-1 and IGF-2 and which may contribute to the tumour growth.[30]

CEREBRAL GIGANTISM

In Sotos' syndrome of cerebral gigantism the birth length is above the 90th centile and there is rapid linear growth during the first four years of life after which time the growth rate slows to normal. Although the head is large there is usually mental retardation.(31)

Hemimegalencephaly is a rare developmental disorder characterised by early onset seizures and skull asymmetry. The increased brain mass on the affected large side is associated with an increased number of cortical neurones and glial elements and with an increase in size of all cerebral layers and loss of the normal architecture.(32) The DNA and RNA content may be increased by 40–50% on the affected side.(33) It can be speculated that an abnormal increase in growth factor receptors on the neurones of the affected side might be a cause for this unusual example of fetal tissue overgrowth.

An understanding of the factors which control fetal growth and the growth of individual tissues within the fetus is a matter of great importance. Fetal overgrowth is rare and is usually related to abnormalities of insulin or insulin-like growth factors or their receptors promoting tissue growth and development. Study of the infant of the diabetic mother is beginning to help us understand some of the factors which control fetal growth, the development of congenital malformations and the development and control of tumours.

"Mary, Mary, quite contrary
How does your fetus grow?"
"Just like my garden, Sir" she said,
"You've told me now I know,
With silver bells and cockle shells
and pretty maids all in a row."

With apologies to Tommy Thumb's Pretty Song Book (c1744).

REFERENCES

1. Walton A, Hammond J. The maternal affects on growth and information in Shire horse – Shetland pony crosses. *Proc Roy Soc London, Series B – Biological Sciences* 1938; **125**: 311-335.
2. Penrose LS. Data on the genetics of birthweight. *Ann Eugen* 1952; **16**: 378-380.
3. Saugstad LF. Birth weights in children with phenylketonuria and in their siblings. *Lancet* 1972; **i**: 809-813.
4. Boyer PH. Low birth weight in fibrocystic disease of the pancreas. *Pediatrics* 1955; **16**: 778-784.
5. Karn MN, Penrose LS. Birth weight and gestation time in relation to maternal age, parity and infant survival. *Ann Eugen* 1951; **16**: 147-164.
6. Pedersen J. Weight and length at birth of infants of diabetic mothers. *Acta Endocrinol* 1954; **16**: 330-342.
7. Farquhar JW. The child of the diabetic woman. *Arch Dis Child* 1959; **34**: 76-96.

8. Liggins GC. The influences of the fetal hypothalamus and pituitary on growth. In: *Size at Birth*. Eds. K Elliott, J Knight. Ciba Foundation Symposium 27. Amsterdam: Elsevier. 1974; pp.165-184.
9. Kalkhoff RK, Kandaraki E, Morrow PG, Mitchell TH, Kelber S, Borkowf HI. Relationship between neonatal birth weight and maternal plasma amino acid profiles in lean and obese non-diabetic women. *Metabolism* 1988; **37**: 234-239.
10. Hernandez T, Coulson RA. Effects of insulin on extracellular and intracellular amino acid pools in the Cayman. *Am J Physiol* 1969; **217**: 1846-1852.
11. Lundholm K, Scherstén T. Protein synthesis in human skeletal muscle tissue: influence of insulin and amino acids. *Eur J Clin Invest* 1977; **7**: 531-536.
12. Fulks RM, Li JB, Goldberg AL. Effects of insulin, glucose, and amino acids on protein turnover in rat diaphragm. *J Biol Chem* 1975; **250**: 290-298.
13. Yang JW, Fellows RE. Characterisation of insulin stimulation of the incorporation of radioactive precursors into macromolecules in cultured rat brain cells. *Endocrinology* 1980; **107**: 1717-1724.
14. Winick M, Coscia A, Noble A. Cellular growth in human placenta. 1. Normal placental growth. *Pediatrics* 1967; **39**: 248-251.
15. Lai WH, Guyda HJ, Branchaud CL, Goodyer CG. Insulin-induced receptor regulation in early gestation and term human placental cell cultures. *Placenta* 1985; **6**: 505-517.
16. Carson SA, Chase R, Ulep E, Scommegna A, Benveniste R. Ontogenesis and characteristics of epidermal growth factor receptors in human placenta. *Am J Obstet Gynecol* 1983; **147**: 932-939.
17. Panigel M, Myers RE. L'éffet de la foétectomie et celui de la ligature des vaisseaux foétaux interplacentaires sur l'ultrastructure des villosités placentaires chez Macaca mulatta. *CR Académie Science Série D* (Paris) 1971; **272**: 315-318.
18. Wegmann TG, Fotedar A, Green D. Immunotrophism and fetal survival. In: *Perspectives in Immunoreproduction*. Eds. S Mathur, R Fredericks. Hemisphere Publications, 1986.
19. Beer AE, Billingham RE, Scott JR. Immunogenetic aspects of implantation and fetoplacental growth rates. *Biol Reprod* 1975; **12**: 176-189.
20. Winick M, Noble A. Cellular growth in human placenta. II. Diabetes mellitus. *J Pediatr* 1967; **71**: 216-219.
21. Salafia C. The fetal, placental, and neonatal pathology associated with maternal diabetes mellitus. In: *Diabetes Mellitus in Pregnancy*. Eds. EA Reece and DR Coustan. New York: Churchill Livingstone, 1988; pp.143-181.
22. Bhaumick B, Danilkewich AD, Bala RM. Altered placental insulin and insulin-like growth factor-1 receptors in diabetes. *Life Sci* 1988; **42**: 1603-1614.
23. Naeye RL. Infants of diabetic mothers: a quantitative morphologic study. *Pediatrics* 1965; **35**: 980-988.
24. Susa JB, Grupposo PA, Widnes JA, Domenech M, Clemens GK, Sehgal P, Schwartz R. Chronic hyperinsulinemia in the fetal rhesus monkey: Effects of

physiologic hyperinsulinemia on fetal substrates, hormones and hepatic enzymes. *Am J Obstet Gynecol* 1984; **150**: 415-420.
25. Breitweser JA, Meyer RA, Sperling MA, Tsang RC, Kaplan S. Cardiac septal hypertrophy in hyperinsulinemic infants. *J Pediatr* 1980; **96**: 535-539.
26. Joassin G, Parker ML, Pildes RS, Cornblath M. Infants of diabetic mothers. *Diabetes* 1967; **16**: 306-311.
27. Wiedemann HR. Complexe malformatif familial avec hernie umbilicale et macroglossie – un "syndrome nouveau"? *J Genet Hum* 1964; **13**: 223-232.
28. Beckwith JB. Macroglossia, omphalocele, adrenal cytomegaly, gigantism and hyperplastic visceromegaly. *Birth Defects* 1969; **5**: 188-196.
29. Pettenati MJ, Haines JL, Higgins RR, Wappner RS, Palmer CG, Weaver DD. Wiedemann-Beckwith syndrome: presentation of clinical cytogenetic data on 22 new cases and review of the literature. *Hum Genet* 1986; **74**: 143-154.
30. Gansler T, Allen KD, Burant C *et al.* Detection of Type 1 insulin-like growth factor (IGF) receptors in Wilms' tumours. *Am J Path* 1988; **130**: 431-435.
31. Sotos JF, Dodge PR, Muirhead D, Crawford JD, Talbot NB. Cerebral gigantism in childhood. *N Engl J Med* 1964; **217**: 109-116.
32. Bignami A, Palladini G, Zapella M. Unilateral megalencephaly with nerve cell hypertrophy. *Brain Res* 1968; **9**: 103-114.
33. Manz HJ, Phillips TM, Rowden G, McCullough DC. Unilateral megalencephaly, cerebral cortical dysplasia, neuronal hypertrophy and heterotopia: cytomorphometric, fluorometric, cytochemical, and biochemical analyses. *Acta Neuropathol (Berl)* 1979; **45**: 97-103.

Mechanisms of overgrowth

Professor R.D.G. Milner

INTRODUCTION

Human fetal growth is not uniform and its control is complicated. The first level of control is genetic, the second resides in feto-placental homeostatic mechanisms and the third is by the maternal environment acting through the placenta. Tissue patterns and organ primordia are established during embryogenesis, then from the end of the first trimester and throughout the second the fetus undergoes massive cellular hyperplasia. The third trimester is characterised more by cellular hypertrophy, though some hyperplastic development continues. There are the equivalent of some 42 successive mitotic divisions in pregnancy in progressing from a fertilised ovum to a term infant, with only five more divisions being necessary to achieve adult size. Maximal growth velocity in length occurs at approximately 20 weeks of gestation, and in weight at 34 weeks.

In models that partition the contribution of genetic and environmental factors to birthweight, roughly one third of the variation is due to genetic factors, one third to environmental factors and one third is unknown.[(1)] It is noteworthy that of the 38% which is genetic, the maternal genotype (20%) is more important than the fetal genotype (15%), probably reflecting the maternal uterine constraint to fetal growth in later pregnancy.

When things go wrong for the fetus undergrowth is a much commoner outcome than overgrowth. Overgrowth is an unusual kind of pathology and to understand it requires attention to the semantics of the word. The synonym "macrosomia" is often applied inappropriately, since the excess weight of an overgrown baby is more likely to be the consequence of adiposity than an increase in lean body mass. Adipocyte lipid becomes an important contributor to body weight in the last trimester. It is worth remembering that the first 1.5 kg of the 3.0 kg term infant takes two-thirds of pregnancy to develop. In the first 1.5 kg there is about 50 g fat, whereas the second 1.5 kg acquired in the last 12 weeks of gestation includes 500 g fat. Lipid accumulation in the third trimester, which is largely controlled by glucose-sensitive insulin secretion, is the most important single contributor to a term infant being overweight. Adequate cellular delivery of nutrient is a prerequisite for both normal and excessive intrauterine growth. Nutrient oversupply is not known to influence growth before 28 weeks but may modulate weight gain thereafter by stimulating pancreatic β cell ontogeny and insulin secretion.

Each aspect of organ modelling requires orchestrated intercellular signalling at two levels. The release of peptide growth factors and the modulation of extracellular matrix represent paracrine actions that occur within cell populations and between adjacent germ layers. In contrast, endocrine hormones may stimulate growth non-specifically or promote specific maturational events. The relationships between paracrinology, endocrinology and the environment in fetal growth have been reviewed in detail recently[(2)] and this paper is a synopsis of the parts of that more general treatise which are relevant to overgrowth.

EXPERIMENTAL EVIDENCE

Insulin

Insulin and other peptides involved in fetal growth originate in the fetus or from the fetal side of the placenta which is impermeable to peptide hormones. Although insulin is present in the human fetal pancreas from 10 weeks' gestation, insulin secretion appears to be glucose insensitive until approximately 28 weeks' gestational age.[3] Recent experiments have added to our sparse knowledge of human fetal insulin secretion. Perfusion of isolated islet clusters from fetuses of less than 16 weeks caused a small monophasic rise in insulin secretion within 30 min of a glucose challenge.[4] The response increased at 17 to 20 weeks but only became biphasic in the perinatal period. Other secretogogues such as amino acids, which may be more physiologically important, were not tested.

There are several pathways by which insulin can act as a fetal growth factor. First, it may alter cellular nutrition to increase nutrient uptake and utilisation. Second, insulin may exert a direct anabolic action via either the insulin or the type 1 insulin-like growth factor (IGF) receptor. Third, insulin may modulate the release of IGF or other growth factors from fetal tissues. Insulin and IGF receptors have been identified in human fetal tissues from at least 15 weeks' gestation; insulin receptor number increased with gestational age until 25 weeks, after which time binding capacity was enhanced by an increase in receptor affinity only.[5] While we found no direct mitogenic action of insulin on human fetal fibroblasts or myoblasts obtained from fetuses of less than 20 weeks' gestation (DJ Hill, personal communication), it is conceivable that later in fetal development insulin may exert a direct growth-promoting action. We demonstrated this in isolated fetal rat myoblasts which incorporate tritiated thymidine at an enhanced rate in the presence of physiological amounts of insulin for a short time at the end of gestation.[6]

There have been several attempts to reproduce in animal models the overgrowth seen in the human infant of a diabetic mother. Injection of the fetal rat with insulin in late gestation, after extension of pregnancy by treatment of the dam with progesterone, resulted in increased fetal weight and nitrogen content.[7] The postmature fetus was capable of laying down adipose tissue, and this was greater in fetuses exhibiting an induced hyperinsulinaemia than in fetuses from control animals. However, the model is unavoidably unphysiological since the rat does not normally lay down subcutaneous fat until after birth.

Susa *et al.* implanted osmotic minipumps containing insulin into monkey fetuses. Three weeks of pharmacological hyperinsulinaemia resulted in a 34% increase in fetal body weight associated with enlargement of the heart, liver and spleen, but not the lung, kidney or brain. Despite serum insulin levels in excess of 20 nM the fetuses remained euglycaemic. In subsequent studies[8] a less extreme fetal hyperinsulinaemia was produced, causing a 23% increase in body weight. However, the only organ found to be enlarged was the heart, suggesting that most of the excess weight was due to large deposits of adipose tissue which were observed but not quantitated. Insulin infusion caused a fall in plasma free fatty acids and an increase in hepatic lipogenic enzyme activity. Circulating IGF-1 levels were elevated in animals with gross hyperinsulinaemia but not in those with moderately elevated levels. No acceleration of skeletal development was noted in either group of fetuses. Osmotic minipumps have also been used to make fetal pigs hyperinsulinaemic for two weeks late in gestation.[9] No increase in total body weight or length was found, but the experimental animals did manifest an increase in tissue glycogen stores and in the RNA/DNA ratio of skeletal muscle. The susceptibility of different species to fetal hyperinsulinaemia may be related to the stage of development at which insulin secretion becomes glucose responsive and tissue insulin sensitivity occurs. These events happen shortly after birth in the pig and in late fetal life in the monkey.

The growth hormone family

The placenta is a hormone factory and the hormones considered here, placental lactogen (PL) and growth hormone (GH), are chosen for consideration because there is experimental and theoretical evidence respectively that they could play an important part in fetal growth control.

Human placental lactogen (hPL). hPL has 85% homology in amino acid sequence with GH and is released into both maternal and fetal compartments. A role for hPL in fetal development seemed unlikely because of its low somatotropic activity in classical GH bioassays such as tibial growth in the hypophysectomised rat. Such test systems may be inappropriate because they measure hPL interaction with GH receptors and take no account of the possibility of specific hPL receptors in fetal tissues. Random measurements of fetal serum hPL in the second trimester are between 50 and 200 ng/ml. hPL in this concentration range promotes DNA synthesis and cellular anabolism in isolated human connective tissues and hepatocytes.[10] The actions on DNA synthesis were mediated by a paracrine release of IGF peptides. Specific binding sites for hPL are present on cell membranes from second trimester fetal liver and skeletal muscle, and receptor numbers increase with body weight between 12 and 19 weeks.[11] Although the mechanisms for hPL to potentiate fetal growth are there, the role of hPL *in utero* remains uncertain since reports exist of healthy term infants born to women with placentae lacking the two hPL genes. In these circumstances other related peptides such as placental GH may play a compensatory role.

Placental and pituitary growth hormone (GH). The human placenta contains a GH-like molecule which differs from pituitary GH at 13 amino acids and is a product of the variant GH gene, hGH-v, which remains dormant in the pituitary. Placental GH is secreted copiously into the maternal circulation towards term, but disappears within one hour of delivery.[12] Attempts to measure placental GH in the fetus have been bedevilled by the abundance of pituitary GH and it is not yet appropriate to speculate on its role in fetal life.

Pituitary GH is found in the human fetal pituitary and circulation from at least 10 weeks' gestation and by mid-pregnancy plasma GH levels are at peak of more than 200 mU/l. Despite this plethora pituitary GH appears to have little influence on fetal development, possibly because GH receptors do not appear in connective tissue before birth in the mouse, rat or sheep and not until at least the second trimester in man. GH is without effect on human fetal muscle cell growth *in vitro* but stimulates DNA synthesis together with release of IGF-1 by isolated human fetal hepatocytes from as early as 12 weeks.[10]

Tissue growth factors and fetal nutrition

The fetus grows in response to the actions of a wide spectrum of tissue growth factors some of which have a general stimulating action, whereas others are specific. The insulin-like growth factors (IGF) and epidermal growth factor (EGF) are described here as illustrating the two modes of action, but the reader wishing to have a realistic idea of the growth factor jungle should consult a more general review.[13]

Insulin-like growth factors (IGF). There are two predominant classes of insulin-like growth factors: IGF-1 otherwise known as somatomedin C (SmC), and IGF-2. The analogous peptide to IGF-2 in the rat is called multiplication stimulating activity (MSA). The IGFs are so called because they have structural and functional similarities with insulin and proinsulin. This relationship helps explain the limited biological cross-reactivity: insulin being a weak growth factor for fibroblasts while the IGFs enhance glucose oxidation in isolated adipocytes.[14]

In the fetus most if not all tissues synthesise IGFs which are released to act locally in a paracrine or autocrine fashion. IGF-1 has been recovered from all tissues tested from human fetuses of 9 to 19 weeks' gestation.[15] Lung and intestine had the highest concentration and liver the lowest. Complementary evidence of human fetal tissue IGF has been obtained by immunohistochemistry.[16] The circulation therefore probably represents a sump receiving IGF overflow from all the tissues and there seems to be little of biological import to be gained from analysing blood IGF concentrations. This has not inhibited investigators one jot.

The concentration of IGF-1 in human cord blood is one half or less of that present in the normal adult[17] despite the rapid rate of fetal growth. But cord IGF-1 levels do correlate with both fetal age and body weight whereas those of IGF-2 do not. IGF-2 levels in cord blood are the same as or slightly lower than those in the adult. But there are further obstacles to a biological link between cord IGF levels and fetal growth. The total IGF concentration in the blood does not reflect the IGF free to react with receptor since most IGF is bound to a carrier protein. In the adult and in neonates of 30 weeks' or more gestation this has a molecular weight of approximately 150 K daltons, whereas in infants of under 27 weeks' gestation it is approximately 40 K daltons in size.[18] The ontogeny of binding protein form and affinity may control the amount of IGF available to the tissues.

The actions of IGF and other growth factors depend as much on the ontogeny of receptors as on the messenger peptide. The apparent paradox of rapid fetal growth in the face of low circulating levels of IGF could be resolved if fetal tissues were more sensitive than postnatal tissues to the action of IGF. Most human fetal tissues possess receptors for both IGF-1 and IGF-2 though the liver is said to have IGF-2 receptors only.[5]

There is indirect evidence that hPL also stimulates maternal IGF synthesis and release. Normal women have elevated IGF-1 levels in late pregnancy which fall following parturition. A GH-deficient woman was shown to have normal circulating levels of IGF-1 and IGF-2 at 35 weeks' gestation, which fell rapidly post partum in parallel with the disappearance of circulating hPL.[19] Recent work suggests that hPL may also have a direct action on IGF synthesis and release in the fetal compartment. We have shown that hPL is capable of stimulating amino acid uptake and thymidine incorporation by human fetal fibroblasts and myoblasts,[20] and that this can be inhibited but not abolished by IGF-1 antibody. We have also shown that hPL, but not GH, stimulates human fetal fibroblasts and myoblasts to release IGF-1 into the culture medium in a dose dependent manner.[21] A possible direct link between hPL and insulin has been suggested by the observation that insulin stimulated hPL is released from isolated trophoblasts in a dose dependent manner.[22,23]

Epidermal growth factor (EGF). By early second trimester EGF is found in the human fetus in the gastrointestinal tract, kidney, pituitary, trachea and placenta.[24] In the fetus, EGF affects growth, differentiation and function of epithelial cells.[25] When given parenterally to the fetal lamb, EGF stimulates skin hypertrophy and growth of the viscera. In both the rabbit and lamb EGF causes lung epithelial maturation and surfactant production. *In vitro*, EGF is mitogenic and can influence differentiation; EGF inhibits glucocorticoid-induced keratinisation of embryonic chick skin. Receptors for EGF are abundant in human placenta, especially on the microvillous plasma membranes facing the maternal circulation and the basolateral membranes facing the fetal circulation. It is not surprising therefore that studies with isolated trophoblasts or placental cultures have shown that EGF modulates trophoblast differentiation and function. In homogenous cultures of term trophoblasts EGF caused a dose related release of hPL and hCG.[26] Trophoblasts differentiated into a syncytium of cytotrophoblasts but did not increase in number. It is not known if the EGF acting on placenta *in vivo* is placental or comes from elsewhere in the fetus or mother.

Fetal nutrition. The difficulty in dissecting variables is seen particularly when fetal growth is considered from a nutritional viewpoint. There is good evidence linking failure of cellular delivery or uptake of nutrient in the fetus with hypoinsulinaemia and a fall in circulating IGF levels.[2] All three go together and the result is undergrowth. The corollary has been much more difficult to demonstrate. Chronic glucose infusion in the pregnant rat leads to fetal hyperinsulinaemia and raised circulating IGF levels[27] but no increase in body size. Hyperalimentation of pregnant rats by gavage had no effect on body weight, plasma insulin or IGF levels of normal fetuses, but interestingly reduced the mortality of fetuses growing in a uterine artery-ligated horn.[28] The difficulty in producing fetal overgrowth probably reflects the fact that the fetus normally grows at a near-maximal rate *in utero*.

CLINICAL EVIDENCE

Clinical examples of generalised fetal overgrowth, be it overweight or true macrosomia, act as catalysts to scientific thought and experiment. Most pathologies that produce a big baby are associated with fetal hyperinsulinaemia or "hyperinsulinism" as it is sometimes called. This leads us to consider those categories of infant who are hyperinsulinaemic and analyse the aetiology of the excess insulin secretion and its effect on fetal growth. Two diagnoses are particularly interesting: Beckwith-Wiedemann syndrome (BWS) and the infant of the diabetic mother (IDM), because genetics may be involved in the aetiology of the former whereas the latter is environmental in origin.

Beckwith-Wiedemann syndrome (BWS)

The following is culled from a recent comprehensive review of BWS.[29] BWS is a rare congenital anomaly with a prevalence of approximately 1:12 000 births. Classical clinical stigmata are exomphalos, macroglossia and gigantism. There is pancreatic hypertrophy, hyperplasia of the islets of Langerhans, hyperinsulinaemia and a tendency to hypoglycaemia. Organ examination shows the overweight to be the consequence of cellular hyperplasia and hypertrophy of most viscera and the lean body mass. Fetal organomegaly may be the cause of secondary features such as exomphalos, inguinal and diaphragmatic hernia, bowel malrotation and facial dysmorphism. There is an increased risk of developing specific tumours in long term survivors.

The fascination of BWS as one of nature's experiments comes from our incomplete understanding of its genetic aetiology. Classical genetic analysis suggests that BWS is an autosomal dominant trait with varying expressivity and incomplete penetrance, and recent studies have shown a chromosomal abnormality in some cases of BWS which involves duplication of part or most of chromosome 11. This evoked interest because the gene for IGF-2 is on chromosome 11, but where the gene was examined no amplification was found. Since only a minority of patients studied have shown a chromosomal abnormality we are left with the possibility that either the structure around the chromosome breakpoint at 11p might be important or that other genes could be involved. Alternative pathways could involve abnormality of the genetic control of signal transduction or the cell surface receptor for growth factors.

Infant of a diabetic mother (IDM)

Fetal hyperinsulinaemia is accepted to be the cause of overgrowth in the IDM and in turn is the consequence of the metabolic disturbances which characterise diabetic pregnancy. The proof of this aetiology lies in the fact that when maternal diabetic metabolic homeostasis is fully corrected the IDM becomes indistinguishable from normal. In addition to hyperglycaemia other classes of metabolites, notably amino acids, have a trophic effect on β cell development, as well as being stimuli of insulin secretion. In addition, the ontogeny of insulin receptors may be abnormal in the IDM. Monocytes from the cord blood of normal human infants had five times the insulin-binding capacity of adult cells, and those taken from the cord blood of IDM had an even greater capacity to bind insulin.(30)

Too many β cells secreting too much insulin either individually or collectively cause a modest increase in lean body mass(31) and a gross excess of fat accumulation, but no precocious osseous development. Insulin excess has not only structural but functional consequences, causing neonatal hypoglycaemia, and respiratory distress as a result of inhibition of fetal surfactant biosynthesis.(32) Whether insulin is responsible for the polycythaemia and subsequent circulatory problems and jaundice of the IDM is controversial. Some think that the polycythaemia is due to increased erythropoietin production as a result of chronic fetal hypoxaemia,(33) but an alternative is that insulin is a direct stimulant of erythroid progenitor cell growth in the presence of erythropoietin.(34) Possibly both are true.

Other examples of fetal hyperinsulinaemia.

The third classical example of fetal hyperinsulinaemia causing overgrowth is nesidioblastosis. The pathological anatomy and physiology of such an infant is largely indistinguishable from that of the IDM, but the aetiology is different; in nesidioblastosis the cause of the abnormal β cell development is unknown.(35) It is not environmentally produced and may have its origins, along with BWS, in disturbed genetic control of pancreatic organogenesis. Erythroblastosis fetalis and transposition of the great vessels are conundra. In erythroblastosis there is hyperinsulinaemia and neonatal hypoglycaemia but no body overgrowth. A plausible interpretation is that the haemolytic aetiology of the erythroblastosis has an overall growth retarding effect, but this does not help to explain the β cell hyperplasia which mysteriously occurs in the ventral but not the dorsal pancreas.(36) Transposition of the great vessels is commonly associated with fetal overgrowth and islet hyperplasia has also been described,(37) but it is not clear if the overgrowth and β cell abnormality are due to abnormal fetal circulation or to unrecognised maternal gestational diabetes.

COMMENT

Fetal overgrowth can only be understood in the context of mechanisms controlling normal fetal growth. Opinion is shifting from the view that one or more class of signals such as endocrine or paracrine messengers or the delivery of nutrient, acting alone or in concert, control growth, to the view that they modulate growth which is ultimately under the control of the fetal and maternal genome. Generalised overgrowth is much rarer than undergrowth, but when it occurs, is associated with fetal hyperinsulinism. Abnormal β cell development and insulin secretion may arise from genetic or environmental causes.

REFERENCES

1. Polani PE. Chromosomal and other genetic influences on birth weight variation. In: *Size at Birth*. Eds. K Elliott and J Knight. Ciba Foundation Symposium 27. Amsterdam: Elsevier. 1974; pp.127-164.
2. Milner RD, Hill DJ. Interaction between endocrine and paracrine peptides in

prenatal growth control. *Eur J Pediatr* 1987; **146**: 113-122.
3. Milner RDG. Fetal growth: the role of insulin and related peptides. In: *Paediatric Endocrinology in Clinical Practice*. Ed. A Aynsley-Green. Lancaster: MTP Press, 1984; pp.125-148.
4. Otonkoski T, Andersson S, Knip M, Simmell O. Maturation of insulin response to glucose during human fetal and neonatal development. Studies with perifusion of pancreatic islet-like cell clusters. *Diabetes* 1988; **37**: 286-291.
5. Sara VR, Hall K, Misaki M, Fryklund L, Christensen L, Wetterberg L. Ontogenesis of somatomedin and insulin receptors in the human fetus. *J Clin Invest* 1983; **71**: 1084-1094.
6. Crace CJ, Hill DJ, Milner RDG. Mitogenic actions of insulin on fetal and neonatal rat cells *in vitro*. *J Endocrinol* 1984; **104**: 63-68.
7. Ktorza A, Nurjhan N, Girard JR, Picon L. Hyperglycaemia induced by glucose infusion in the unrestrained pregnant rat: effect on body weight and lipid synthesis in postmature fetuses. *Diabetologia* 1983; **24**: 128-130.
8. Susa JB, McCormick KL, Widness JA, Singer DB, Zeller WP, Schwartz R. Chronic hyperinsulinaemia in the fetal rhesus monkey: effects of physiological hyperinsulinemia on fetal growth and composition. *Diabetes* 1984; **33**: 656-660.
9. Spencer GSG, Hill D, Garsson H, MacDonald A, Collenbrander B. Somatomedin activity and growth hormone levels in body fluids of the fetal pig: effect of chronic hyperinsulinaemia. *J Endocrinol* 1983; **96**: 107-114.
10. Strain AJ, Hill DJ, Swenne I, Milner RDG. The regulation of DNA synthesis in human fetal hepatocytes by placental lactogen, growth hormone and insulin like growth factor I/somatomedin-C. *J Cell Physiol* 1987; **132**: 33-40.
11. Hill DJ, Freemark M, Strain AJ, Handwerger S, Milner RDG. Placental lactogen and growth hormone receptors in human fetal tissues: relationship to fetal plasma hPL concentrations and fetal growth. *J Clin Endocrinol Metab* 1988; **66:** 1283–1290.
12. Hennen G, Frankenne F, Closset J, Gomez F, Pirens G, El Khayat N. A human placental GH: increasing levels during second half of pregnancy and pituitary GH suppression as revealed by monoclonal antibody radioimmunoassay. *Int J Fertil* 1985; **30**: 27-33.
13. Hill DJ, Strain AJ, Milner RDG. Growth factors in embryogenesis. *Oxf Rev Reprod Biol* 1987; **9**: 398-455.
14. King GL, Kahn CR, Rechler MM, Nissley SP. Direct demonstration of separate receptors for growth and metabolic activities of insulin and multiplication-stimulating activity (an insulin-like growth factor) using antibodies to the insulin receptor. *J Clin Invest* 1980; **66**: 130-140.
15. D'Ercole AJ, Hill DJ, Strain AJ, Underwood LE. Tissue and plasma somatomedin-C/insulin like growth factor I (SM-C/IGF-1) concentrations in the human fetus during the first half of gestation. *Pediatr Res* 1986; **20**: 253-255.
16. Han VKW, Hill DJ, Strain AJ, Towle AC, Lauder JM, Underwood LE,

D'Ercole AJ. Identification of somatomedin/insulin like growth factor immunoreactive cells in the human fetus. *Pediatr Res* 1987; **22**: 245-249.
17. Gluckman PD, Johnson-Barrett JJ, Butler JH, Edgar BW, Gunn TR. Studies of insulin-like growth factor-I and -II by specific radioligand assays in umbilical cord blood. *Clin Endocrinol* 1983; **19**: 405-413.
18. D'Ercole AJ, Wilson DF, Underwood LE. Changes in the circulating form of somatomedin-C during fetal life. *J Clin Endocrinol Metab* 1980; **51**: 674-676.
19. Merimee TJ, Zapf J, Froesch ER. Insulin-like growth factor in pregnancy: studies in a growth hormone-deficient dwarf. *J Clin Endocrinol Metab* 1982; **54**: 1101-1103.
20. Hill DJ, Crace CJ, Milner RDG. Incorporation of [^{3}H] thymidine by isolated fetal myoblasts and fibroblasts in response to human placental lactogen (HPL): possible mediation of HPL action by release of immunoreactive SM-C. *J Cell Physiol* 1985; **125**: 337-344.
21. Strain AJ, Hill DJ, Swenne I, Milner RDG. Regulation of DNA synthesis in human fetal hepatocytes by placental lactogen, growth hormone and insulin-like growth factor I/somatomedin C. *J Cell Physiol* 1987; **132**: 33-40.
22. Hochberg Z, Perlman R, Brandes JM, Benderli A. Insulin regulates placental lactogen and estradiol secretion by cultured human term trophoblast. *J Clin Endocrinol Metab* 1983; **57**: 1311-1313.
23. Bhaumick B, Dawson EP, Bala RM. The effects of insulin-like growth factor-I and insulin on placental lactogen production by human term placental extracts. *Biochem Biophys Res Commun* 1987; **144**: 674-682.
24. Kasselberg AG, Orth DN, Gray ME, Stahlman MT. Immunocytochemical localization of human epidermal growth factor/urogastrone in several human tissues. *J Histochem Cytochem* 1985; **33**: 315-322.
25. Gospodarowicz D. Epidermal and nerve growth factors in mammalian development. *Ann Rev Physiol* 1981; **43**: 251-263.
26. Morrish DW, Bhardwaj D, Dabbagh LK, Marusyk H, Siy O. Epidermal growth factor induces differentiation and secretion of human chorionic gonadotrophin and placental lactogen in normal human placenta. *J Clin Endocrinol Metab* 1987; **65**: 1282-1290.
27. Heinze E, Thi CN, Vetter U, Fussganger RD. Interrelationship of insulin and somatomedin activity in fetal rats. *Biol Neonate* 1982; **41**: 240-245.
28. De Prins FA, Hill DJ, Milner RDG, Van Assche A. Effect of maternal hyperalimentation on intrauterine growth retardation. *Arch Dis Child* 1988; **63**: 733-766.
29. Engstrom W, Lindham S, Schofield P. Wiedemann–Beckwith Syndrome. *Eur J Pediatr* 1988; **147**: 450-457.
30. Neufeld ND, Kaplan SA, Lippe BM. Monocyte insulin receptors in infants of strictly controlled diabetic mothers. *J Clin Endocrinol Metab* 1981; **52:** 473-476.
31. Naeye RL. Infants of diabetic mothers: a quantitative morphological study. *Pediatrics* 1965; **35**: 980-988.
32. Smith BT, Giroud CJP, Robert M, Avery MP. Insulin antagonism of cortisol

action on lecithin synthesis by cultured fetal lung cells. *J Pediatr* 1975; **87**: 953-955.

33. Widness JA, Susa JB, Garcia JF, Singer DB, Sehgal P, Oh W, Schwartz R, Schwartz HC. Increased erythropoiesis and elevated erythropoietin in infants born to diabetic mothers and in hyperinsulinemic rhesus fetuses. *J Clin Invest* 1981; **67**: 637-642.
34. Perrine SP, Greene MF, Lee PDK, Cohen RA, Faller DV. Insulin stimulates cord blood erythroid progenitor growth: evidence for an aetiological role in neonatal polycythemia. *Br J Haematol* 1986; **64**: 503-511.
35. Kloppel G, Heitz PU. Nesidioblastosis: A clinical entity with heterogenous lesions of the pancreas. In: *Evolution and Tumour Pathology of the Neuroendocrine System*. Eds. S Falkmer, R Hakanson, F Sundler. Amsterdam: Elsevier, 1984; pp.349–370.
36. Milner RDG, Dinsdale F. Wirdnam PK, Van Assche FA. Pancreatic endocrine cell fractions in erythroblastosis fetalis. *Diabetes* 1983; **32**: 313-315.
37. Naeye RL. Transposition of the great arteries and prenatal growth. *Arch Pathol* 1966; **82**: 412-418.

Discussion

Chairman: Mr M.D.G. Gillmer

GILLMER: Could you please clarify one point? On two or three occasions during your talk you mentioned lipids. Could you clarify whether you are talking about storage, structural or both?

MILNER: Intra-adipocyte storage fat. I do not know of any evidence that would relate anything I have said to structural lipids.

CHARD: You centred quite a lot of what you said around hPL and its potential role. What is your comment on hPL-absent pregnancies? They are quite a well known phenomenon which do not seem to be associated with any known abnormality of the fetus or its growth or metabolism, or the metabolism of the mother.

MILNER: It is probably because hPL is a member of a family. In those pregnancies where the hPL gene is missing, another family member stands in. Would you accept that conceptually?

CHARD: Such as...? You said "another member of the hPL family" — do you mean the *v* gene or the human growth hormone variant?*

MILNER: Yes, hGH-v.

HILL: I thought that I might elaborate a little on that. It is true that there are infants who have deletion of the hPL A and B genes, but with perfectly normal birthweights, and they are perfectly normal infants. There are even infants who have deletions of hPL A and B and the growth hormone variant gene and are perfectly normal. But when their placentae were examined there was hPL immunoreactive material present. There is another hPL gene, that is the hPL L gene, which is not normally expressed in the placenta. But if you chalk out part of the genome which takes in the hPL A, B, and *v* gene, it is possible that the remaining hPL L gene could come under the control of the normal growth hormone gene promoter. So in that circumstance when you chalk out certain members of the family you may switch on one that is normally dormant. That could account for the residual hPL immunoreactive material which is in that placenta. So, while I would agree that the clinical evidence suggests that you really do not need hPL A and B gene products, it is not clear that you have wiped out all growth hormone peptide family members from that type of placenta.

CHARD: The product of the L gene would presumably have to be non-immunoreactive in the circulation because the methodology to demonstrate the deficiency is an immunoassay.

HILL: That observation depended on using monoclonal antibodies raised against members of the growth hormone family. The placental lactogen L (if that is what it

*(hGH-v)

is) peptide was not picked up by the conventional hPL antibodies. This work was done mainly in Liège and some of their other antibodies did pick up this material.

CHARD: The concept of alternatives being brought on stage because of the absence of some of the others is a perfectly reasonable one. But it perhaps begins to stretch credibility after a certain point when one has got a lot of deletions. One ought to consider alternative hypotheses, among which are that hPL or related compounds do not have very much to do with metabolism in human pregnancy.

HILL: To qualify our statements, the mechanisms for hPL to exert an anabolic action exist as far as we can see in defined culture conditions. We cannot comment on the degree to which hPL is active *in vivo*.

LEVENE: Thyroxin and other thyroid hormones clearly have an important role in maturation of the nervous system and in skeletal maturation. Do they have any role at all in fetal somatic growth?

HAN: I think that there is no evidence that thyroxin has any role in the fetal size or the infant size at birth. There is ample evidence that absence of thyroid gland makes no difference in the birth size of the infant. What one can observe at that time is retardation in skeletal maturation, by looking at the ossification centres of the femur at birth.

LEVENE: What is the releasing factor whereby growth hormone and thyroxin become important growth mediators in older children? You showed that there are plenty of receptors for growth hormone, but why is it that they do not actually appear to work?

HILL: We do not actually know when growth hormone receptors appear in human fetal tissue. We have found growth hormone receptors in the liver in early second trimester, but at that stage there were no growth hormone receptors in muscle. If we can take muscle as a representative connective tissue (which may not be the case) we could postulate that the skeletal tissues did not recognise growth hormones until at the earliest late in the second trimester. In fact the clinical data would suggest that growth does not really suffer until after birth in the absence of growth hormone. So it could be that growth hormone receptors do not appear on connective and skeletal tissues until very late in fetal development, or perhaps even postnatally in some tissues.

SNOW: I would like to reinforce what Dr Hill is saying. Experimentally in the mouse one knows that epidermal growth factor receptors are present at around about primitive streak stages. But there is no epidermal growth factor produced in the embryo until birth. The feeling is that that receptor may use some other peptide growth factor.

LEVENE: I thought that Dr Hill showed that there is a lot of growth hormone and there are growth hormone receptors within the liver at least.

MILNER: Within the liver, yes, but not within the muscle. I was somewhat constrained in my presentation by being asked to talk about overgrowth. The obverse takes you into fetal decapitation experiments and anencephaly, and that takes you into the mainstream of the argument of human pituitary growth hormone not being essential for normal intrauterine development. That is also a rather more complicated sub-plot than appears from the didactic single statement.

WIGGLESWORTH: I would like to discuss macrosomia in the infant of the diabetic mother. One assumes that is the model for hyperinsulinaemia in the fetus. The model clearly shows, if you get a really gross example, the organs or tissues that are affected are limited. Brain growth is, if anything, limited. Clearly there are differences in what causes the CNS to grow normally and what is going to affect the growth of the liver, the heart and some of the skeletal tissues.

GILLMER: I thought that studies, including your own, had shown a symmetrical macrosomia apart from the brain. I was interested in something that Professor Cockburn said about a demonstration that insulin produced brain cell growth in either the mouse or the rat. That is the first time that I had ever heard of insulin having an effect on brain growth.

COCKBURN: I did say that. That was the work of Yang and Fellows, whose article "Characterisation of insulin stimulation and incorporation of radioactive precursors of macromolecules into cultured rat brain cells" appeared in *Endocrinology* in 1980. (1)

GILLMER: It is contrary to what one might call conventional wisdom on that subject.

COCKBURN: It is true that there is a relatively reduced size of brain and this is what I found in the infant of the diabetic mother.

CAMPBELL: It is not my impression that the infant of the diabetic mother measured *in utero*, has a head circumference below the mean. In fact it is slightly above the mean. The abdominal circumference, of course, is symmetrically excessively grown, but the head circumference is not small.

MILNER: It brings out this concept of secondary and tertiary consequential abnormalities. If you start off with the infant of the diabetic mother and you say either on the basis of fetal hypoxia or fetal hyperinsulinaemia that you get increased fetal erythropoiesis you have immediately explained why you have got a big liver and a big spleen. Once you have fetal polycythaemia you explain why you get a big heart because you get increased fetal viscosity and all the consequences. If you come back to the Beckwith-Wiedemann syndrome and say that there is something genetically wrong which actually increases the lean body mass, that explains why you have got the macroglossia, the facial dysmorphism and the abdominal visceral enlargement. That explains why you consequentially get the diaphragmatic hernia and the inguinal hernia.

GILLMER: You mentioned erythroblastosis and the fact that the ventral pancreas only was affected. You also hinted that you had views as to why this was not characteristic macrosomia. You felt that it was due to other aspects of this condition. Would you like to elaborate?

MILNER: The root of the pathology of erythroblastosis is maternal antibody coming into the fetal compartment causing fetal haemolysis which in turn causes increased fetal erythropoiesis. It does not have to be Rhesus disease; it can be from any of the causes. That has got to be one of the things that would make Sherlock Holmes' ears prick up, because why with that kind of pathophysiology should you get abnormal pancreatic development, bona fide hyperinsulinaemia and neonatal hyperglycaemia as a transient phenomenon? It affects only one of the two embryonic parts of the pancreas.

NICOLAIDES: Because of the consequent anaemia and hyperdynamic fetal circulation with a normal perfusion you would expect that the uptake of glucose would be increased.

MILNER: It is an explanation which has been proffered before, and it has a certain plausibility.

NICOLAIDES: We have evidence from Doppler that the mean velocity of blood in the descending thoracic aorta is increased with progressive fetal anaemia. This could explain why the fetuses are hyperinsulinaemic.

MILNER: That is in erythroblastosis?

NICOLAIDES: Yes. There is usually normal placental perfusion and the glucose levels are slightly elevated even when you correct for the way you measure glucose because they are anaemic.

HAN: Why should it affect only one part of the pancreas and not the other?

COCKBURN: Why in the Beckwith-Wiedemann should it affect only one half of the child and not the other?

SNOW: We find macrosomia in our reduced size embryos in that depending on when you reduce the size and trigger the accelerated growth we produce animals which have significantly longer limbs than normal both in absolute and in comparative terms — comparative to preaxial column length. Within limits we can put that increase in length either into the forelimbs or the hindlimbs. With rather less accuracy we can put it into the femur or into the foot. How that is controlled, I have not the vaguest idea. It is totally counterintuitive because these embryos during all of these formative stages are significantly smaller than usual, but they have longer limbs.

HALL: This seems an appropriate point to ask if there is a definition for fetal overgrowth, and is there a definition of macrosomia?

STEER: The international classification of diseases does not define fetal macrosomia.

WIGGLESWORTH: It is pretty variable in infants of diabetics. There are a very small proportion now who would have the most gross effects. Big hearts are common, big livers are common, but for the whole picture it is a relatively small proportion.

GILLMER: We think a lot about diabetes as the cause of macrosomia or the classical form of overgrowth, but I am fond of saying that the least common cause of fetal overgrowth is diabetes. Obesity is the most common, something which we have not discussed. Based on studies which were done in 1981 or 1982 looking retrospectively at 6000 or so singleton pregnancies all of which had booked before 20 weeks' gestation at certain dates, we looked at body mass index in the mother and birthweight centile in the baby, reporting < 10th, 11th to 90th and > 90th. There were about 600 patients > 90th and < 10th, and just under 5000 in the middle range. In the obese group you have a surfeit of babies above the 90th centile in women who are above the 90th centile (and that was corrected for height), and a deficit that you would expect in the numbers of those less than the 10th centile. I raise this question because this is probably the commonest cause of apparent overgrowth relative to what you would expect. The converse is seen in women who are lean for their body height who produce less than the expected 10% of babies above the 90th centile. The other question is going back to the perinatal data which Richard Naeye collected.(2) They are based on a negroid population with birthweight compared to maternal weight gain during pregnancy. If the woman starts pregnancy obese or within the normal range then there is a fairly symmetrical relationship of maternal weight gain to birthweight. But if she starts the pregnancy significantly underweight there is a cut-off above which you see quite a relatively large increase in birthweight. Presumably this must relate in some way to substrate availability, although probably it is much more complex. Other growth factor activity must be involved. Does anyone have any comment?

HOWIE: Had you done glucose tolerance tests on all these obese women to know that they were not latent diabetics?

GILLMER: No, but we have done other studies looking at unselected populations. We looked at 500 women considering their glucose tolerance. The problem of course with pregnancy is that as it advances there is an alteration in glucose tolerance, as was shown in using Professor Lind's data from the early 70s. I would be happy to say from other studies, although not from this retrospective analysis, that this change is not simply a consequence of metabolic abnormality in the offspring of these women. Obese women are more likely to produce babies that are larger, and create potential clinical problems. The mechanism remains unexplained.

LIND: The question that was asked was "What is macrosomia?" We have not actually tried to answer the question. My anxiety is that in Europe people who have been interested in diabetic pregnancy universally say that any baby of 4.5 kg or more is macrosomic. In my view that is nonsense because 5% of the normal population will have a baby at term which will be 4.5 kg or more. Therefore, many more people are going to have "macrosomic" babies who are actually normal. Diabetics then, would contribute a very tiny proportion of macrosomic babies. So I think it would be useful if a group like this could come up with a working definition of the difference between macrosomia and a heavy baby.

WIGGLESWORTH: That is not particularly difficult. In macrosomia the organs are abnormally large for the overall size of the baby.

LIND: How do you assess organ size in large babies?

CLAPP: If you wanted to spot overgrowth and undergrowth as abnormalities they must be defined by something else other than weight. What you really need is either better functional or morphometric criteria upon which to base a firm diagnosis of an abnormal growth pattern.

FRASER: Do you have information from these groups of overweight babies above the 90th centile concerning the distribution of hyperinsulinaemia? It might very well be that there was hyperglycaemia in some of these obese women which was not picked up.

GILLMER: I am trying to emphasise the point which has been made by many before me, that tall obese women have the largest babies in all population groups, while short lean women have the smallest babies. In part, that is the constraint of the Hammond-Wolff situation, but the adiposity of the human mother does seem to have an effect. In other studies I have been unable to demonstrate it being due to the hyperinsulinaemia of the offspring or the significant glucose intolerance of the mother.

COCKBURN: If you asked me to define macrosomia in the infant after birth I would like to bring in the concept of time. In other words it is growth velocity that one would take into account. I just wanted to throw the challenge back to the obstetricians. Can you measure the growth velocity in the infants of diabetic mothers, for example, and come up with a factor? What we are talking about is a very rapid rate of growth.

BRUDENELL: That is what you were talking about, Professor Campbell, is it not? You were talking about a take-off from about 30 weeks.

CAMPBELL: Yes. Weight gain took off from about 26 weeks in the study which I analysed of the diabetic fetus. Growth before that was similar to that of appropriately grown fetuses.

BRUDENELL: You can actually measure the growth velocity; Flynn did that in twins between 16 and 20 weeks and showed that there is an increase in the velocity of growth during that period.[3] The take-off thereafter becomes clinically obvious at about 30 weeks. The end point is a big, heavy baby. I do not think that you could end up by defining fetal macrosomia in terms of velocity of growth.

COCKBURN: If you have a child going along the 97th centile from 12 weeks that is different from one who has gone along the 50th centile until 26 weeks and then goes up over the 90th centile. It is that velocity between the mid point and the end point. The first part is presumably what his genetic potential is giving him, but then there is something else coming in, insulin let us say, that is causing the macrosomia; you can only get that by a velocity measurement.

BRUDENELL: In dealing with the newborn baby and looking at its growth thereafter what would you measure? Presumably, you would use something like a ponderal index.

COCKBURN: Length velocity.

BRUDENELL: So you would measure the rate at which the baby gets longer?

LEVENE: I do not necessarily agree with that. If we take macrosomia as indicating excessive soft tissue mass, which I believe it to be, then we have a very simple index of that. It is skin fold thickness or mid-arm circumference. That surely is the gold standard we can measure in newborn infants to decide whether they are macrosomic. There are normal standards for this in full term babies, although perhaps not in premature babies. Is it possible to measure skin fold adipose tissue with ultrasound?

CAMPBELL: Yes, it has been attempted with varying degrees of success. I do not think that you get very accurate predictions of macrosomia or even weight from these measurements. I think that the problem is knowing exactly where on the bone you are measuring to get a consistent measuring point. You would have to take a transverse section of the arm and it is very difficult to know in different fetuses that you are at exactly the same level, and indeed if the arm is flexed or extended you will get different skin fold thicknesses.

LEVENE: It can certainly be done retrospectively once the baby is born.

COCKBURN: You can get, let us say, a short trisomy 21 which is a short very fat macrosomic.

LEVENE: If you are considering subcutaneous fat, whichever way you measure it, then you would not necessarily relate that to the birthweight of the baby or to the length of the baby. That is a function on its own. I am not sure where Down syndrome babies would come in the range of normal skin fold thicknesses. I am not sure that it is particularly relevant to the definition of macrosomia. I think that they would be sufficiently dissimilar to exclude them.

NICOLAIDES: In trisomy 21 some of the increased abdominal circumference is caused by oedema. It is sonolucent, and it may be possible to differentiate it from increased fat deposition as a cause of increased abdominal circumference in macrosomia. In trisomy 21 an important marker on antenatal ultrasound is an oedematous thickening on the back of the neck observed as a "halo".

PATEL: Concerning velocity of growth, I thought that Professor Persson had shown and commented on the velocity of growth in babies over a certain weight who ended up over the 90th centile.

PERSSON: It is true among the known diabetic "big babies" there are certainly two groups. There are those who are large throughout the pregnancy, say 2 SDs above the mean, growing at 37 g per day. They will end up slightly above 2 SDs, say 4 kg. Then there are the macrosomic babies. They are often within the normal range at 32 weeks or even 36 weeks, but then they start growing much faster. The pregnancy usually goes on a week or so beyond 280 days, and they grow with a velocity of 60, 90 or even 100 g per day post-term. These are the ones who end up in the 6 to 6.5 kg class, and you can only diagnose the increased growth at about 38 or 40 weeks.

MILNER: Do they have a tendency to hypoglycaemia neonatally?

PERSSON: Yes, they are not only fat but also very large fetuses; they are at least 56 cm long.

LIND: This comes back again to Professor Cockburn's point that if you are going to do slopes you are going to need at least three points; ideally you would want four or five points.

CLAPP: Is there a change in the fat distribution pattern in the macrosomic infant?

Is the difference between central body fat and extremity fat marked? Could there be something related to thigh circumference, as an example, versus abdominal circumference, which might let you pick these things up? Does anyone know about the fat distribution in the infant of the diabetic mother?

NICOLAIDES: Steve Gabbe who was in our department tried to look at the subscapular deposition of fat as the earliest sign. But it is not an easy technique.

HOWIE: Is it true that mothers who eat too much throughout the pregnancy will make their babies large? One of the most difficult things we found was measuring dietary intake in caloric terms during pregnancy. An important practical issue is whether or not the mother who simply overeats is having an impact on her baby.

GILLMER: The data is cross-sectional and retrospective so it is impossible to answer that.

COCKBURN: It is an important practical issue for mothers because if they do eat too much and they make their babies big, then...

GILLMER: We reported the reverse in the *Nutrition in Pregnancy* Study Group Proceedings,(4) where we actually dieted women, and we found no difference in birthweight, although we were able to demonstrate substantial reductions in their stored body fat as measured by skin fold thickness and fat cell volume.

HOWIE: But the other end of the scale may be totally different.

GILLMER: It may well be.

COCKBURN: It may also be a result of a pattern of eating. Someone who nibbles constantly maintains a high blood glucose continuously and is different from someone who is fat but eats only at mealtimes.

STEER: If you are more than 20% above your ideal body weight, right up to 20 kg, the fetal weight gain does not correlate very well at all with maternal weight gain.

GILLMER: Again, that is cross-sectional data.

CLAPP: There is some evidence to suggest that this can be related to the caloric mix that the woman ingests, and that the more simple sugars that she ingests the greater the birthweight. A lot of the data is cross-sectional and deals with cultural changes in diet in Eskimos. The average birthweight of the Eskimo populace was increased by some 600 g when the trading store came to be in North America. Traditionally before that they ate a very low simple sugar diet and after that they ate a very high simple sugar diet.

HALL: It was reported a few years ago that Faroëse women had unusually large babies, but this was interpreted to be due to a high consumption of fish which they thought would have an effect of prolonging gestation by producing prostaglandins.(5) We are presently working on this because it is also the case that Orkney and Shetland women have unusually large babies and they do not eat a particularly large amount of fish. So, it is a complicated field.

STEER: This is in the Faroe Islands?

HALL: Yes. They have unusually large babies, but the authors suggest that it was due to the prolongation of gestation. I think that it was probably not the explanation, but rather something to do with maternal size.

COCKBURN: The children in Orkney at the age of $10^1/_2$ years are 3 cm taller than those in Glasgow so it is a maintained thing.

ALBERMAN: There is plenty of literature on differences in fetal growth velocity in different societies. For instance, in the Irish, in Italian births and in Chinese births it seems to be faster than in other groups. I have always wondered whether it was due to the high carbohydrate diet.

REFERENCES

1. Yang JW, Fellows RE. Characterization of insulin stimulation of the incorporation of radioactive precursors into macromolecules in cultured rat brain cells. *Endocrinology* 1980; **107:** 1717-1724.
2. Naeye RL. Infants of diabetic mothers: a quantitative morphologic study. *Pediatrics* 1965; **35:** 980–988.
3. Flynn MD. *Increased fetal growth in macrosomic diabetic pregnancy: a new observation.* Presentation to the British Diabetic Association, 1986.
4. Campbell DM, Gillmer MDG. *Nutrition in Pregnancy.* Proceedings of the Tenth RCOG Study Group. London: RCOG, 1983.
5. Olsen SF, Hansen HS, Sorensen TIA, Jensen B, Secher NJ, Sommer S, Knudsen LB. Intake of marine fat, rich in (n-3) polyunsaturated fatty acids may increase birth weight by prolonging gestation. *Lancet* 1986; **ii:** 367–369.

Obstetric problems of fetal macrosomia

Mr J.M. Brudenell

INTRODUCTION

Fetal macrosomia may be defined in terms of birthweight percentile (> 90 or > 95) or actual birthweight. For the obstetrician it is probably most useful to consider any baby whose birthweight is equal to, or greater than, 4000 grams as being macrosomic, because it is in this group that most obstetric difficulties will arise.

INCIDENCE

The incidence of macrosomia varies with the population studied. In England and Wales in 1980, 46 036 babies were born with a birthweight of 4000 g or more, an incidence of 8%.[1] At King's College Hospital, London in 1986/7, 7% of babies born came into this category. The incidence of babies weighing 4500 g or more at King's during this period was 1%. In the USA, the incidence of this birthweight is also quoted as 1%[2-4] and on this basis some 66 000 babies weighing 4500 g or more will be delivered there annually.

PERINATAL MORTALITY AND MORBIDITY

Vaginal delivery of a big baby may result in maternal injury but the greater risk is to the baby. The perinatal mortality rate for macrosomic babies in England and Wales in 1980 was 39 per 1000 compared to 32 per 1000 for the 3000 – 3999 g group. The corresponding stillbirth rate was 22 per 1000 and 17 per 1000, indicating a slightly greater risk of stillbirth over first-week death in the macrosomic group. Older studies quoted perinatal mortality rates five times higher for those babies weighing 4500 g or more,[5-7] but with modern management of labour and an increased use of Caesarean section the risk to the large baby has been much reduced. Thus the perinatal mortality from birth trauma, intrauterine hypoxia and birth asphyxia in England and Wales in 1980 was not increased for the macrosomic baby.[1] Perinatal morbidity, however, remains an increased hazard for the big baby. Prolonged labour, intrapartum asphyxia, shoulder dystocia and birth trauma are all more likely to occur in association with fetal macrosomia.[4]

DIAGNOSIS OF FETAL MACROSOMIA

The dangers of fetal macrosomia are much reduced if the condition can be diagnosed before the onset of labour. This is particularly true of the complications of labour and delivery, especially shoulder dystocia.[8] Maternal obesity, excess weight gain in pregnancy, previous big baby, not smoking, post-maturity and maternal diabetes have all been reported to be associated with fetal macrosomia, and the obstetrician must take these factors into account when considering the diagnosis. The clinical diagnosis of fetal macrosomia before labour is made on the basis of abdominal palpation and the measurement of the symphysis fundal height. A symphysis fundal height measurement of 42 cm or more is strongly suggestive of fetal macrosomia as is the presence of an excess of liquor. The clinical diagnosis of disproportion before the onset of labour has tended to fall into disuse at the present time in favour of a policy of "wait and see what happens". Although this is satisfactory in most cases, a diagnosis of serious disproportion as a result of the combination of fetal macrosomia and a small maternal pelvis should still be made by the obstetrician as a result of abdominal assessment and engagement of the fetal head, and a pelvic examination to assess the size of the maternal pelvis. The use of X-ray pelvimetry seems almost to have disappeared from current obstetric practice except in breech presentations, but a lateral, erect X-ray of the pelvis can still be helpful when serious disproportion is suspected and a decision is to be taken on elective Caesarean section or trial of labour.

Once labour has started fetal macrosomia, if not detected previously, should be suspected whenever there is secondary arrest in the first stage of labour or prolongation of the second stage. It must be considered particularly before commencing oxytocin augmentation or embarking on a mid-pelvic forceps delivery, especially when the occiput is in the posterior or transverse position. Experience is an important factor in the clinical diagnosis of fetal macrosomia, both before and during labour but even the most experienced obstetrician may be mistaken in his estimate of the size of the baby. An important point about fetal macrosomia, from the clinician's point of view, is that the diagnosis should be considered whenever fetal/pelvic disproportion seems to be present at any stage in late pregnancy or labour.

ULTRASOUND

Ultrasound scanning is the most commonly used investigation to determine fetal weight *in utero*. In most centres the fetal weight estimation is based on a single measurement of the fetal abdominal circumference. However, even in skilled hands this method is not very accurate in detecting macrosomia. At King's, of 35 infants of diabetic mothers with a birthweight between 4000 and 4499 g, 17 were detected by ultrasound; none of the 3 infants weighing 4500 g or more were detected. A sensitivity in detecting fetal macrosomia of approximately 50% is better than average but does not compare with the accuracy of the method in the lower weight ranges. In all cases success in estimating fetal weight depends on the skill and accuracy with which the abdominal circumference is measured, and the time at which the scan is performed in relation to the time of delivery. The nearer to the time of delivery that the scan is performed the more accurate the estimate is likely to be. In our hands using our present abdominal circumference/weight chart there is a definite tendency to underestimate fetal weight when the fetus is macrosomic. The need for greater accuracy in the antenatal diagnosis of macrosomia has led to investigators combining different measurements of a fetus such as the femur length and abdominal circumference.(9) This has a sensitivity of 63%, but a rather low specificity (85%) and many false positives were detected.

In another study, femur length and abdominal circumference measurements were combined to calculate an *in utero* ponderal index.(10) Although the index was found to be highly correlative with fetal overgrowth and was highly specific (93%) it was not sensitive (24%) and therefore was not clinically very useful in predicting birthweights of 4000 g or more. In commenting on the general use of ultrasonic weight estimation procedures, Deter and Hadlock[11] point out that the errors in such estimations range up to 15%(± 2SDs), and conclude that current ultrasonic weight estimation procedures are not accurate enough to be used effectively in the detection of macrosomia. This rather depressing conclusion should nevertheless not stop the clinician from taking the ultrasound findings into account when attempting to detect fetal macrosomia antenatally.

The concept of a fetal-pelvic index was introduced[12] as a method of identifying a presence or absence of fetal/pelvic disproportion. The method combines ultrasound measurements of the head and abdomen with X-ray measurements of the anterior, posterior and transverse diameters of the maternal pelvic inlet and mid-pelvis. The presence of disproportion as judged by the mode of delivery was accurately predicted in 32 out of 34 macrosomic babies (4000 g). The method does involve antenatal radiography of women with clinically suspected disproportion and macrosomia, and seems unlikely to gain general acceptance in the present climate of antipathy to antenatal X-rays. It might be helpful in a woman thought to have a macrosomic baby and disproportion but who was anxious to avoid a Caesarean section.

MANAGEMENT OF FETAL MACROSOMIA

Since the antenatal diagnosis of macrosomia is difficult the clinical decision on how the baby should be delivered is somewhat arbitrary. Parkes and Ziel[3] proposed that all babies with an antenatal estimated fetal weight of > 4500 g should be delivered by elective Caesarean section. Other authors have supported this view. The number of additional Caesarean sections that this would entail was computed by Gross *et al.*[13] who concluded, on the basis of the need to avoid shoulder dystocia, that such a policy was justified. The contrary view has been taken in other studies which could not demonstrate that an increased use of Caesarean section and other obstetric advances reduced the risk of fetal asphyxia and trauma associated with large fetal size.[14] In Lobb and Beazley's series of babies weighing > 4500 g,[15] 65 out of 86 were delivered vaginally without perinatal mortality or significant morbidity. It would seem reasonable at present to take other factors into account when deciding how best to deliver an apparently macrosomic baby. Malpresentation or position, suspected disproportion, maternal age and past obstetric history, and other complicating factors such as diabetes all deserve consideration. Planned Caesarean section is generally preferable to emergency Caesarean section after a long labour. From the patient's point of view the latter combination generally represents the worst of both worlds.

When the patient with a suspected macrosomic fetus is allowed to go into labour, careful monitoring of the progress of labour and fetal wellbeing is essential. Secondary arrest in a primigravid patient requires careful assessment. Emergency Caesarean section at this stage may be a better alternative than oxytocin augmentation. The effect of planned and emergency Caesarean sections on total rates of Caesarean section in fetal macrosomia varies, from 14% for 4000 g babies and 25% for 4500 g babies at King's to 34% in a series from Chicago reported by Gross for the > 4500 g group.[13]

FORCEPS DELIVERY

It is self evident that instrumental delivery of a macrosomic baby requires great care and skill on the part of the obstetrician and "difficult" forceps delivery from the mid-pelvis is to be avoided. It is not always as self evident to the less experienced obstetrician that the alternative emergency Caesarean section may also be very difficult when the head of a macrosomic baby is deeply impacted in the pelvis.

SHOULDER DYSTOCIA

Although shoulder dystocia is more common when the baby is macrosomic most authorities hold that its occurence cannot be predicted.[13] Modanlou *et al.*[16] considered the anthropometric reasons for shoulder dystocia and concluded that macrosomic neonates who had experienced this condition had significantly greater shoulder to head, and chest to head proportions than macrosomic babies delivered without it. The infant of a diabetic mother who is macrosomic is especially likely to have disproportionately large shoulder and trunk measurements. The incidence of shoulder dystocia varies widely from series to series, probably due to differences in population studied, the extent to which Caesarean section is used, and a variation in recording practices such as the degree of traction necessary to qualify for a diagnosis of shoulder dystocia. A figure of 8.6% shoulder dystocia for babies in the 4000 g range and 35.7% for babies in the 4500 g group is quoted in one large series, and is fairly typical.[13] In practice, the majority of cases of shoulder dystocia occur in babies who are not macrosomic. At King's in 1986/7 there were 23 cases of shoulder dystocia in macrosomic (> 4000 g) and 30 cases in babies who were not macrosomic by this definition, a reminder that shoulder dystocia can occur at almost any birthweight. Nevertheless, most series relate shoulder dystocia to fetal weight[16-18] and most agree that weight alone is an unreliable predictor. Considerable interest centres on the predictability or otherwise of shoulder dystocia in the USA where the complications of this condition, particularly brachial plexus damage, are a not uncommon cause for litigation.[13,19] Whilst it is true that significant risk factors can be identified no clinically useful risk profile for shoulder dystocia has been developed.[13] It seems important therefore that every obstetrician is prepared to deal with this complication. Turning the patient onto her left side and performing a generous episiotomy is the traditional method employed in the UK, delivery being effected by traction sometimes combined with suprapubic pressure. Although this manoeuvre often succeeds it is very important not to use excessive traction if nerve damage to the brachial plexus is to be avoided. If moderate traction does not succeed two alternative manoeuvres are suggested. The Woods manoeuvre[20] consists of rotating the posterior shoulder through 180 degrees in a corkscrew fashion so releasing the anterior shoulder posteriorly. The McRoberts manoeuvre[21] has the patient lying on her back with her hips fully flexed. The resulting rotation of the symphysis pubis frees the anterior shoulder. Symphysiotomy[22] and cephalic replacement followed by Caesarean section[23,24] have been reported, but would seem only to be measures of last resort.

MACROSOMIA IN DIABETIC PREGNANCY

Fetal macrosomia is a common complication of diabetic pregnancy and merits a brief separate consideration. The weight distribution curve of the infants of diabetic mothers shows a shift to the right.[25] Fetal hyperinsulinaemia seems to be the major cause of macrosomia in diabetic pregnancy.[26] This is more likely to occur when the control of the maternal diabetes has been poor, but good control does not protect against the development of fetal macrosomia.[27] No constant relationship has been found between mean blood glucose levels in pregnancy and birthweight, although a correlation was found between haemoglobin A1 levels at term and birthweight.[28,29] Roberts and Baker[30] found a relationship between maternal fructosamine levels in the first trimester and fetal growth, and concluded that maternal diabetic control in early pregnancy may contribute to fetal macrosomia, a finding supported by an earlier study.[31] Developing macrosomia can be detected by serial ultrasound scans and is usually readily apparent in the third trimester. Characteristically a rapid acceleration of growth occurs in the last 2 or 3 weeks before full term. Induction of labour at 38 weeks is indicated in this situation and may avoid the intrapartum and neonatal problems associated with the macrosomic diabetic fetus as well as avoiding the risk of intrauterine death from hypoxia.[32]

CONCLUSIONS

Fetal macrosomia poses considerable problems to the obstetrician. Antenatal detection is not very accurate and the risk of increased perinatal mortality and morbidity, especially when the diagnosis is made late in labour, may be considerable. Careful antenatal assessment and monitoring in labour with the judicious use of planned and emergency Caesarean section is needed if the risks are to be avoided. Shoulder dystocia is a particular hazard when the fetus is macrosomic and requires prompt effective treatment. In diabetic pregnancy developing fetal macrosomia can be detected by serial ultrasound scans and appropriate steps taken to avoid the associated complications.

REFERENCES

1. MacFarlane A, Mugford M. *Birth Counts. Statistics of Pregnancy and Childbirth 1984*. Vol 134. London: HMSO, 1984.
2. Modanlou HD, Dorchester WL, Thorosian A, Freeman RK. Macrosomia—maternal, fetal and neonatal implications. *Obstet Gynecol* 1980; **55**: 420-424.
3. Parks DG, Ziel HK. Macrosomia — a proposed indication for primary Caesarean section. *Obstet Gynecol* 1978; **52**: 407.
4. Spellacy WN, Miller S, Winegar A, Peterson PQ. Macrosomia—maternal characteristics and infant complications. *Obstet Gynecol* 1985; **66**: 158-161.

5. Nathanson JN. The excessively large fetus as an obstetric problem. *Am J Obstet Gynecol* 1950; **60**: 54-63.
6. Posner AC, Freidman S, Posner LB. The large fetus. A study of 547 cases. *Obstet Gynecol* 1955; **5**: 268-278.
7. Sack RA. The large infant. A study of maternal, obstetric, fetal and newborn characteristics; including a long-term pediatric follow-up. *Am J Obstet and Gynecol* 1969; **104**: 195.
8. Benedetti TJ, Gabbe SC. Shoulder dystocia—a complication of fetal macrosomia and prolonged second stage of labour with midpelvic delivery. *Obstet Gynecol* 1978; **52**: 526-529.
9. Hadlock FP, Harrist RB, Sharman RS, Deter RL, Park SK. Estimation of fetal weight with the use of head, body and femur measurements — a prospective study. *Am J Obstet Gynecol* 1985; **151**: 333-337.
10. Miller JM Jr, Korndorffer FA Jr, Kissling GE, Brown HL, Gabert HA. Recognition of the overgrown fetus: In-utero ponderal indices. *Am J Perinatol* 1987; **4**: 86-89.
11. Deter RL, Hadlock FP. Use of ultrasound in the detection of macrosomia: a review. *J C U* 1985; **13**: 519-524.
12. Morgan MA, Thurnau GR. Efficacy of the fetal-pelvic index for delivery of neonates weighing 4000 grams or greater: A preliminary report. *Am J Obstet Gynecol* 1988; **158**: 1133-1137.
13. Gross TL, Sokol RJ, Williams T, Thompson K. Shoulder dystocia: A fetal-physician risk. *Am J Obstet Gynecol* 1987; **156**: 1408-1418.
14. Boyd ME, Usher RH, McLean FH. Fetal macrosomia: Prediction, risks, proposed management. *Obstet Gynecol* 1983; **61**: 715-722.
15. Lobb MO, Beazley JM. Big babies — an analysis of 118 consecutive cases of birth weight more than 4.5 kg. *J Obstet Gynaecol* 1984; **4**: 181-184.
16. Modanlou HD, Komatsu G, Dorchester W, Freeman RK, Bosu SK. Large-for-gestational-age neonates. Anthropometric reasons for shoulder dystocia. *Obstet Gynecol* 1982; **60**: 417-423.
17. Acker DB, Sacks BP, Freidman EA. Risk factors for shoulder dystocia. *Obstet Gynecol* 1985; **66**: 762-768.
18. Gross SJ, Shime J, Farine D. Shoulder dystocia: Predictors and outcome. *Am J Obstet Gynecol* 1987; **156**: 334-338.
19. Iffy L, Goldsmith LS. Obstetric background of malpractice claims involving fetal damage. In: *Second Perinatal Practical and Malpractice Symposium.* Ed. L Iffy. New York: Healthmark Communications, 1985; p.95.
20. Woods CE, Westbury NY. A principle of physics as applicable to shoulder delivery. *Am J Obstet Gynecol* 1943; **45**: 796-804.
21. Gonick B, Stringer CA, Held B. An alternate manoeuvre for management of shoulder dystocia. *Am J Obstet Gynecol* 1983; **145**: 882-884.
22. Lee CY. Shoulder dystocia. *Clin Obstet Gynecol* 1987; **30**(1): 77-82.
23. Sandberg EC. The Zavanelli manoeuvre: A potentially revolutionary method for the resolution of shoulder dystocia. *Am J Obstet Gynecol* 1985; **152**: 479-484.

24. O'Leary JA, Gunn D. Option for shoulder dystocia – cephalic replacement. *Contemporary Obstetrics and Gynaecology* 1986; **27**(1): 157-159.
25. Bradley RJ, Nicolaides KH, Brudenell JM. Are all the infants of diabetic mothers "macrosomic"? *Br Med J* 1988; **297:** 1583-1584.
26. Susa JB, Schwartz R. Effects of hyperinsulinemia in the primate fetus. *Diabetes* 1985; **34**(Supplement 2): 36-41.
27. Knight G, Worth RC, Ward JD. Macrosomy despite well-controlled diabetic pregnancy. *Lancet* 1983; **ii:** 1431.
28. Small M, Cameron A, Lunan CB, MacCuish AC. Macrosomia in pregnancy complicated by insulin-dependant diabetes mellitus. *Diabetes Care* 1987; **10**: 594-599.
29. Stubbs SM, Leslie RDG, John PN. Fetal macrosomia and maternal diabetic control in pregnancy. *Br Med J* 1981; **282**: 439-440.
30. Roberts AB, Baker JR. Relationship between fetal growth and maternal fructosamine in diabetic pregnancy. *Obstet Gynecol* 1987; **70**: 242-246.
31. Lin C, River J, River P, Blix PM, Moawad AH. Good diabetic control in early pregnancy and favorable fetal outcome. *Obstet Gynecol* 1986; **67**: 51-56.
32. Brudenell JM. Diabetic pregnancy: some continuing problems. *William Meredith Fletcher Shaw Memorial Lecture*. London: RCOG, 1987.

Discussion

Chairman: Mr M.D.G. Gillmer

GILLMER: Should not the practice of managing the large baby be changing now that there is such an awareness of the danger of litigation?

BRUDENELL: There is no question that in the United States this is a problem because there is a view taken by some obstetricians, who are not particularly popular with their colleagues, that shoulder dystocia can be predicted. Of course, as long as you have got someone to stand up in court and say that, then the lawyers tend to employ these people to give evidence when litigation occurs. I think that there is no doubt that the fear of litigation would mean that any baby that was suspected of being macrosomic might well be delivered by planned Caesarean section.

GILLMER: You mentioned a paper from the US looking at bisachromial diameters on computerised tomography scans which states that a bisachromial diameter of more than 14 cm is an indication for abdominal delivery. I believe that there are people in the US trying to replicate this work using nuclear magnetic resonance.

BRUDENELL: One does have to say that big babies are usually not diabetic. Most big babies deliver vaginally without serious complications. The difficulty is to pick up those that are likely to run into difficulties, particularly delay in labour and shoulder dystocia in the second stage.

CAMPBELL: I think that if one was certain that it was 4.5 kg one would be heading towards Caesarean section but the evidence has shown that the rate of dystocia is 34%, is that correct?

BRUDENELL: Yes.

CAMPBELL: I think that is a risk that few of us would be prepared to take. I think that the great problem is predicting the weight of these babies. Even before Deter(1) said that there is a constant percentage error throughout the prediction range, I said it. It was 16% when I did the original study on predicting weight. We still use that same prediction line, and it is clearly inappropriate for the large fetus. It was designed to pick up small-for-dates fetuses. For small babies of 1 kg you can get to within ± 150 g when predicting the actual weight, and that is good. But for a 4 kg baby it is ± 600 g, so you have got a huge distribution. Clearly our mean error is below the actual one so we should change our line on the big ones. Even if we got our mean prediction spot on the average mean weight of the fetus for big babies the distribution would still be ± 600 g at 4 kg. It seems you are going to miss most of them and that is the greatest problem.

CLAPP: We are trying to look at this problem now because we are very upset when we section somebody for macrosomia and they turn out to have a baby that weighs 3800 g at 41 weeks. That does happen with embarrassing frequency. The real question is whether one can do any better than we do right now in predicting the macrosomic infant ultrasonically by combining different measurements. The problem is with the prediction lines that you use for normally grown pregnancies which do not seem to hold for those babies that accelerate in late pregnancy.

CAMPBELL: The literature is heavy with formulas combining every parameter that you can think of.

CLAPP: If the best you can get is ± 10% you are never going to get there.

CAMPBELL: Few of them are as good as that. Most predictions are ± 15%, and that is 2 SDs.

HALL: If you could predict them that would certainly be an indication to have an obstetrician in the delivery room. Usually, the baby can quite easily be delivered by the obstetrician when they get there, but the midwife has got stuck in getting the baby out. Of course, that would not be true in the United States where you usually do have an obstetrician present. But then, you also have the lawyer just outside the door!

GILLMER: You mentioned fetal monitoring which obviously is a very controversial area. I think that most of us would agree that it should be used routinely for the fetus of the diabetic mother. Were you saying that in any patient where macrosomia was suspected that continuous fetal heart monitoring was advisable or even mandatory?

BRUDENELL: We do have fairly good evidence now that all infants of diabetic mothers tend toward hypoxia as they approach full term. So clearly they are going to be at particular extra risk. I do not know that you can draw the conclusion that it is appropriate for all women with macrosomic babies. Macrosomia clearly occurs without any abnormality in carbohydrate metabolism or associated hypoxia. In general, one looks to see in a big baby having a big placenta that the big placenta will work well. It does not do so in diabetes probably because of the morphological changes in the placenta. Cordocentesis evidence certainly suggests that there is a tendency toward hypoxia in these babies particularly as they approach term. Certainly they need monitoring, and I do not mean just CTGs; I mean fetal blood sampling as well.

COCKBURN: One of the things you did not mention was the timing of clamping of the cord in delivery. Many of these babies are very plethoric, and they could be made even more plethoric if 200+ ml of blood from the large placenta is entered into them. Have you any advice on what to do about the placenta in relation to the delivery of these large fetuses?

BRUDENELL: No, we simply clamp the cord in the ordinary way. Interestingly enough, Harold Gamsu, a paediatrician who has had a good deal of experience in dealing with these, used quite often to have to venesect them and replace the plasma back to the baby. He says that nowadays that is much less common and I suppose that it might be to some extent perhaps because we are controlling their maternal blood sugars rather better. We certainly do not delay cord clamping but we do not rush to clamp it.

PATEL: Why are they plethoric?

BRUDENELL: If they are hypoxic then that explains why they are plethoric.

PATEL: Are you suggesting that all these babies who are born plethoric are hypoxic? If they are then we are not able to detect it.

BRUDENELL: It is very unusual to find a simple cause and effect anywhere in nature. But if you have hypoxia, and we do have evidence to support that, then you would expect the babies to become plethoric.

GILLMER: Has anyone theorised that for the diabetic infant it is an effect of hyperinsulinaemia on the haemopoietic system?

COCKBURN: There is certainly a lot more haemopoietic tissue in the liver. Whether that is due to a chronic hypoxaemia is arguable. I do not know how much marrow there is in other haemopoietic areas but certainly there is more haemopoietic tissue in the liver of the largest of the babies of diabetic mothers than in the normal sized ones. Whether it is hypoxia or whether it is some growth factor that is resulting in this extra red cell mass I do not know.

PATEL: Is the baby that is macrosomic likely to be the one that is plethoric, or is it seen in non macrosomic babies of diabetic mothers?

COCKBURN: It only occurs with the macrosomia. There could be another factor as these babies also tend to have large kidneys.

PATEL: Is doing haematocrit one way of diagnosing the condition?

BRUDENELL: Postnatally?

PATEL: No, intrapartum. You suggested that we should monitor them and also do scalp pH, and I wonder if haematocrit can be checked on a scalp blood sample.

BRUDENELL: I think that is probably a bit too esoteric for me. Clearly the degree of plethora which they have can be very considerable and it may be that hypoxia alone is not the cause. It is tempting to think that if they are hypoxic over a period of time they would produce more red blood cells to try and help out. There may be other factors.

NICOLAIDES: It is interesting that in Rhesus disease, for example, you have to become extremely anaemic before you develop hepatic erythropoiesis. You have to have an anaemia of less than 7 g; you are about to die before you develop hepatic erythropoiesis. Looking at this aspect of hepatic erythropoiesis in babies, if it is true in all macrosomic babies, it would give a better idea as to the pathogenesis of macrosomia.

CAMPBELL: Why do you think that it is hepatic erythropoiesis in the diabetic?

NICOLAIDES: Because somebody suggested that the livers of these babies have an excess of erythropoietic tissue.

WIGGLESWORTH: I have not actually counted. I have seen relatively few such babies over the years. But I think it is generally so that babies of diabetics do have a lot of erythropoietic tissue. If there is going to be increased erythropoietic tissue it would be likely to be in the liver because that forms such a major site of erythropoiesis in the fetus in any case.

NICOLAIDES: But not at that gestation. At 20 weeks the major erythropoietic tissue in the fetus is the marrow. If I can turn back to the model of Rhesus disease where you have to develop extreme degrees of anaemia before you develop hepatic erythropoiesis, in spite of the fact that the oxygen content is low the pO_2 is maintained. Therefore if erythropoietin is released in response to a low pO_2 we will not get very high levels of erythropoietin until there is severe anaemia. Perhaps in the diabetic if for one reason or another you have a chronic low grade mild hypoxia then you may have release of erythropoietin.

PATEL: Define a "mild low grade hypoxia".

NICOLAIDES: Around the 10th percentile of the normal range. In fetal blood from diabetic pregnancies the mean pO_2 is significantly lower than the normal range. There is a statistically significant decrease in the whole population.

CLAPP: Where in the fetal circulation is the pO_2 lower?

NICOLAIDES: In fetal blood taken either from the umbilical vein or from the umbilical artery obtained by cordocentesis.

CLAPP: It makes a big difference because if it is lower in the umbilical vein that indicates a problem with placental transfer of oxygen. If it is lower in the umbilical artery that could mean a variety of things. I am very surprised then that the pO_2 cannot be normal in this condition. If it is lower in the umbilical vein then it is lower throughout the fetal carcass. It would have to indicate a deficit in placental transfer of oxygen at normal atmospheric pressures.

NICOLAIDES: Or increased placental consumption of oxygen. It is commonly held that the placenta in these pregnancies enlarges to improve fetal nutrition. They also argue that the placenta enlarges as a by-product of the metabolic disturbances in the mother and that the big placenta is compromising the fetus through its increased metabolic activity and therefore increased oxygen consumption. The blood that is presented in the intervillous space will have a residual decrease in its pO_2 because it is taken up by the placenta.

BRUDENELL: The other factor in diabetic pregnancy is that although the blood flow through the myometrium is normal, uteroplacental blood flow by various studies has always been shown to be markedly reduced in diabetes. There are morphological changes in the placenta which would account for a poor transfer of oxygen across to the fetus. So you have got a number of factors that may operate and make the baby hypoxic.

COCKBURN: And yet it is odd that we always argue that that is the cause of the small-for-dates baby.

BRUDENELL: And it is, but the bottom line is that every now and again out of the blue in late pregnancy, as we all know, the baby dies. You do have to have an explanation for that because it is a well described and established phenomenon of diabetic pregnancy. It is much less common now than it was, but our experience of diabetic pregnancy up to full term and certainly in post maturity is relatively limited. This is why I am anxious that we do not get too much experience of that because I do think that the further we go on the more likely it is that we get a return to late intrauterine death. Hypoxia is made worse by things like pre-eclampsia and so on, and certainly poor diabetic control makes it worse. You can envisage a combination of circumstances where the hypoxia would be sufficiently severe to kill the baby.

MARSAL: I would like to follow up the remarks of Mr Brudenell on the changes in the placental flow in diabetic pregnancy. We have been measuring volume flow in the aorta of diabetic fetuses and have calculated a proportional distribution taking the thoracic aortic flow as 100% and then measuring the abdominal aorta and the umbilical vein flow. We also studied some normal non-diabetic pregnancies. It was a longitudinal study with three or four measurements between the 26th and 40th week of gestation and included 41 relatively well controlled diabetics. In the last eight weeks of pregnancy there was a larger proportion of blood flow going to the central body and the periphery of the fetus, and less to the placenta than in normal pregnancies. This is in agreement with your report on intraplacental flow and placental changes.

CAMPBELL: I was under the impression that late intrauterine death in macrosomic fetuses was extremely rare now, and it was usually the small diabetic fetus that died.

BRUDENELL: You can get intrauterine growth retardation in the diabetic pregnancy just as you can get it in any other and it is most often associated with diabetic angiopathy. The classic late intrauterine death is not of a small baby; it is of a macrosomic baby.

GILLMER: I think that the studies of lactate accumulation due in part to hyperglycaemia, with coexistent hypoxia, seem to offer the best explanation for what occurs.

BRUDENELL: That is absolutely right, but if you have got hypoxia as well as hyperglycaemia we showed some years ago that there is an increase in the incidence of fetal distress in labour in diabetic pregnancies. This has also been documented by others. We showed that when we controlled maternal glucose with intravenous insulin during labour we showed an immediate decrease in the incidence of fetal distress. If you get hyperglycaemia it is going to make any effect of hypoxia worse in terms of lactic acid and low pH.

COCKBURN: I am just going to remind Professor Wigglesworth of a question that was posed to him by Professor Milner regarding the transposition of great arteries in these big fetuses.

WIGGLESWORTH: Yes, I remember Naeye's paper on all this.[2] Although we have had a number over the years we have never actually counted islets or β cells in these babies. The idea was that alteration of the circulation meant that the abdominal organs would be perfused with more glucose and this might stimulate insulin production. I am not particularly impressed by the large size of the babies; they are obviously larger than most perinatal deaths which is not quite the same as these are not a normal population.

GILLMER: One of my diabetic patients who had poorly controlled diabetes for most of her pregnancy produced a baby with transposition of the great vessels and it was not macrosomic. So it broke all the rules.

REFERENCES

1. Deter RL, Hadlock FP. Use of ultrasound in the detection of macrosomia: a review. *JCU* 1985; **13:** 519–524.
2. Naeye RL. Transposition of the great arteries and prenatal growth. *Arch Pathol* 1966; **82**: 412-418.

SECTION 4

FETAL UNDERGROWTH

Epidemiology

Professor E.D. Alberman

INTRODUCTION

The first stage of any epidemiological study is to reach an agreement on the definition of the condition being reviewed. The term fetal undergrowth implies undergrowth for a given gestational age, and the first problem is that of measurement of gestational age. Even if this can be established, it is not obvious that norms of birthweight for gestational age for babies born pre- or post-term are representative of all conceptions that have reached that gestational age. They are likely to have characteristics associated with their gestational age at birth which may confound the epidemiology of any apparent undergrowth. These are points which will be discussed elsewhere in this volume.

However even if we consider only term births which constitute the majority of deliveries, variations of birthweight distribution between different socio-biological and population subgroups are such that it is problematical to arrive at an agreed "norm" from which to assess the associations and consequences of deviation. Stein and Susser(1) have pointed out the distinction, in this context, between the statistical "norm", which delimits the modal area of variation of a measure, and the "clinical norm", which distinguishes "all that is unimpaired, functioning and well from all that is impaired, malfunctioning and ill", and certainly this is a useful distinction to make. Unfortunately adverse consequences of undergrowth may not be perceived at birth, and again questions of definition of what is a malfunction or impairment would arise. In practice one is left with a definition which is largely statistically based, although many attempts have been made to render this more pragmatic. One cannot therefore escape some discussion of the statistical background of the definition of fetal undergrowth.

In addition it is becoming clear that fetal undergrowth takes many different forms, stunting and wasting being two such forms which are described. As yet the epidemiology of the different forms is not well worked out, and will not be further referred to in this paper.

THE DISTRIBUTION OF BIRTHWEIGHTS

There is general agreement that birthweight distributions, whether for all gestational ages or for a given gestational age, are of a shape that resemble, but are not strictly a Gaussian, or "normal" form. One particular departure from the normal is a tendency towards an excess in the tail of babies of low birthweight, which can be reduced but not eliminated by restricting the curve to a specific gestational age. It is the births in these tails which represent, for a given gestational age, those babies who are undergrown, and there are two main ways of defining these statistically. One is to express them in terms of a given percentile of all birthweights for that gestational age, and cut-off points used have been the 3rd, 5th or 10th. The other is to express them in terms of the deviation from the mean, making the assumption that the distribution is basically Gaussian, and defining them as under two standard deviations from the mean, a measure which in a Gaussian distribution corresponds to just under the 3rd percentile. In practice, since the distributions can be shown to depart in several ways from the Gaussian form, the use of percentiles is probably the better choice.

BIOLOGICAL INFLUENCES ON THE DISTRIBUTION

There are certain biological influences on the distribution which are marked and consistent. These include sex, plurality, birth order, and maternal height, weight and birthweight. These are each of a different nature and it is worth considering them separately.

Sex and plurality

Fetal sex seems to have its own independent effect on fetal growth, birthweight of males being higher on average than that of females of the same gestational age. In effect it means that the "norms" for males and females differ and, as Stein and Susser(1) pointed out, the importance of this is illustrated by the fact that at a given weight for gestational age girls have an advantage over boys in terms of perinatal survival and neonatal course. A similar situation pertains in the case of multiple births but in this case the relative retardation of growth in multiple births is secondary to a cause extrinsic and not intrinsic to the fetus.

Birth order

Relative growth retardation is also seen in first births, although it may be mitigated if preceded by a spontaneous abortion.(2) In this case also it may be presumed that the cause is extrinsic to the fetus, but this time it seems that no fetal benefit is gained in relation to later births of the same birthweight and gestational age. It may be that the benefit is a negative one, in the sense that the dangers to large first babies may be greater than for other birth orders. However, Stein and Susser(1) argued that, in contrast to the situation with fetal sex and plurality, we should not use different norms for first and later births from which to assess fetal undergrowth.

Social and economic deprivation

Fetal growth rate is slowed under conditions of social and economic deprivation(3) whether this is measured using occupational, educational, or financial classifications. The mechanisms through which this slowing is mediated are certainly in part nutritionally based, both through maternal lifelong nutritional status, which may permanently stunt growth, and through nutritional or general health status around the time of conception and pregnancy, reflected by maternal weight. These will be discussed in depth elsewhere in this volume, but they bear directly or indirectly on much of the epidemiology of fetal undergrowth in relation to other factors.

Adverse factors other than nutrition are also more common under conditions of deprivation: maternal infections, often the smoking habit, alcohol and drug abuse and occupational hazards, and close pregnancy spacing. The effects of these hazards will be discussed further later, but first one should consider the overall confounding effect of deprivation on apparently biological variables such as maternal height and ethnic group.

Parental height

Although both parents contribute towards the eventual height of their offpsring it is the maternal influence which is predominant in the case of birthweight. At least three mechanisms have been suggested through which this influence may reduce birthweight for gestational age. One is the purely genetic effect;[4,5] one is an immediate effect of severe maternal malnutrition which can be palliated with nutritional supplementation;[6] and finally there seems to be an effect which Ounsted and Ounsted[7] have termed "maternal constraint", which they have shown to be familial through the female line. Any or all of these are likely to be associated with

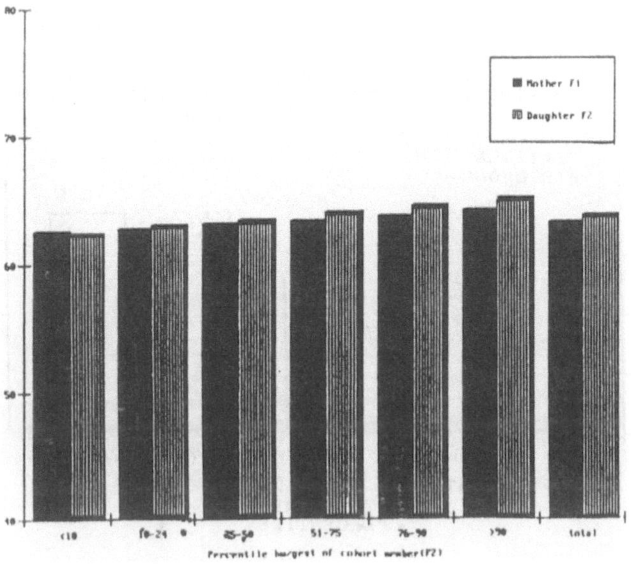

Figure I
Mean height in inches of female cohort member at 23 yrs and her mother by percentile bw/gest for cohort member – 1958 cohort
(Alberman *et al.* in preparation)

short maternal stature, and/or low maternal weight.

However there is potential circularity in these effects, since adult height in its turn is influenced by maternal birthweight. Figure I is taken from preliminary findings from an ongoing study oi intergenerational effects in the 1958 National Birthday Trust Fund birth cohort[8] (Alberman *et al.* in preparation). Increasing birthweight for gestational age in the cohort members is associated on the one hand with an increase in the height of their mothers, and on the other with an increase in the height of cohort members at the age of 23 years. Interestingly, although the increases in height of the mothers and their adult daughters are closely associated, in those whose birthweight was less than the 10th percentile mean adult height was actually less than that of their mothers, while in all other groups it was greater.

Presumably this overall increase of height in the second generation is reflecting the steady secular increase in height that has been recorded in the developed countries. The exception in the case of the cohort members born small-for-dates may be reflecting maternal constraint, or a direct adverse effect of fetal undergrowth. These results are closely related with those of other studies relating birthweight in one generation to birthweight in the next.[9-11] This we are also able to look at in the 1958 cohort, and Figure II shows how the mean birthweight of the female children of the cohort members rises consistently as their mothers' birthweight for ges-

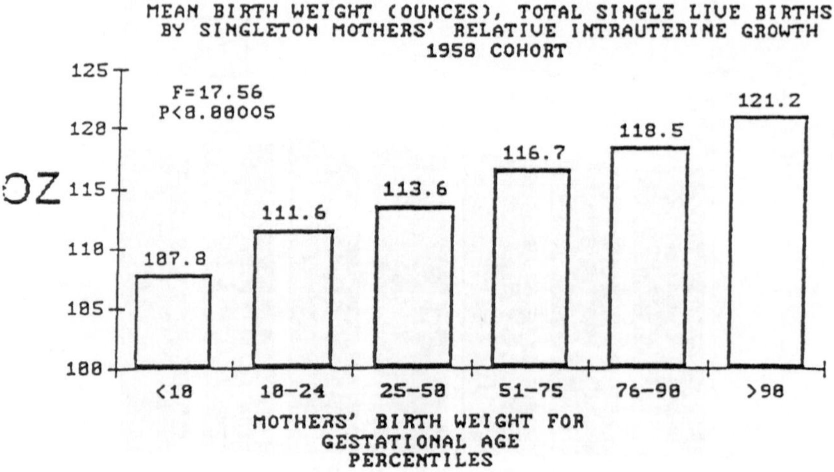

Figure II
Mean birthweight (ounces), total single live births by singleton mothers' relative intrauterine growth – 1958 cohort.
(Emanuel *et al.* in preparation)

tational age rises, and this was true also of the male children (Emanuel *et al.* in preparation). Unfortunately information on the gestational age of the children of the cohort is lacking, so we do not know which of those who were of low birth-weight were growth retarded. It is hoped to collect this information at a later sweep. We do know from the literature that within sibships there tend to be recurrences of preterm births, and fetal growth retardation.

Important also in this respect is the evidence from Norway showing the tendency within sibships to repeat fetal growth retardation, and preterm birth.(12)

Ethnic group

As with maternal height, genetic factors must play some part in effecting the well known differences in birthweight distribution between ethnic groups.(7) However, as with maternal height, the situation is confounded by the close inter-relationships between ethnic group and social class, for until recently socio-economic advantage has been largely confined to white populations. This needs to be taken into account when comparing fetal growth rates in different populations.

Table 1. Percentage low birthweight and infant mortality rates in different ethnic groups

Singapore: 1967–74 Single live births % < 2500 g			
Gestational group	Chinese %	Malay %	Indian %
Pre term	32.4	28.1	40.4
Term	5.0	6.5	9.8
Post term	4.6	8.4	6.7
All	6.1	8.1	11.5
ENMR	11.6	14.3	12.1
NMR	13.8	17.6	14.7
PNMR	4.8	12.3	7.8

(Hughes *et al.*, reference 14).
ENMR = early neonatal mortality rate
NMR = neonatal mortality rate
PNMR = perinatal mortality rate

However there are some clear-cut comparisons; for instance the consistently high rate of low birthweight births in US blacks compared with US whites has long been recognised, and there are annual vital statistical reports showing that among blacks birthweight for gestational age is consistently lower than among whites.[13] Hoffman and his colleagues[13] and many others, have shown that they have a mortality advantage over white babies at low gestational ages. However the socio-economic status of the blacks in the US overall is markedly lower than that of the white population and the raised mortality rates of the black babies overall at term testifies to the effect of that disadvantage.

However there is data from Singapore[14] where, it is maintained, three ethnic groups, Chinese, Malay and Indian, live in the same social environment with total health care coverage. Table 1 shows the proportion of low birthweight live births born preterm, at term, and post-term in each of these ethnic groups, showing a marked excess of small-for-date births (≤ 2500 g at term) in the Indian group. However the overall mortality rates, early neonatal, neonatal and perinatal are persistently highest in the Malay group, and intermediate in the Indians, in spite of their apparently disadvantageous weight distribution, 10% of their term births weighing 2500 g or less. It should be noted that overall the mortality rates, which were the average of those occurring between 1967–74, are relatively favourable compared with other countries for those years.

It seems that these weight differences may truly reflect genetic, or possibly intergenerational differences. However it would have been interesting to know the birthweight/gestational specific mortality rates, and also something of the adult heights in the different generations.

In general, as in the case of maternal height, it is important to be able to distinguish between apparently genetically determined relatively slow fetal growth in certain ethnic groups, and that determined by environmental disadvantage, for this raises the question of the choice of appropriate "norms" for different ethnic groups, and the selection of outcome measures to assess their appropriateness. A large number of different statistical strategies have been proposed to try to produce international norms which take into account ethnic environmental differences. This is discussed in some detail in a series of review papers edited by Wharton and Dunn[15] but it is fair to say that no simple solution has yet been proposed.

There are of course also very interesting questions as to the long term benefit or otherwise of striving to equalise birthweight distributions in different populations. In addition, little is known about the natural history of secular anthropometric changes, whether these start with increases in birthweight, or with increases in parental height. Certainly a change in a rate of fetal growth must be a part of this process.

Abnormal genetic effects

As well as the apparently subtle genetic effects which have been described there are some more clear-cut causes of fetal undergrowth.[4] Certain chromosomal anomalies, the most important of which is Down Syndrome, are known to cause fetal growth retardation, and there are also some single gene defects which cause dwarfing. There have been interesting comments as to the relationship of some fetal malformations to generalised or localised growth retardation.[1] Certainly these are related, but whether causally or not, and, if not, which preceded the other is an important question. Thus congenital heart defects may be due to a slowing of certain development pathways.

Fetal or placental infection

It is well known that fetal infections lead to growth retardation, babies with rubella embryopathy, or cytomegalo virus infection commonly being small-for-dates. Worldwide, possibly the most important infective cause of low birthweight is malaria, which seems to act largely through infestation of the placenta.[16] There are probably very large numbers of other infections that contribute directly or indirectly to fetal growth retardation.

Maternal smoking and alcohol consumption

In the developed countries much of the fetal growth retardation that we see is attributable to maternal smoking, which can retard fetal growth to the extent that at term the babies of mothers who smoke may be on average 100–170 g lighter than those who do not.[17] Moreover the literature[18] on the effects of alcohol consumption in pregnancy is also pointing to the importance of drinking as an agent of fetal growth retardation (Table 2), with odds ratios of being small-for-dates rising con-

Table 2. Odds ratio for a small-for-gestational age birth by alcohol consumption adjusted by multiple logistic regression.

No. of drinks per day	Odds Ratio	95% confidence intervals
≤ 1	1.11	1.00 – 1.23
1 – 2	1.62	1.26 – 2.09
3 – 5	1.96	1.16 – 3.31
≥ 6	2.28	0.91 – 5.77

(Mills *et al.*, reference 18).

sistently with the number of drinks consumed.

Occupational hazards

There is an increasing body of literature on the effect of work in pregnancy in relation to fetal growth. Many data sets have looked at birthweight alone, but a recent paper looking at pregnancy amongst obstetricians[19] has shown an excess of births of a weight under the 10th percentile for a given gestational age (standard used not given). According to this, primiparous obstetricians delivering during their residency were significantly more likely to produce growth retarded babies compared with 8.2% in those born before and 1.0% born after, but this is a highly selected sample.

Altitude

Another circumstance under which fetal growth rate is retarded is pregnancy at high altitudes. It can be shown that birthweight distribution shifts in a systematic way to lower levels as altitude rises.[20] This effect has been compared by Meyer[21] to that of smoking, for under both circumstances relative placental weight is not reduced and similar structural changes occur, predisposing to antepartum haemorrhage.

Spacing of pregnancies

It has been shown that babies born after a short interval from a previous birth are likely to be of low birthweight.[22] Certainly in one population we have recently studied this seems to be due to fetal undergrowth rather than preterm birth. In births between 1978 and 1984, all of 37 weeks or later, to Bangladeshi mothers living in Tower Hamlets, birthweight is closely associated with length of the interval between the date of one birth and the next. Except at extremely long intervals it rises steadily as interval lengthens (Hilder, in preparation). This group of mothers is exceptional in the close spacing between pregnancies, but the picture seems to be consistent with the literature.

CONCLUSION

An attempt has been made to review some of the most important aspects of the epidemiology of fetal undergrowth, with the exception of the effects of pregnancy pathology, of which hypertensive disease is probably the most important, and which would warrant a chapter on its own. The whole subject is enormously complex, but its study is exciting and rewarding. It provides many clues to the genetic and environmental patterns of fetal and adult growth, as well as being associated with numerous different pathological conditions. We have much to learn yet, and a necessary prerequisite for a fuller understanding is better data on a population scale of reliable gestational age as well as birthweight data.

ACKNOWLEDGEMENTS

Preliminary reports have been included from a study of intergenerational effects on reproduction funded by the National Institutes of Health and the Thrasher Research Fund.

REFERENCES

1. Stein ZA, Susser M. Intrauterine growth retardation: epidemiological issues and public health significance. *Semin Perinatol* 1984; **8**: 5-14.
2. Alberman E, Roman E, Pharoah POD, Chamberlain G. Birthweight before and after a spontaneous abortion. *Br J Obstet Gynaecol* 1980; **87**: 275-280.
3. Baird D. Epidemiologic patterns over time. In: *The Epidemiology of Prematurity*. Eds: DM Reed, FJ Stanley. Graz: Urban and Schwarzenberg 1977: pp.5-15.
4. Polani PE. Chromosomal and other genetic influences on birth weight variation. In: *Size at Birth*. Eds: K Elliott, J Knight. Ciba Foundation Symposium 27. Amsterdam: Elsevier. 1974: pp.127-164.
5. Morton NE. Genetic aspects of prematurity. In: *The Epidemiology of Prematurity*. Eds: DM Reed, FJ Stanley. Urban and Schwarzenberg, 1977: pp.213-230.
6. Rush D, Alvir JM, Garbowski GC *et al*. The National WIC Evaluation; evaluation of the special supplemental food programme for women, infants and children. *Am J Clin Nutr* 1988; **48**:
7. Ounsted M, Ounsted C. *On Fetal Growth Rate*. Clinics in Developmental Medicine, No 46. London: Spastics International Medical Publications, 1973.
8. Butler NR, Bonham DG. *Perinatal Mortality*. Edinburgh: E and S Livingstone, 1969.
9. Klebanoff MA, Graubard BI, Kessel SS, Berendes HW. Low birth weight across generations. *JAMA* 1984; **252**: 2423-2427.
10. Hackman E, Emanuel I, van Belle G, Daling J. Maternal birth weight and subsequent pregnancy outcome. *JAMA* 1983; **250**: 2016-2019.
11. Carr-Hill R, Campbell DM, Hall DM, Meredith A. Is birth weight determined genetically? *Br Med J* 1987; **295**: 687-689.
12. Hoffman HJ, Bakketeig LS. Heterogeneity of intrauterine growth retardation and recurrence risks. *Semin Perinatol*, 1984; **8**:15-24.
13. Hoffman HJ, Stark CR, Lundin FE, Ashbrook JD. Analysis of birth weight, gestational age, and fetal viability. *Obstet Gynecol Surv* 1974; **29**: 651-681.
14. Hughes K, Tan NR, Lun KC. Low birthweight of live singletons in Singapore. *Int J Epidemiol* 1984; **13**: 465-471.
15. Wharton B, Dunn PM. Perinatal growth: The quest for an international standard for reference. *Acta Pediatr Scand* Supplement 319, 1985.
16. McGregor IA, Wilson E, Billewicz WZ. Malaria infection of the placenta in The Gambia, West Africa; its incidence and relationship to stillbirth, birthweight and placental weight. *Trans R Soc Trop Med Hyg* 1983; **77**: 223-244.
17. Butler NR, Alberman ED. *Perinatal Problems*. Edinburgh: E and S Livingstone, 1969.
18. Mills JL, Graubard BI, Harley EE, Rhoads GG, Berendes HW. Maternal alcohol consumption and birth weight. How much drinking during pregnancy is safe? *JAMA*; **252**:1875-1879.
19. Grunebaum A, Minkoff H, Blake D. Pregnancy among obstetricians: a comparison of births before, during and after residency. *Am J Obstet Gynecol*, 1965; **15**:329-352.

20. Grahn D, Kratchman J. Variation in neonatal death rate and birth weight in the US and possible relations to environmental radiation, geology and altitude. *Am J Hum Genet* 1965; **15:** 329–352.
21. Meyer MB. Effects of maternal smoking and altitude on birth weight and gestation. In: *The Epidemiology of Prematurity.* Eds: DW Reed, FJ Stanley. Baltimore, Munich: Urban and Schwarzenberg, 1977: pp.81-104.
22. Federick J, Adelstein P. Influence of pregnancy space on outcome of pregnancy. *Br Med J* 1973; **4**:753-756.

Aetiology of fetal undergrowth

Professor J. S. Wigglesworth

INTRODUCTION – DEFINING THE PROBLEM

To make sense of aetiology in fetal undergrowth it is important to know what we mean by the term. It is usually defined in terms of fetal growth charts; however, there are considerable differences between growth charts derived from different populations as discussed by other contributors to this volume. The heterogeneity of many populations now, particularly in Britain, means that a standard growth chart applicable to a particular hospital or district may be difficult or impossible to construct. Birthweight for gestation also differs by sex and differs between first and later pregnancies. If a small-for-gestational-age (SGA) infant is to be defined in terms of a growth chart it is by no means easy to decide which chart to use and what corrections should be applied.

Definitions vary markedly between workers. SGA infants are variously defined as those below the 10th, 5th or 3rd centiles as defined by different growth charts or two standard deviations (SD) below the mean for gestation. How the SGA infant is defined may depend on the purpose for which it is defined. Thus the clinician intent on preventing any of the potential problems of fetal growth retardation, i.e. hypoglycaemia, may prefer an inclusive definition such as the 10th centile, whereas a researcher wishing to study the problems might well prefer a selected population below the 3rd centile, or 2 SD below the mean, where each infant could be regarded as significantly small in terms of the normal birth population at the gestation in question. However it may not be adequate to consider the problem purely in terms of growth charts. To determine what represents undergrowth and what may have caused it demands some consideration of the major factors controlling normal fetal growth and the interplay between them.

FACTORS CONTROLLING NORMAL FETAL GROWTH

Although control of cell multiplication and differentiation within different organs may be a complex process involving many different forms of stimulus from endocrine and paracrine factors, the process as it concerns the fetus as a whole can be summed up as the "inherent growth potential" of the fetus and is, of course, genetically determined. The optimal expression of this growth potential is dependent on substrate availability via the placenta. Unlike growth in infancy and childhood there is no essential requirement for pituitary growth hormone or thyroid hormones to modulate overall body growth.(1)

There is no predetermined fixed size which the fetus must attain to allow organ maturation and live birth. For a particular genetic growth potential the size actually attained by the fetus will vary widely according to nutrient availability, growth allowance or constraint. If nutrient supply is suboptimal the fetus will not achieve maximum potential. Within quite wide limits this may be regarded as a highly effective means of adaptation allowing birth of healthy infants over a wide range of birthweights, without interfering with their potential eventual adult size. How one defines fetal growth retardation within this spectrum of biological adaptation is largely a matter of personal philosophy.

However the situation is more complex, as growth potential will have its own variation,[2] and fetuses growing within a given environment would be expected to display a birthweight distribution round a mean. An infant of a particular birthweight below the mean may be one of low growth potential within a normal uterine environment, one of average growth potential subject to mild intrauterine growth restraint, or one of high growth potential subject to severe intrauterine growth restraint. Either low growth potential alone or high growth potential with severe growth restraint might cause the infant to present with significant problems, whereas the infant with average growth potential would be well adapted to its mild growth restraint.

TYPES OF GROWTH RETARDED FETUS

In studies on fetal and newborn rats, later extended to human fetuses, Winick divided early growth into an initial cell proliferation stage followed by an intermediate stage with both cell proliferation and cell growth and a final stage of mainly cell growth.[3] In the human the phase of cell proliferation has been assumed to last up to 16 weeks, the phase of intermediate growth from 16–32 weeks and the phase of cellular hypertrophy from 32 weeks onwards.[4] The most cursory examination of developing organ structure would reveal that different organs develop over quite separate time courses and that within each organ there are a variety of tissues developing and maturing at different rates. Thus in the human brain the main proliferation of neurones within the cerebral hemispheres appears to occur in the period from 12–18 weeks,[5] while the cerebellar neurones proliferate over the first year of life.[6] However the simple model proposed by Winick, although it may readily be disproved in detail,[7] does accord with the observation that a growth retarding stress operating in early pregnancy has a permanent effect on growth potential, whereas one operating in late pregnancy interferes mainly with fetal nutrition.

To some extent this seems to apply even to the fetal rat which should, according to the Winick hypothesis, be in the pure cell proliferation stage until the end of the first neonatal week.

CLASSIFICATION OF FETAL UNDERGROWTH

In considering the causes of fetal undergrowth it is preferable to classify the problem visually in terms of possible sites of fetal growth impairment working from the fetus itself out to the maternal environment (Figure I).

It will be seen from the diagram that the picture is bound to be complicated by variations in the site at which the growth retarding influence is applied and that where it acts, as exemplified in particular for smoking (see below). However we do not have any logical means of considering aetiology which avoids such problems.

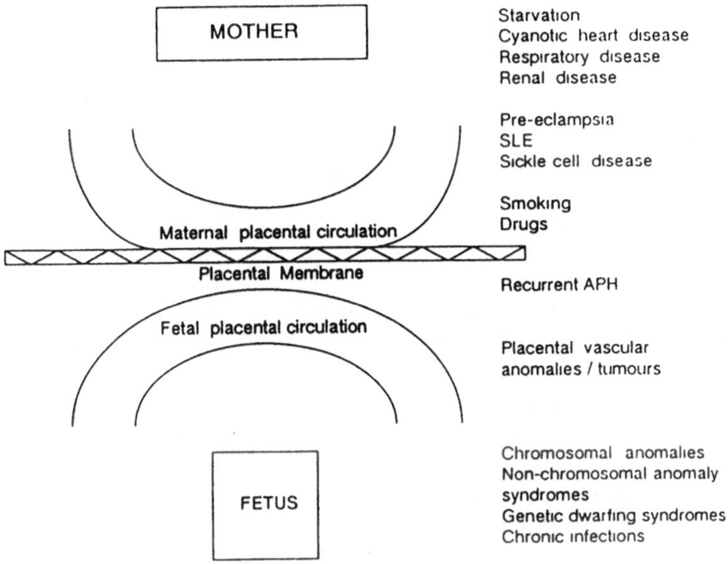

Figure I.
Diagrammatic representation of causes of fetal undergrowth and their sites of action.

CAUSES OF IMPAIRED GROWTH POTENTIAL

Genetic–chromosomal

It has been estimated that some 40% of total birthweight variation is genetically determined.[8] Thus the true frequency of genetically determined fetal growth retardation cannot be determined.

Fetal growth is impaired in a high proportion of chromosomally abnormal fetuses. In Turner's syndrome the average weight at term is 84% of normal, in trisomy 13 birthweight is 80% of normal, while in trisomy 21 birthweight is 80–90% of normal.[8] More severe retardation is seen in fetuses with trisomy 18, with an average birthweight only 62% of normal. Unbalanced autosomal anomalies such as chromosomal deletions are also associated with reduced birthweight.[8] Severe growth retardation is also a feature of fetuses with triploidy.[9]

In addition there are a number of genetically determined syndromes with severe dwarfing apparent by birth, including Seckel and Russell Silver syndromes.[10]

Many non-chromosomal malformation syndromes are associated with fetal growth retardation. Anencephalic fetuses are usually significantly growth retarded even if allowance is made for the missing cerebral tissue.(11)

Infants affected by a number of skeletal abnormalities such as osteogenesis imperfecta are growth retarded,(12) as are those with renal agenesis or severe cystic dysplasia with oligohydramnios.

Infection

The most characteristic form of infection to cause fetal growth retardation is the rubella virus.(13) Studies by Naeye and Blanc(14) indicated that rubella infection was associated with a reduced number of small cells within the fetal organs. About 30% of infants with cytomegalovirus infection are growth retarded.(15) Growth retardation as a result of other congenital viral infections is rather poorly documented,(16) although it has been reported in herpes simplex and varicella zoster. Among bacterial infections listeriosis is sometimes associated with growth retardation. Congenital syphilis and toxoplasmosis may also cause growth retardation.

Irradiation and therapeutic drugs

High dose irradiation is known to cause fetal growth retardation, although few women should be exposed to this hazard.(17) A variety of drugs which are known to have teratogenic effects on experimental animals will cause fetal growth retardation in association with the specific anomalies, or growth retardation alone if administered at a slightly later time. Such drugs include folic acid antagonists (aminopterin and methotrexate), antiepileptics (trimethadione), anticoagulants (Warfarin), and tetracyclines. Maternal administration of immunosuppressive drugs such as cyclophosphamide and azathioprine has been shown to cause fetal growth retardation in rats,(18) and a review of the literature by the same author suggested that these agents were also associated with SGA infants in human pregnancies.

Maternal addictions

Heroin. Maternal heroin addiction is well established as being associated with both preterm and SGA infants. The effect persisted when allowance was made for differences in maternal nutrition,(19) and growth retardation of rabbit fetuses also results from heroin administration.(20) However the possibility that infections, other drugs or adulterating agents may play a role in the effect cannot be excluded.

Smoking. The adverse effect of maternal smoking on fetal growth has been repeatedly demonstrated over the last 30 years. Most studies agree that the infants of mothers who smoke average about 200 g less than those of non-smoking mothers.(21) In many of the earlier studies it was not apparent to what extent the lower mean birthweight reflected preterm birth rather than fetal growth retardation as there is a higher frequency of short gestation among pregnancies to smoking mothers. Miller and Hassanein(22) showed that maternal smoking was associated with reduction in birthweight and crown–heel length in infants born at term, but there was no effect on ponderal index (ratio of body weight to body length). This supports the view that smoking results in decreased growth potential rather than impaired fetal nutrition. Further support for decreased growth potential in these cases comes from the observations on 7 and 11 year follow-up of the children in the National Child Development Study.[23] There was a reduced height and delay in educational attainment in the children of mothers who smoked, after adjusting for other sociobiological factors. A more recent study showed that increasing maternal age was associated with increased severity of fetal growth retardation.[24]

One of the problems of investigating the mechanism of fetal growth retardation produced by smoking is the plethora of possible candidates.[21] Thus nicotine when injected into pregnant rhesus monkeys caused a rise in maternal blood pressure, and a fall in maternal heart rate, an immediate fall in fetal blood pressure and fetal heart rate associated with a fall in pH, a rise in base deficit and fall in oxygen tension, followed by persistent fetal hypotension and tachycardia.[25] It was concluded that the effect was due to vasoconstriction of uterine vessels with reduced perfusion of the intervillous space.

Carbon monoxide destroys the oxygen combining power of haemoglobin and myoglobin and effectively causes hypoxia which may compromise fetal growth. The low concentration of hydrocyanic acid within tobacco smoke is partly detoxicated by combination with thiosulphate to form thiocyanate, which is a hypotensive agent. The cyanide may cause cellular anoxia by inactivating cytochrome oxidase. Either or both these mechanisms could impair fetal growth.

Finally there may be a decrease in carbonic anhydrase activity within the red cells of both mother and fetus due to inhibition by cyanide, thiocyanate and carbon monoxide. This may in turn interfere with cellular respiration in the fetus with resultant tissue hypoxia, acidosis and retarded growth.

Alcohol. Growth retardation is a prominent feature of the fetal alcohol syndrome.[26–28] The severity of growth retardation is related to the quantity of alcohol consumed, and is marked in cases where alcohol intake exceeds 45 ml pure alcohol per day.[27] The common association of heavy smoking with heavy drinking may impose some problems in analysis. It remains unclear whether the fetal effects are due to alcohol itself, to its metabolite acetaldehyde or indirect through impairment of fetal placental circulation.[3]

THE PLACENTA AND FETAL GROWTH IMPAIRMENT

The relationship which can generally be observed between placental and fetal size has long raised the question as to whether a small placenta causes impairment of fetal growth, whether it is a consequence of reduced need by a smaller fetus, or whether the size of both is determined in parallel by genetic or environmental factors. As pointed out by Keirse,[17] the answer is more complex than the question because weight and size are poor reflections of function and because several adaptations may occur. Experimental reduction of the endometrial caruncles before pregnancy to reduce placental mass in sheep results in fewer cotyledons, but each may be larger.[29] Maternal smoking in pregnancy may cause an increase in placental weight despite a lower birthweight.[30] The low oxygen saturation of high altitudes may have a similar effect.

Most growth retarded fetuses have a higher fetal/placental weight ratio than seen in normally grown fetuses. Fetal/placental weight ratio may vary from 4.5 in the highest placental weight groups to 7.3 in the lowest.[31] The fetus appears to outgrow its small placenta, possibly by improving the efficiency of exchange. A similar occurrence has been recognised in animal experiments.[32]

Specific abnormalities of the fetal placenta resulting in IUGR

Vascular abnormalities of the fetal side of the placenta may cause fetal growth retardation. Analysis of data from the Collaborative Study of Cerebral Palsy showed that single umbilical artery was significantly associated with low birthweight,[33] this was later confirmed in a British study.[34] Ligation of an umbilical artery at 100 days' gestation caused fetal growth retardation in the fetal lamb, but ligation at an earlier stage had no effect on fetal growth.[35]

Large chorioangiomas of the placenta may be associated with fetal growth retardation, presumably due to extensive short circuit of the placental villi with impaired placental exchange.[36] The donor twin of a twin–twin transfusion pair is usually growth retarded despite having, characteristically, a larger placental area than the recipient co-twin. The precise mechanism of growth retardation in this situation remains unclear. Of abnormalities of placental development only circumvallate placenta is accepted by Fox[36] as associated with fetal growth retardation.

Abnormalities on the maternal side of the placenta

The major placental abnormalities which impair fetal growth involve the maternal aspect of the placenta, that is the uteroplacental circulation. Thus recurrent antepartum haemorrhage in the first and second trimesters is strongly associated with fetal growth retardation.[37,38] This presumably is related to impairment in development of uteroplacental circulation. In contrast, placenta praevia shows no association with fetal growth retardation. [39]

MATERNAL CONDITIONS AND FETAL GROWTH RETARDATION

The subject of maternal nutrition is largely beyond the scope of this paper and is dealt with elsewhere. However, acute maternal starvation in women who were well fed prior to pregnancy was shown in the Dutch wartime experience to cause a reduction in birthweight of about 200 g.[40] The effects of nutrition in pregnancy on birthweight in chronically malnourished women may be different and may be influenced by additional factors such as physical work load.[41]

In developed countries the major factor in pregnancy causing inadequate fetal nutrition is impairment in uteroplacental circulation, most commonly due to pre-eclampsia or hypertension. The relationship between pre-eclampsia and fetal growth retardation has been debated for many years. The problem appears to have been the large proportion of women who present with signs of mild pre-eclampsia late in pregnancy and usually have well grown infants. Recent studies have confirmed that early onset or severe pre-eclampsia is associated with fetal growth retardation, while late onset or mild pre-eclampsia has no such association. [37,42]

Utero–placental lesions in early onset pre-eclampsia and unexplained fetal growth retardation

The characteristic and primary vascular lesions in pre-eclampsia are those of the spiral arteries at the myometrial–decidual junction and extending into the decidua. In normal pregnancy the cytotrophoblast cells invade the myometrial and decidual segments of the spiral arteries in successive waves during the first and second trimesters and transform the musculoelastic walls of the vessels into fibrinoid tubes to form the uteroplacental arteries of pregnancy. In pre-eclampsia there appears to be failure of the trophoblast to migrate normally into the myometrial segments of the spiral arteries early in the second trimester so that these vessels fail to undergo the expected physiological changes.[43] At a later stage, after pre-eclampsia has become clinically recognisable, the decidual spiral arteries show the changes of acute atherosis,[44,45] comprising fibrinoid necrosis of the wall with invasion by lipid-containing macrophages. The damaged arteries may then show development of thromboses and aneurysms, with consequent placental infarction and haematoma formation.[46] There has been continuing argument as to whether the spiral artery changes of pre-eclampsia or hypertension with albuminuria, can occur in the absence of maternal hypertension and be a cause of fetal growth retardation in non-hypertensive pregnancies.[47,48]

Morphometric studies of the placenta have shown reductions in total volume, volume of parenchyma and villous surface area in cases of severe pre-eclampsia and in cases of fetal growth retardation without hypertension.[49] Both groups had a high incidence of multiple placental infarcts.

I would however accept the views of Robertson,[48] that it is doubtful whether a satisfactory explanation for the pathogenesis of unexplained fetal growth retardation can be found solely in lesions of the uteroplacental blood supply.

Maternal illness

There are a number of forms of maternal illness which can limit fetal growth by hypoxia or nutritional impairment.

Hypertension. Essential hypertension may pose no increased risk of fetal growth retardation,[37] and placental growth is normal.[49] Fetal growth retardation is a problem only with superimposed proteinuria when the effects merge with those of pre-eclampsia.

Congential heart disease. Fetal growth retardation occurs most frequently in cases of maternal cyanotic heart disease and was reported in 52% of pregnancies in this group as compared with 9% of pregnancies in the acyanotic group.[50] The cyanotic group with growth retarded infants included mainly patients with complex lesions unamenable to surgical correction.

Chronic respiratory disease. Maternal asthma has been reported to be associated with an increased rate of fetal growth retardation in older studies but with modern therapy may be a complication only of occasional cases with poor control.[51]

Similarly, in cases of cystic fibrosis, the severity of maternal hypoxaemia and hypercapnia may determine the adequacy of fetal growth, although severity of pancreatic involvement and intestinal malabsorption may also be significant.[52]

Bronchiectasis,[53] and kyphoscoliosis,[54] have also been reported to be associated with fetal growth retardation.

Chronic renal disease. Chronic renal disease of moderate severity is associated with fetal growth retardation in up to 24% of cases.[55] However it is difficult to distinguish between any direct effect of the renal impairment and that of associated hypertension. It has however been shown that uraemia in experimental animals can be associated with fetal growth retardation without maternal hypertension, although the effect is probably due to decreased maternal food intake.[56]

Collagen diseases. Systemic lupus erythematosus (SLE) is associated with retarded fetal growth.[57] It may be difficult to differentiate the influence of renal lesions and treatment with steroids and immunosuppressive drugs from those of the decidual bed vasculitis caused by the SLE.

Anaemia. Most severely anaemic pregnant women have associated nutritional problems which make assessment of the effect of the anaemia *per se* impossible to establish. There is doubt whether pure anaemia is associated with retardation of fetal growth. [37,57]

Women with sickle cell disease have an increased incidence of growth retarded infants as may those with sickle-thalassaemia and sickle-haemoglobin C disease .[58] The basis for growth retardation in sickle cell disease is almost certainly impaired uteroplacental circulation due to obstruction by sickled cells with resultant placental microinfarcts.

REFERENCES

1. Parkes MJ. Endocrine factors in fetal growth. In: *Fetal and Neonatal Growth*. Ed. F Cockburn. Chichester: John Wiley and Sons, 1988: pp.33–48.
2. Yates JRW. The genetics of fetal and postnatal growth. In: *Fetal and Neonatal Growth*. Ed. F Cockburn. Chichester: John Wiley and Sons, 1988: pp.1–10.
3. Winick M, Noble A. Cellular response in rats during malnutrition at various ages. *J Nutrition* 1966; **89**: 300-306.
4. Brar HS, Rutherford SE. Classification of intrauterine growth retardation. *Semin Perinatol* 1988; **12**: 2–10.
5. Dobbing J, Sands J. Timing of neuroblast multiplication in developing human brain. *Nature* 1970; **226**: 639–640.
6. Dobbing J, Sands J. Quantitative growth and development of human brain. *Arch Dis Child* 1973; **48**: 757–767.
7. Sands J, Dobbing J, Gratrix CA. Cell number and cell size: organ growth and development and the control of catch-up growth in rats. *Lancet* 1979; **ii**: 503–505.
8. Polani PE. Chromosomal and other genetic influences on birth weight varia-

tion. In: *Size at Birth*. CIBA Foundation Symposium 27. Amsterdam: Elsevier, 1974: pp.127–160.
9. Doshi N, Surti U, Szulman AE. Morphologic anomalies in triploid liveborn fetuses. *Hum Pathol* 1983; **14**: 716–723.
10. Smith DW. *Recognizable Patterns of Human Malformation*. 3rd edition. Philadelphia: WB Saunders, 1982; pp.82–96.
11. Honnebier WJ, Swaab DF. The influence of anencephaly upon intrauterine growth of fetus and placenta and upon gestation length. *J Obstet Gynaecol Br Commonw* 1973; **80**: 577–588.
12. Elias S, Simpson JL, Griffin LP. Intrauterine growth retardation in osteogenesis imperfecta. *JAMA* 1978; **239**: 23.
13. Alford CA. Rubella. In: *Infectious Diseases of the Fetus and Newborn Infant*. Eds. JS Remington, JO Klein. Philadelphia: WB Saunders, 1976: pp.71–106.
14. Naeye RL, Blanc W. Pathogenesis of congenital rubella. *JAMA* 1965; **194**: 1277–1283.
15. McCracken GH, Shinefield HR, Cobb K, Rausen AR, Dische MR, Eichenwald HF. Congenital cytomegalic inclusion disease. *Am J Dis Child* 1969; **117**: 522–539.
16. Waterston AP. Virus infections (other than rubella) during pregnancy. *Br Med J* 1979; **2**: 564–566.
17. Kierse M. Aetiology of intrauterine growth retardation. In: *Fetal Growth Retardation*. Eds. FA Van Assche, WB Robertson. Edinburgh: Churchill Livingstone, 1981:pp.37–56.
18. Scott JR. Fetal growth retardation associated with maternal administration of immunosuppressive drugs. *Am J Obstet Gynecol* 1977; **128**: 668–674.
19. Naeye RL, Blanc W, Leblanc W, Khatamee MA. Fetal complications of maternal heroin addiction: abnormal growth, infections, and episodes of stress. *J Pediatr* 1973; **83**: 1055–1061.
20. Taeusch HW, Carson W, Wang NS, Avery ME. Heroin induction of lung maturation and growth retardation in fetal rabbits. *J Pediatr* 1973; **82**: 869–875.
21. Pirani BB. Smoking during pregnancy. *Obstet Gynecol Surv* 1978; **33**: 1–13.
22. Miller HC, Hassanein K. Maternal smoking and fetal growth of full term infants. *Pediatr Res* 1964; **8**: 960–963.
23. Butler NR, Goldstein H. Smoking in pregnancy and subsequent child development. *Br Med J.* 1973; **4**: 573–575.
24. Cnattingius S, Axelsson O, Eklund G, Lindmark G. Smoking, maternal age, and fetal growth. *Obstet Gynecol* 1985; **66**: 449–452.
25. Suzuki K, Horiguchi T, Comas-Urrutia AC, Mueller-Heubach E, Morishima HO, Adamsons K. Pharmacologic effects of nicotine upon the fetus and mother in the rhesus monkey. *Am J Obstet Gynecol* 1971; **111**: 1092–1101.
26. Olegärd R, Sabel KG, Aronsson B, Sandin B, Johansson PR, Carlsson C, Kyllerman M, Iverson K, Hrbek A. Effects on the child of alcohol abuse during pregnancy. *Acta Pediatr Scand* (Suppl) 1979; **275**: 112–121.
27. Ouellette EM, Rosett HL, Rosman NP, Weiner L. Adverse effects on offspring of maternal alcohol abuse during pregnancy. *N Engl J Med* 1977; **297**:

528–530.
28. Little RE. Moderate alcohol use during pregnancy and decreased infant birth weight. *Am J Public Health* 1977; **67**: 1154–1156.
29. Robinson JS, Kingston EJ, Jones CT, Thorburn GD. Studies on experimental growth retardation in sheep. The effect of removal of endometrial caruncles on fetal size and metabolism. *J Dev Physiol* 1979; **1**: 379–398.
30. Naeye RL. Effects of maternal cigarette smoking on the fetus and placenta. *Br J Obstet Gynaecol* 1978; **85**: 732–737.
31. Thomson AM, Billewicz WZ, Hytten FE. The weight of the placenta in relation to birthweight. *J Obstet Gynaecol Br Commw* 1969; **76**: 865–872.
32. Alexander G. Studies on the placenta of the sheep (ovis aries L.). Effect of surgical reduction in the number of caruncles. *J Reprod Fertil* 1964; **7**: 307–322.
33. Froehlich LA, Fujikura MD. Significance of a single umbilical artery. *Am J Obstet Gynecol* 1966; **94**: 274–279.
34. Bryan EM, Kohler HG. The missing umbilical artery. *Arch Dis Child* 1974; **49**: 844–852.
35. Emmanouilides GC, Townsend DE, Bauer RA. Effects of single umbilical artery ligation in the lamb fetus. *Pediatrics* 1968; **42**: 919–927.
36. Fox H. Placental malfunction as a factor in intrauterine growth retardation. In: *Fetal Growth Retardation.* Eds. FA Van Assche, WB Robertson. Edinburgh: Churchill Livingstone, 1981:pp.117–125.
37. Federick J, Adelstein P. Factors associated with low birth weight of infants delivered at term. *Br J Obstet Gynaecol* 1978; **85**: 1–7.
38. Funderburk SJ, Guthrie D, Meldrum D. Outcome of pregnancies complicated by early vaginal bleeding. *Br J Obstet Gynaecol* 1980; **87**: 100–105.
39. Gabert HA. Placenta praevia and fetal growth. *Obstet Gynecol* 1971; **38**: 403–406.
40. Smith CA. The effect of wartime starvation in Holland upon pregnancy and its product. *Am J Obstet Gynecol* 1947; **63**: 599–609.
41. Hytten FE. Nutrition in relation to fetal growth. In: *Fetal Growth Retardation.* Eds. FA Van Assche, WB Robertson. Edinburgh: Churchill Livingstone, 1981: pp.57–62.
42. Long PA, Abell DA, Beischer NA. Fetal growth retardation and pre-eclampsia. *Br J Obstet Gynaecol* 1980; **87**: 13–18.
43. Brosens I, Robertson WB, Dixon HG. The role of the spiral arteries in the pathogenesis of pre-eclampsia. In: *Obstetrics and Gynecology Annual.* New York: Appleton-Century-Crofts, 1972: pp.177–191.
44. Zeek PM, Assali NS. Vascular changes in the decidua associated with eclamptogenic toxemia of pregnancy. *Am J Clin Pathol* 1950; **20**: 1099–1109.
45. Robertson WB, Brosens I, Dixon HG. The pathological response of the vessels of the placental bed to hypertensive pregnancy. *J Pathol Bact* 1967; **93**: 581–592.
46. Wigglesworth JS. Vascular anatomy of the human placenta and its significance for placental pathology. *J Obstet Gynaecol Br Commonw* 1969; **76**:

979–989.

47. Sheppard BL, Bonnar J. The ultrastructure of the arterial supply of the human placenta in pregnancy complicated by fetal growth retardation. *Br J Obstet Gynaecol* 1976: **83**: 948–959.
48. Robertson WB. Maternal blood supply in fetal growth retardation. In: *Fetal Growth Retardation*. Eds. FA Van Assche, WB Robertson. Edinburgh: Churchill Livingstone. 1981: pp.126–138.
49. Boyd PA, Scott A. Quantitative structural studies on human placentas associated with pre-eclampsia, essential hypertension and intrauterine growth retardation. *Br J Obstet Gynaecol* 1985; **92**: 714–721.
50. Shime J, Mocarski EJM, Hastings D, Webb GD, McLaughlin PR. Congenital heart disease in pregnancy: short and long term implications. *Am J Obstet Gynecol* 1987; **156**: 313–322.
51. Greenberger PA, Patterson R. Beclomethasone diproprionate for severe asthma during pregnancy. *Ann Inter Med* 1983; **98**: 478–480.
52. Palmer J, Dillon-Baker C, Tecklin JS, Wolfson B, Rosenberg B, Burroughs B, Holsclaw DS Jr, Scanlin TF, Huang NN, Sewell EM. Pregnancy in patients with cystic fibrosis. *Ann Inter Med* 1983; **99**: 596–600.
53. Thaler I, Bronstein M, Rubin AE. The course of pregnancy associated with bronchiectasis. *Br J Obstet Gynaecol* 1986; **93**: 1006–1008.
54. Kopenhager T. A review of 50 pregnant patients with kyphoscoliosis. *Br J Obstet Gynaecol* 1977; **84**: 585–587.
55. Katz AI, Davison JM, Hayslett JP, Singson E, Lindheimer MD. Pregnancy in women with kidney disease. *Kidney Int* 1980; **18**: 192–206.
56. Nitzan M, Orloff S, Chrzanowska BL, Schulman JD. Intrauterine growth retardation in renal insufficiency:. An experimental model in the rat. *Am J Obstet Gynecol* 1979; **133**: 40–43.
57. Carlson DE. Maternal diseases associated with intrauterine growth retardation. *Semin Perinatol* 1988; **12**: 17–22.
58. Powars DR, Sandhu M, Niland-Weiss J, Johnson C, Bruce S, Manning PR. Pregnancy in sickle cell disease. *Obstet Gynecol* 1986; **67**: 217–228.

Discussion

Chairman: Dr M.J. Whittle

NICOLAIDES: In spite of these complications and the various adverse effects of specific things like smoking, their effect upon growth is very marginal. All the maternal diseases other than the ones that affect the blood supply to the placenta appear to have a very marginal effect. These environmental factors appear to be maximal after 37 weeks. Is there a significant decrease from all of these environmental factors at gestations below 37 weeks?

ALBERMAN: The best example that we have is from smoking. All the evidence shows that as far as birthweight is concerned, it is only in the last trimester, in effect, that smoking seems to have an effect. However, we also have shown that smoking causes spontaneous abortion. But there is no evidence that if you smoke in early pregnancy and the fetus survives, it will have retardation in growth. Whether this is simply a statistical effect or what, I am uncertain.

WIGGLESWORTH: Surely the other thing about smoking, although its effect is relatively minor on birthweight, is that its effect does seem to be relatively prolonged. In one study there was a significant impairment in growth rate for a long period of time. This would suggest that the influence is operating relatively early and interfering with growth potential.

RUSH: I would like to make three points. Firstly, small differences are actually very important. The American black/white difference in birthweights is about 150 g. If you fiddle statistically and make believe that black birthweights are the same as white birthweights the entire perinatal mortality difference among blacks would disappear. In other words, you can attribute the totality of a doubling of perinatal mortality to that 150 g difference. So from the individual child's point of view you are right; these differences may be marginal. But if one could change distributions by this much in large populations they could have profound effects on survival.

The second point concerns what Professor Alberman said about the Japanese in the United States. It reminds me of studies from 20 years ago. The Japanese post-Second World War had shifted the national birthweight distributions upwards by some 300 g. I know of no large groups where there have been shifts of that size, and they remain as testimony that environmental conditions whatever their specific elements can have profound effects. In the 1958 cohort of children, it would be interesting to look at social class change, those who were upwardly and downwardly mobile, and also a change in any other element such as cigarette usage, for example, to see whether one could get larger than the overall intergenerational effects.

Finally, we have just completed the 10-year follow up analysis of the 1970 cohort. We see at 10 years of age about 1.25 cm difference in height for children of smokers of average amounts during pregnancy versus children of non-smokers. If you adjust for social class factors this halves to about 0.6 cm. If we could adjust for everything that we do not know about we do not know how much it would fall, but I guess that it might be to 0.3 cm or thereabouts. We were most interested in the head circumferential differences. Head circumference and brain growth are probably quite distinct from linear growth. We see a complete catch up in head circumferential growth in the children of the smokers by age 10. This is not true at age 5. Unfortunately, it is complicated, but the long term effects of smoking I begin to believe more and more are probably insignificant functionally.

WHITTLE: We were shown very high perinatal mortality rates in babies weighing less than the 10th centile. My question would be whether it is possible to tease out the major cause from all those different factors that we were talking about. This comes back to Mr Nicolaides' point that it might be that in that group there are a lot of babies dying of some sort of placental disease which might be fundamentally of maternal origin. That makes us feel that all these small babies are really at risk. There may be lots of different reasons why the babies are small, but how many of those reasons are associated with loss of a baby?

ALBERMAN: What is most important from all this work is to distinguish between babies that are at the lower tail for statistical reasons. Someone has got to be at the top and someone has got to be at the bottom and there are all sorts of reasons why they are, given that there is any normal variation. The question of whether there is an increased risk related to the absolute birthweight is very interesting; I suspect that there is not. I suppose that if we were able to do what the Swedes have done, that is to remove from the lower tail all the babies that should not be there, we probably would not find a difference. In fact, if you look only at the fifth centile of different populations then the increase in mortality drops off very quickly if you once allow for the fact that different populations have different standards. This leads us back to macrosomia too because while I am sure that you are right to say that as a practising clinician in this country, an absolute value of 4000 g or 4500 g is dangerous, I am sure that that is right in this context. The problem is that probably in Sweden this would not be right. In Japan, for instance, maybe one should say 3500 g. So I think that this question of trying to tease out what is normal and physiological variation and the question of what norm you are going to use is perhaps to a practising clinician the most important thing to do. But it is difficult.

RUSH: I will make one minor argument for an absolute birthweight independent of the aetiology. I mentioned the remarkable perinatal statistics of the Amerindian population in the United States, who are short, economically deprived and who have infants of surprisingly large birthweight. Forgetting the diabetes issue, they have very low perinatal mortality. Within the first week the mortality of the children begins to express itself in terms of their economic status. After the first week or so, even after the first couple of days, it begins to look like the American Black population which is a very deprived population. So you have a group which has very high birthweights, almost certainly on a genetic basis, and this confers very strong advantage and protection at least for a short period of time.

CLAPP: I would argue that they need a different growth curve and that they are a different population. If you take the lowest 10th centile and the largest 10th centile of that population, or any population , that is where you are going to find the morbidity. The real question is what is the optimal birthweight for any given population as defined.

RUSH: Their curve is shifted to the right and at each given birthweight their survival is the same as that of the overall white population. In other words, their lowest 10th percentile does much better than other people's lowest 10th percentile, and it is heavier.

CAMPBELL: It is this lower 10th percentile and the tail of the normal distribution which interests me. We are always told that to make it more realistic we have to correct for various factors such as parity, maternal weight and height as well as the sex of the child. Effectively, we are programmed to be told to correct. I have never made corrections for maternal weight and height because I think that the small baby of a small woman is still at risk. Some think that the small baby of a primigravida is at risk. So should we be making corrections at all, apart from sex?

ALBERMAN: Sex and multiple birth are the two where the mortality of the smaller group is lower. You have got to correct for multiple births because that is such a different distribution. In fact, weight-for-weight they do better.

LIND: There are a couple of points, firstly the physiological. I am always fascinated by people who quote the Denver work(1) and say that at 5000 feet above sea level all the babies are smaller. But surely, the function of physiology is to return people to their optimum norm. If you live at 5000 feet then presumably you have adapted to that and have done so over many generations. So why do we still presume that the babies are therefore smaller because of presumed oxygen deprivation or whatever? If you conceive at sea level and rapidly go and spend the rest of your pregnancy in Denver I understand it. But as a generation thing I am sure that someone can give me an answer.

HALL: As far as height and weight are concerned I think that it is a mixed picture. Amongst small women there will be a group who are programmed to be small and have reached their full genetic height; in respect of them you should correct because you should expect that their babies would be smaller than normal. But if you have a woman who is small because she herself was deprived either in intrauterine life or in her childhood, then she is a woman who is at risk of producing a baby which is at risk. The same thing applies to some extent to weight.

STEWART: I have a comment in response to your remarks about the Denver growth charts. A colleague and I had so many arguments about this that he took Kloosterman's data(2) which were related to sea level and he drew the curves out on the same scale. In fact, they are absolutely identical — the Kloosterman sea level data and the Denver data.

STEER: There was a lot of discussion earlier this year following our publication of the fact that women who are underweight and have ovulation induced are much more likely to have small-for-gestational-age babies, since most of these babies show catch-up growth and do quite well afterwards. The fact remains that small babies are more vulnerable. If you look at the North East region survey 50% of all unexpected stillbirths at term were less than the 10th centile. That is certainly our consistent finding.

In terms of the parity effect the higher birthweight of second and third babies is simply related to the higher maternal weight. If you look at the relationship between weight of pregnancy and birthweight, if you correct for that, then the difference between first babies and second babies simply disappears. We know that perinatal mortality for first babies is higher because there are more small babies. So I agree with Professor Rush that very small shifts in mean birthweight and therefore shifts in the tail of distribution can actually make very important differences in terms of rare events such as perinatal mortality on a public health basis.

HAY: It seems to me that we are mixing a lot of apples and oranges. We are talking about birthweight contributing to perinatal mortality and in selected cases we are forgetting the morbidity. If we focus on what causes the birthweight and we say that that has a particular effect on mortality or morbidity, that is useful information. But we keep coming back to saying low birthweight causes mortality and morbidity or at least is associated with it. We forget that if we just keep on lumping these things together we are going to miss out on the selective pathology. The Denver issue keeps coming up. It really does not show an effect of altitude at all. This is a very selected population of lower socioeconomic mixed white and black. There was also about a 10% population of Chicanos in the group. If at the same time you compare the population of babies delivered at Leadville, Colorado, a population that lives at 10 000 feet, their birthweight distribution is exactly the same per matched population in Denver of the same socioeconomic status and racial background. That population has not yet shown a specific effect of altitude. Other population studies in my understanding have shown an effect of altitude, but that one does not.

NICOLAIDES: What is the mechanism of death in these small babies? If it is asphyxia or reduced oxygen supply and hypoxia you cannot surely equate that group with the group of small Indian women who somehow through hormonal factors are reducing the size of their babies, and not through placental insufficiency.

BRUDENELL: From a practical point of view we have babies who have a genetic potential. Some will overperform as in the case of diabetics and some will underperform. In the two groups of overperformers and underperformers we must identify those who are at risk. If we take the macrosomic babies, most of them are going to be all right. Some will not for a variety of reasons, and the other way around. Does it in the end come down to a factor like blood supply, as Mr Nicolaides suggested? We need to identify the members of these two groups at either end of the scale who need special attention.

GILLMER: Is there a separate pathology that is killing these babies or producing morbidity?

CLAPP: I would suggest approaching the subject a bit differently, and that is from the point of view that any given fertilisation has a given genetic potential for growth which can either be fostered or restricted by a variety of factors, either normal or pathological. The trick is to decide not what low birthweight is or high birthweight is, but what is optimal birthweight per given potential. That is what one should strive for knowing that morbidity and mortality are least, I think, at that middle ground. You cannot do that by talking about absolute birthweights; you have to look at the individual genome. Relative to the risk at birth and the perinatal period there is an optimal birthweight for any infant. What we see and where we find the mortality and morbidity is in the true pathologic process that influences the growth and causes the low birthweight. For one populus that may be a birthweight of 2500 g, for another it may be 1800 g, and for another it might be closer to 3000 g.

CAMPBELL: I would agree with Mr Nicolaides that certainly in Western societies impaired blood supply to the placenta seems to be pre-eminently the cause of hypoxic intrauterine growth retardation and mortality. But globally maternal undernutrition is the biggest cause of small-for-dates babies or intrauterine growth retardation. These women have babies with a high perinatal mortality. The Guatemalan studies have shown that when they have supplements to their diet they have babies of a higher birthweight. Therefore there may be a different mechanism of death in Third World countries. It may be poor perfusion of the placenta, but there may be nutritional factors again. Therefore, perhaps on the world scale blood flow to the placenta is not the main cause.

GILLMER: When we talk about perinatal mortality rate, that includes neonatal death. Maybe the vascular deaths are occurring and we are having stillbirths. The first week deaths are occurring because of some major nutritional problems with the baby soon after birth.

CAMPBELL: In Guatemala there are more stillbirths than neonatal deaths.

LEVINE: There is no evidence that the neonatal death rate is any higher in growth retarded babies. I think that excess mortality is all antenatal and not postnatal. If anything, the mortality rate may be lower amongst growth retarded infants.

STEER: A clinical observation that I have often made is that some women seem to have a premature delivery on one occasion, the next time they will have a term baby who is growth retarded and then another premature baby who is quite well grown. Perhaps it is that the baby that is going to grow, whatever happens in the face of a constraint, is thrown out early and the baby that can adapt and grow more slowly will hang in longer. It would be interesting to know if there are any women you have been following up who have had both a preterm delivery and a term growth retarded baby, and what the effect would be on their babies. Is it that we are seeing a separation of the genetic potential reflected in the way they behave?

ALBERMAN: There is a small but select literature on this, particularly on Norwegian births where they have linked together siblings. They have shown that there is a difference in outcome between women who have repeated small-for-dates babies where the outcome is much better than where one of the sibship is unexpectedly small for dates where the outcome is much worse. The Australians are looking at the same thing, not in regard to mortality outcome but morbidity outcome. It seems that outcomes such as cerebral palsy may be more common where just one of the babies is small-for-dates. They have done the same for preterm.

STEER: In the same mother?

ALBERMAN: Yes, within sibships. They have followed through mothers who have had three or four births. They can show that there is a relationship between the gestational age between babies, and between the birthweight for gestational age between babies, of the same mother. The ones at highest risk are the ones that step out of the pattern, which is exactly what one would expect.

RUSH: It goes the other way as well. There is an optimal birthweight which you can exceed once the pattern is established. Within a particular mother there is an expressed biological optimum.

COCKBURN: Richard Naeye would explain this in African women in the part of Africa where there is a chronic amnionitis associated with insufficiency. You get preterm deliveries and then growth retarded babies. He would relate this to chronic placentitis or amnionitis. In one of his studies he showed that this could be reversed in these same women by giving them zinc supplements.

REFERENCES

1. Lubchenko LO, Hansman C, Dressler H, Boyd E. Intrauterine growth as estimated from liveborn birth-weight data at 24 to 40 weeks of gestation. *Pediatrics* 1963; **32:** 793–800.
2. Kloosterman GJ. On intrauterine growth. *Int J Gyn Obstet* 1970; **8:** 895.

Effects of changes in maternal energy and protein intake during pregnancy, with special reference to fetal growth

Professor D. Rush

INTRODUCTION

The relationship between the diet of the mother and the wellbeing of the fetus and infant continues to be a matter of great importance, uncertainty and controversy. A great deal of information has become available since the RCOG study group on nutrition during pregnancy.(1)

Since observational studies have generated conflicting and uncertain results this review will be limited to studies in which there has been change in diet, whether intended or not. A longer and more detailed version will be appearing elsewhere.(2)

STUDIES OF THE EFFECTS OF FAMINE IMPOSED ON PREVIOUSLY WELL NOURISHED POPULATIONS

During acute famine, while dietary restriction is inevitably accompanied by other insults, the effects of severe deprivation of food probably are dominant, especially when the deprivation has been abrupt and the affected population has been previously well nourished. The best documented reports were those which described the effects of the seige of Leningrad from 1941 to 1943(3,4) following the original report which studied the acute starvation during the winter of 1944–45 in Holland(5) and Dean's report which studied the residents of Wuppertal in 1945–46 and reviewed the earlier literature.(6) These studies were described in detail in a previous review (Table 1).(7)

Even though data collected under these devastating conditions have inherent limitations some conclusions seem warranted. The Leningrad experience probably represents the outer limits of endurance of a population which was previously well nourished, and a fall in mean birthweight of 550 g was observed. With very severe famine, the Dutch experienced a 300 g depression. In Wuppertal, shortage of food was great and there were long periods during which rations were down to half the usual intake. However, birthweight was depressed by 227 g at most, and by considerably less among private patients or when food shortage was intermediate. At this time the official rations were still under 1500 calories per day.

STUDIES OF IATROGENIC DIETARY LIMITATION

There are surprisingly few systematic studies of the formerly widespread medical practice of advising women to limit their diet and weight gain during pregnancy (Table 2). Several of these studies were described in detail in a previous review.(7)

The investigators in Aberdeen who performed one of the earlier studies(8) have since readdressed this issue, with somewhat different results.(9) Heavy primigravi-

Table 1. Studies of the effects of famine on a previously well nourished population

Study	Population	Assignment method/ Research design	Study no.	Group description	Control no.
Antonou, 1947[3]	Leningrad, 1941–43	Comparison with pre- and post-famine births in one clinic	414	Born at height of famine	11 319
Stein *et al.*, 1975 Smith, 1947[45]	Holland, 1944-45	Comparison with period before and after famine, and with areas not exposed	2411	Born in famine area	2439
Dean[6]	Wuppertal, 1945–46	Comparison with pre-scarcity births in one clinic	1906	Born during 1945: severe shortages	2434
			2438	Born during 1946: official rations – 1052–1550 Kcal/d	

dae were pair matched for height, weight gain from 20 to 30 weeks' gestation, and smoking, and half placed on 1250 calories reducing diets from 30 weeks' gestation to term. Although mean birthweights were similar in the two groups, 25% of the women who had been prescribed restricted diets had infants with birthweights under the 25th centile of weight for gestational age, as opposed to 18% of controls, and twice as many treated women had durations of gestation over 40 weeks (32% versus 15%). Whether this difference in duration of gestation was a treatment effect is uncertain, but it would certainly be associated with higher birthweight. Thus the rate of fetal growth was probably impaired by dieting in this trial, as in the earlier study.

The first study had demonstrated significantly depressed size at birth[8] and in early childhood[10] among children exposed either to third trimester maternal dietary restriction or diuretic therapy. The second trial did not demonstrate as great an effect of dietary restriction on fetal growth.

Grieve *et al.* compared the birthweights to primigravidae in the practice of a consultant obstetrician in Motherwell who counselled a diet high in animal protein and low in carbohydrates and calories with those of similar pregnant women in Aberdeen.[11] Both the weight gains of the mothers and the birthweights of the babies in Motherwell were lower than those in Aberdeen. Calculated from the data presented, the median weight gain in the Motherwell women was 0.32 kg per week, compared with 0.46 kg per week in Aberdeen. Birthweights in Motherwell were more than 400 g lower than in Aberdeen, a remarkable difference. While

Group description	Results					Comments
Born before and after famine		During famine	Other time			Fertility drastically reduced during famine
	Stillbirth (%)	5.6	2.6			
	Premature live birth (%)	41.2	6.5			
	Neonatal death (%)	21.2	5.2			
	<2500 g (%)	49.2	?			
	Mean birthweight (g)	2789	3338			
Control areas		Date of birth	Birthweight (g) Famine areas	Control areas North	Control areas South	
	Pre-famine	8=11/1944	3358	3385	3324	
	Famine	12/44-6/45	3051	3228	3313	
	Post-famine	7/45-3/46	3320	3228	3313	
Born before scarcities		1945	1944	1937–38		Decrease in amount of breastmilk during scarcity. 20% of local births in clinic in 1937–38. 70% in 1946
	Mean birthweight (%)					
	Private patients	3325	3414	3495		
	Others	3103	3213	3330		
	Median birthweight	3250	3300	3400		
	%≤2400 g	8.2	6.7	4.3		

perinatal mortality in Motherwell was not reported, it has been said not to have been excessive. Some of the difference in birthweight almost certainly was caused by liberal use of induction of labour in Motherwell, but it is also likely that the high protein content of the diet, along with the restriction of calories, contributed to this dramatic depression in birthweight (see Table 2).

Barsa Gregory and Rush(12) studied the relationship of the prescription of a low calorie diet to weight gain and birthweight among women who participated in the United States National Collaborative Perinatal Project from 1959 to 1963. Singleton term infants below the 31st centile in birthweight were matched to higher weight infants for ethnicity, duration of gestation and maternal smoking, parity, and pre-pregnant weight. Women who had given birth to low birthweight babies were somewhat less likely to have been advised to restrict their diet (37% versus 40%) but the difference was not statistically significant.

The outcome was adjusted first for weight gain in early pregnancy, then in mid-pregnancy and finally in late pregnancy. Again, no statistically significant differences between the frequency of prescription of a low calorie diet and birthweight was observed, nor was late pregnancy weight gain significantly related to whether or not a low calorie diet had been prescribed. Since women who were asked to limit caloric intake had gained and continued to gain more weight than others, the discrepancy in the findings between this observational study and those of the intervention studies might be due to poor compliance with the prescribed dietary regimen.

Table 2. Studies of iatrogenic dietary limitation

Study	Population	Assignment method/ Research design	Study no.	Group treatment	Control no.
Naeye *et al.*, 1973(13)	1044 consecutive perinatal autopsies New York City, 1960–1968. Excluding disorders affecting (a) fetal or placental growth (b) amniotic fluid volume (c) mother's extra-cellular fluid volume...'	Retrospective cohort study	123 32 91	1200–1500 cal diet prescribed below WHO standards, wt. for ht. others)	344 181 163
Campbell & MacGillivray 1975(8) Blumenthal, 1976(10)	Primigravidae, at 30 weeks gestation, with < 570 g/wk weight gain between 20–30 wks	Subjects matched with controls on age, height, weight for height at 20 wks gestation, social class, cigarette use and blood pressure	A) 51	1200 cal, low CHO diet	B) 51 C) 51
Barsa Gregory & Rush, 1987(12)	1137 term singleton births, NYC, 1959–63 registered <25 w gest.	Births <31st centile for birthweight, within strata of ethnic group and duration of gestation with babies ≥ 31st centile, matched for ethnicity, gestation, smoking, parity and pre-pregnant weight.	255		255
Campbell, 1983(9)	Aberdeen Primigravidae >75 centile wt for ht, normal GTT at 28 w gest.	Cases matched with controls on height, wt gain from 20 to 30 w gest and smoking.	91	1250 Kcal reducing diet from 30 wks to term.	91
Grieve *et al.*, 1978(11)	Motherwell Maternity Hospital, Scotland	Retrospective evaluation of low carbohydrate, high protein diet from 1938–1977. Comparable group from Aberdeen used as controls.	295 251	(1965) (1975)	1829

Group treatment	Results				Comments
General dietary advice		Birthweight, % of normal value for gestation			No information about whether dietary advice preceded or followed weight gain, nor of duration of diet.
		Low cal diet	Others		
	Total	103	105		
underweight	among underweight only	98	102		
	with low weight gain	78	97		
others	with high weight gain	108	110		
	among overweight only	105	108		
	with low weight gain	101	103		
	with high weight gain	111	118		
Cyclopen-thiazide 2 tabs/d	Weight gain	A	B	C	
	30–38 wks, normotensives only	0.19	0.32	0.52	
No dietary intervention no diuretics	Birthweight <25th centile (%)	32.2	17.6	18.2	
		Low birthweight	Matched controls	Difference	
	Low calorie diet (%)	37.3	40.4	-3.1	No differences statistically significant. Late pregnancy weight gain unrelated to diet, after controlling for prior weight gain.
	Adjusted for wt gain				
	a) in early pregnancy	–	–	-1.7	
	b) - mid pregnancy	–	–	+1.7	
	c) - late pregnancy	–	–	+2.2	
Regular care		Cases	Controls		
	Change, from 30 to 38 wks.				
	Weight (kg)	2.92	4.21		
	Total body water (l)	2.88	3.81		
	Plasma (l)	0.20	0.32		
	Preeclampsia (%)	39.6	37.4		
	Perinatal death (n)	2	0		
	Birth > 40 wks (%)	31.9	15.4		
	Mean birthweight (g)	3291	3285		
	Birthweight <25 centile (%)	25.3	17.6		
	Length (cm)	49.8	49.8		
(1968-70)		Motherwell	Aberdeen		Report limited to effects on primigravidae
	Median weight gain/wk (kg)	0.32	0.46		
	Birthweight (g)				
	1965	3008			
	1975	2940			
	1968–70		3393		

Table 3. Studies of dietary advice without emphasis or restriction.

Study	Population	Assignment method/ Research design	Study no.	Group treatment	Control no.
Cameron & Graham, 1944[14]	Patients in last 3 months of pregnancy, Glasgow Royal Maternity Women's Hospital, 1942–1943	Alternate	500	Dietary advice; encouraged to apply for priority allowance of food	500
Berry & Wiehl, 1952[15]	Prenatal clinic, Morrisania Hospital, New York City, 1948–1950	Prospective intervention counselling; alternate assignment	116 (+21 with unknown outcome)	Instruction only	110 (+ 13 with unknown outcome)
Lundin & Stark, 1980 (personal communication)	Public prenatal clinic, singleton livebirths.	All patients instructed by Dr. Thos. Brewer registering in one clinic, contrasted with a) same clinic, prior to programme, and b) 2 other clinics, same county and same hospital of delivery	584 (black) 638 (white)	...nutrition lectures and prompting by the physician avoiding maternal weight control, salt restriction... saluretic diuretics were not prescribed. The nutritional emphasis was on eating high quality protein, vegetables and fruit and on discouraging high carbohydrate, high 'junk food' and beverages.	155 92 243 1951
Sweney *et al.*, 1985[16]	Tertiary care center patients.Salt Lake City, registered <20w. gestation	Random assignment within strata 'approx equal' number of women with lower weight gain in each group	22	Counselling by "Higgins method"	21

Table 4. Studies in which the decision to supplement was in part controlled by the participant

Study	Population	Assignment method/ Research design	Study no.	Group treatment	Control no.
Habicht *et al.*, 1974[17]	Rural villages in Guatemala supplied with protein–rich gruel (2) or with beverage containing carbohydrate only (2)	Supplement taken *ad libitum*	178	≥20 000 Kcal supplement taken over entire pregnancy	240

Group treatment	Results				Comments
None		Supervised	Control		Numbers of drop-outs not given monitoring of diet implied but not certain; observers probably not blind
	Stillbirth (%)	4.2	7.2		
	Low birthweight (%)	6.2	10.0		
	Neonatal death (%)	1.6	2.0		
None		Instructed	Control		
	Perinatal death (%)	5 2	6.4		
	(excluding early fetal death	3.7	3.7		
	% <2500 g birthweight)	6.2	9.9		
Black <1964 White		1965–70 (Brewer)	1/61-6/63 (Before Brewer)	Other clinics 1965–70	Results unaffected by restricting analysis to patients registered <28 wks gestation, and seen for at least 4 visits, over at least 4 weeks, and under 19 years of age, or in first pregnancy
Black Other clinics White*	Mean birthweight(g)				
	Black	3146	3163	3178	
	White	3321	3359	3301	
	% <2500 g birthweight				
	Black	9.4	8.4	7 8	
	White	6 3	5 4	7 1	
*includes Spanish Americans					
Unspecified		Counselled	Control		Data on comparability of groups not presented: "no significant difference between groups". Numbers inadequate to test hypothesis.
	Birthweight (g).	3255	3243		
	( ) = n	(25)	(18)		

Group treatment	Results	Comments
<20 000 Kcal supplement taken over entire pregnancy	About 110 g higher birthweight with greater supplementation. Decreased perinatal death (NS)	38% of births not weighed Effect on birthweight confounded by duration of gestation: i.e. with longer gestation, more likely to have had chance to take > 20 000 Kcal.

STUDIES OF DIETARY ADVICE WITHOUT EMPHASIS ON RESTRICTION

Two trials of dietary advice without restriction in either diet or weight gain reported lower rates of both low birthweight and perinatal death in the counselled group than in the controls (Table 3).[14,15]

A recent small study had several internal inconsistencies.[16] Twenty-two women were randomly assigned to counselling by the "Higgins method". The estimated experimental effect (calculated from the authors' data) was a 12 g heavier birthweight in the counselled group (personal communication).

Thomas Brewer has been one of the most vocal advocates of the importance of diet during pregnancy. The results of his programme at the prenatal clinic of the Contra Costa County Hospital, Richmond, California, were described in the previous review.[7] Brewer stressed the advisability of eating high quality protein, vegetables and fruits, while discouraging high carbohydrate and high fat "junk" foods and beverages. Weight control was avoided, as was salt restriction. No significant effects of counselling on perinatal outcome could be detected.

Studies in which the decision to supplement (or the level of supplementation) were in part controlled by the participant

The INCAP study in Guatemala began as a controlled trial with random allocation of villages to two different programmes (Table 4); in analysis, the original design was abandoned, and women who chose to consume over 20 000 calories as supplementary food during pregnancy were compared with those who did not.[17] There was a 110 g difference in mean birthweight, favouring those babies whose mothers had eaten more supplement. However there were many potentially confounding factors including self selection, and a further possible confounding factor in that longer pregnancy was associated both with the opportunity to pass the 20 000 Kcal threshold and to have a larger baby.

Studies in which the decision to supplement (or the level of supplementation) were not under the subjects' control

Studies in developed countries. The results of a number of studies of dietary supplementation are summarised in Table 5 and discussed elsewhere.[2,7] These studies are of varying quality and show conflicting results. Supplementation was associated with increases in mean birthweight in some study groups.[18–23] However, there were decreases in mean birthweight in others.[18–26] The results became consistent when arrayed against protein density of the supplements. In general, there were positive effects in studies in which supplements were not overly protein-dense (see below).

The incidence of low birthweight was lower in the supplemented groups in all studies that reported this outcome, [19,20,25,26,30] as was the incidence of preterm birth.[18,24,26] There were small differences in stillbirth rates or perinatal mortality in favour of the supplemented groups reported in some studies,[25,26,31] but not in another.[18] The magnitudes of these differences are reported in Table 5 and in references 2 and 7.

The effect of protein density. Given the unexpected and untoward result of our trial in New York, we arrayed the reported effect of dietary supplements on birthweight in all trials in which the protein density of supplements was either reported, or could be inferred (Table 6).(2,7) The relationship of protein density to birthweight was striking; higher protein densities were associated with lower birthweight among those who were supplemented, whereas lower protein density supplements (under 20% of calories as protein) were uniformly associated with higher mean birthweight among the supplemented. Thus the inconsistency of the results of the supplementation trials is, in large part, explained by the varying protein density of supplements, with reasonably consistent adverse effects from supplements of high protein density and, in general, modest benefit from supplements of protein density similar to that of a freely chosen diet.

Some comments on the studies of Viegas *et al.* who recently reported two supplementation trials among women of Asian origin in Birmingham(28,32) are necessary, since their results appeared to run counter to this pattern. In their first trial women were randomly allocated to one of three treatment groups, 47 to a daily supplement of 26 g of protein and 273 Kcal, 50 to a comparable level of caloric supplementation without protein, and 45 to an unsupplemented control group. It was unclear whether the results were for the total treatment groups, or excluded women with vaginal bleeding, hypertension, or "low compliance". Infants in the control group had 30 g higher mean birthweight than those who received energy supplementation alone and 40 g higher than those receiving protein and energy supplements.

In a second trial(32) pregnant women of Asian origin were stratified by amount of change in triceps skinfold between 20 and 28 weeks gestation. Women with low and high measurements were then randomly allocated supplements of either 425 Kcal and 40 g of protein a day, 425 Kcal a day, or to a control group. The authors found one statistically significant difference: the 14 women who had low prior triceps skinfold gain and received the high protein and energy supplement had infants with mean birthweight of 3340 g, compared to 2950 g in the energy alone group and 3010 g for the control group. However the birthweights in the presumably optimally nourished high triceps gain groups were 2980, 3110 and 3160 g, respectively. Thus the 14 women with low triceps gain and with protein and energy supplementation had infants with mean birthweights much higher than all other groups, including those presumed to be well nourished. There is no reason to expect treatment among those at high risk to do any more than to bring them to parity with those at low risk while, in fact, they did considerably better than those at presumably lower risk. This pattern is less consistent with a coherent treatment effect than with a random event due to very small numbers in the trial. The statistical power of this study was much too low to accept its results without replication.

Watney and Atton(29) did replicate this study and increased the size of the study group to 78, with 78 randomly matched controls. These authors stated that "the babies of supplemented women were lighter than those of unsupplemented women", but presented no quantitative results.

Table 5. Studies in which the decision to supplement (or the level of supplementation) were not under the subjects'

Study	Population	Assignment method/ Research design	Study no.	Group treatment	Control no.
Balfour, 1944[31]	28 areas, South Wales and North of England, 1937–1939; wives of unemployed or low wage earners	Discretion of doctors; controls were others at clinic; parity lower in controls, social status higher	11,618	1lb dried milk, 1/2lb "Ovaltine" plus "Marmite" or 8 ozs "Minadex"	8095 or 9912 (?)
Ebbs *et al.*, 1941[25] Ebbs *et al.*, 1942[26]	Toronto General Hospital ca. 1940; enrolment prior to 7th month gestation	Alternate among patients with poor diet; a third group with good diet also followed.	90	(A) 45 g protein 840 Kcal vitamins minerals and advice given	120 170
Dieckman *et al.*, 1944[18]	Chicago, ca. 1942; low income	"Random"	179	(II) 100 g/d cereal	175
			102	(IV) Cereal and vitamins A and D	98
Tompkins *et al.*, 1955 [30]	Philadelphia Lying-in Hospital, 1948–1952 less than 15 weeks gestation; married; no major complication. 74% white	"Seriatim"; prospective intervention	332	50g protein, 1.5g Ca/d	467
			334	As above, plus vitamins (+ instruction)	477
Ebbs *et al.*,1942[26]	"Low-income" women in hospital prenatal clinic, in Philadelphia.	Subjects recruited after completion of control pregnancies	122	"Meritene" a high protein-mineral supplement. Amount prescribed not stated.	118
Higgins, 1976[19] Rush, 1981[20]	Public patients at Royal Victoria Hospital, Montreal; 1963–1974.	Patients cared for by Montreal Diet Dispensary retrospectively matched on 5 characteristics with other patients from same clinic.	1213	Dietary evaluation, advice, and for 75% of population, milk, eggs and oranges	1213
Rush *et al.*, 1980[21] Rush *et al.*, 1987[22]	Black public clinic populations, New York City, 1970–1974; registered <30 wks gestation, with at least one nutritional risk factor.	Randomised, partially double-blind prospective intervention; treatment from registration to term.	263	Supplement (40g protein, 470 Kcals/d)	272
			272	Complement (6g protein, 322 Kcals/d)	

control in developed countries

Group treatment	Results	Comments
None; however local authorities reserved their milk for controls	Fed / Controls Perinatal deaths (%): 5.9 / 7.1 often: $x^2 = 12.48$ (Birthweight not reported)	Selective assignment; allocation of local authority milk-supplies only to controls in some areas.
(B) Capsules of corn oil (C) Normal good diet	A / B / C Birthweight (%): 3377 / 3462 / 3392 "Prematurity" (%): 2.2 / 4.0 / 3.0 Miscarriage (%): 0.0 / 6.0 / 1.2 Stillbirth (%): 0.0 / 3.5 / 0.6 Infant death <6M(%): 0.0 / 2.8 / 0.0	Prematurity not defined
(I) None (III) Vitamins A and D	Groups: II & IV / I & II Fetal death (%): 5.1 / 3 7 Delivery <37 wks (%): 2.2 / 4.4 Weight gain (g): 494 / 477 Birthweights (g): 3397 / 3352	
None Vitamins + instruction	Protein / No protein % <2500g birthweight White: 3.9 / 5.0 Black: 8.7 / 13.2 Total: 5.2 / 7.0	Those initially assigned to protein supplements who did not use them were transferred to control group
Routine care (92% black)	Subjects / Controls Birthweight (g): 3005 / 3119 Length (cm): 49.0 / 50.0 Head circ (cm): 33.4 / 34 1 Apgar (5 min): 9.4 / 9.7	Subjects had significantly fewer years of school, lower occupational status and lower initial Hgb, but magnitude of differences not reported. Racial composition of subject group not presented.
Regular care Birthweight (g)	Treated / Controls % <2500g birthwt: 5.7 / 6 8 NS 3291: 3251 / p>0.05 No significant difference in mortality or gestation. Effect greater in women <140 pounds at conception and women of lower parity	
Control (routine multi-vitamins/ mineral tablets)	Supp / Comp / Controls Birthweight (g): 2938 / 3011 / 3970 (NS) Increase in very early delivery and neonatal death at margins of significance in supplement group. Significant depression of birthweight among prematures with supplement. Increased duration of gestation, and %>2500g in complement group, versus other two groups combined. Effect on weight gain only in recruits early in pregnancy.	Effects of heavy smoking on weight gain partially reversed, and on birthweight reversed, by both dietary supplements.

Table 5. (continued)

Study	Population	Assignment method/ Research design	Study no.	Group treatment	Control no.
Adams *et al.*, 1978[23]	Kaiser-Permanente group, San Francisco, at high risk, medically, or nutritionally.	Assignment method unstated; prospective trial	36	(A) Supplement, as developed in 21,22	43
			23	(B) Complement, as developed in 21,22	
Elwood (personal communication)	Two small towns, South Wales, from 1972; treatment from booking for half of pregnancy (on average).	Random allocation (20 oz milk/day available at half price).	276	Males	237
			234	Females	204
Viegas *et al.*, 1986[28]	Birmingham, England S. Asian pregnant women living in defined area, 1979	Random allocation	47 (or 33?)	273 Kcal + 26g pro/d	45 (or 34?)
		Treatment from 28–38 wks	50 (or 28?)	273 Kcal/d	
			(Smaller number of subjects excludes those with vaginal bleeding, hypertension, or "low compliance")		
Viegas *et al.*, 1982[32]	Birmingham, England S. Asian pregnant women living in defined area, 1979–80	Random allocation, stratified by change in triceps skinfold between 20–28 wks gest.	Small prior increment in triceps skinfold		
		Treatment from 28–38 wks gest.	14 (or 12)	425 Kcal + 40g pro/d (37% of energy as protein: text states 10%)	14 (or 12)
			17 (or 15)	425 Kcal/d	
			Large prior increment in triceps skinfold		
			30 (or 21)	Protein + cals (as above)	27 (or 19)
			26 (or 23)	Cals (as above)	
Campbell-Brown, 1983[24]	Aberdeen 1975–1980 Primigravidae at 30 wks with low weight or weight gain	First member of matched pair assigned to supplementation. If delivery <37wks, replaced by next matchable recruit	90	276 ml flavoured milk or, 554 ml whole milk or, 75 g cheese, or combinations	90

Group treatment	Results	Comments
(C) Multi-vitamin/mineral tablet	Birthweight (g): Supp 3227; Comp 3365; Controls 3272 (NS)	Distribution of risk characteristics among treatment groups unclear. Only 45% completion rate. BW <2500 g excluded from analysis.
Males Females	Birthweight Treated / Controls / Difference Male: 3460 / 3390 / 70 Female: 3320 / 3240 / 80 More control mothers were smokers. If smoking controlled, advantage drops to approx. 55 g.	
Fe and Vit C.	Treatment groups: Energy & protein / Energy / Controls Wt gain/wks (g) to 28 wks: 465 / 460 / 360 28–35 wks: 360 / 335 / 300 Dur. gest (wks)*: 38.9 / 39.0 / 39.0 Birth wt (g): 3010 / 3020 / 3050 *Viegas (personal communication)	Data analysed both including and excluding those with vaginal bleeding and hypertension. Not specified with results reported in publications. Results not adjusted for initial disparities in study groups. No mention of whether any women delivered preterm. Number of subjects too small to test hypothesis. No dietary assessment during treatment.
"Orovite 7" "Orovite 7"	Treatment groups: Energy & protein / Energy / Controls Wt gain/wk (g) Low triceps gain: 480 / 300 / 310 High triceps gain: 500 / 320 / 340 Birthweight (g) Low triceps gain: 3340 / 2950 / 3010 High triceps gain: 2980 / 3110 / 3160	Results stratified by change in prior triceps skinfolds, but data on comparability only presented for total (unstratified) groups; comparability across treatment groups therefore not established. Numbers too small to test hypothesis. Results inconsistent with authors' interpretations (see text).
Regular care	Cases / Controls Gestation <37wks (%): 7.2 / 8.2 Wt gain/w (kg): 0.40 / 0.36 Dur. gest (wks): 39.7 / 39.6 Birthweight (g): 3032 / 2995 Length (cm): 48.5 / 48.2 Head circ (cm): 34.2 / 34.2	

Table 5. (continued)

Study	Population	Assignment method/ Research design	Study no.	Group treatment	Control no.
Watney & Alton, 1986[29]	W. Bromwich, England. Pregnant women with low 2nd trimester triceps skinfold gain (per criterion of ref 32), half "White" and half Asian.	Half assigned to supplementation, 3rd trimester	78	Milk based supplement comparable to the protein energy supplement of ref. 32	78

Studies in developing countries. Most studies of protein and calorie supplementation in developing countries showed increased mean birthweight with supplementation,[33–41] which is not surprising given that levels of nutrition were often very low. However the magnitude of effects varied widely and reported results were often internally inconsistent. Details of these trials (in chronological order) are presented in Table 7 and were discussed in detail previously.[7]

The studies in the Gambia conducted by Prentice and his colleagues have been widely quoted.[39,40] Baseline birthweights were collected for four years among all births in one village, 86 (or 87) during the wet season, and 96 during the dry season. Supplementation was then instituted in the subsequent two years (1100 Kcal day for six days a week for 51 births during the wet season, and 950 Kcal a day for six days a week for 42 births during the dry season). Supplemented women had infants of higher birthweight compared to the prior control years, but only during the wet season. The investigators interpreted this result to mean that only with the additional stress of the wet season (greater field work, and presumably lower food supply) could any effect of supplementation be detected.

Their initial results are not fully consistent with this interpretation.[39] During the control years reported daily diet intake during the wet season was not lower than in the dry season (1464 versus 1468 Kcal per day), nor was the incremental intake in the years of supplementation greater during the wet season (430 Kcal versus 433 Kcal per day during the dry season). Their interpretation dictates that, prior to supplementation, wet season birthweights should have been markedly lower than those in the dry season, but this was not the case. During the control period dry season mean birthweight was 2889 g, and 2844 g in the wet season. Further, supplementation during the wet season should logically have brought birthweights up to the levels of the dry season. In fact, it was observed that wet season supplemented women had infants with birthweights considerably higher than the three other study groups, including supplemented women in the dry season. This pattern of results is as consistent with a chance finding as with a treatment effect.

Their subsequent report[40] raises several unanswered and at times disturbing questions. In this analysis the control birthweights (increased in number by one) were lower than in the original report in the wet season, and considerably higher in the dry season (by 70 g).[39] The birthweights of the expanded supplemented group were nearly identical.

In this second publication the extent of the dry season is defined in three different ways: climatically, from July through October, as a hunger season from July to

Group treatment	Results	Comments
Unspecified	The babies of supplemented women were lighter than those of unsupplemented women.	

September, and for analysis — presumably after reviewing the results of the study — in order to maximise the relationship of supplementation to birthweight, from July to January. Thus the reported dramatic effect of supplementation on the birthweight did not follow from using in analysis the period of hunger, nor the climatic wet season, but rather an extended period we might call the gestation wet season, i.e. well into the dry season. In addition, the reported energy intakes for this gestational wet season before supplementation were essentially identical to those in the dry season, and the reported levels of supplementation were, again, nearly identical in the two seasons. While the birthweights from the control period reported in the second publication (unlike the results reported in the initial publication) are more coherent than the authors' interpretation, the dietary information is not. Further, the mid- to late pregnancy weight gains, upper arm circumference gains and triceps skinfold gains fall dramatically during the dry season (January to June or July), remain at their worst through the summer and then rise markedly during the period of presumably greatest stress. Further, there were no effects of supplementation on these indices that might have mediated the effects of intervention.

The conclusions from these studies, if the results are credible, are important. Large effects on birthweight might be achievable by maternal supplementation if both basal diets are low, and additional nutritional burdens are placed on the population. However, such conclusions should not be accepted, and certainly not incorporated into public policy, until confirmation is available from other sites, and with other somewhat more secure research designs than these sequential studies. This is particularly true since neither the mediating physiological variables, nor the observed dietary changes, could reasonably account for the effects on birthweight.

The Special Supplemental Food Program for Women, Infants and Children (WIC).

The Special Supplemental Food Program for Women, Infants and Children (WIC) was begun in the United States in 1973, and is available to women with low income and at least one other characteristic that might make them subject to nutritional risk. Currently the programme which also supplements postpartum women and preschool children up to the age of five, has over 3 000 000 enrolled clients and is funded at $1.7 billion a year. Approximately one-third of American pregnant women meet the income eligibility criterion, and in 1980 we estimated that 40% of income eligible women were actually enrolled in the programme.(43) This proportion had risen to about 46% in 1986. The supplements are substantial:

approximately 800 Kcal per day of dairy products, cereals, vitamin C rich juices, and several miscellaneous items such as eggs, peanut butter and lentils. The programme aims not only at an adequate diet, but at coordination and improvement of health care. In 1978 when the US Congress reauthorized the WIC programme, it mandated that a thorough evaluation of the health effects of the programme be carried out. As part of the evaluation, we reviewed some 85 past studies of effects of the WIC programme, both published and unpublished.(44)

Stockbauer and Blount(45,46) studied WIC participation in Missouri during 1980, and the Medicaid recipient subset of the same births(47,48) finding a statistically significant higher mean birthweight of 16 g associated with WIC participation, almost entirely contributed by non-whites for whom the difference was 48 g. A detailed review of each study is included in the final reports of the National WIC Evaluation (NWE).(49) In summary, the array of results, showing supplementation to be associated with modest increases in birthweight and reductions in low birthweight is reasonably consistent with the studies presented in Tables 1 to 7.

Table 6. Controlled trials of dietary supplementation in pregnancy; protein density and birthweight difference between subjects and controls, in rank order by protein density of supplementation.

Site	% of calories as protein	Birthweight diff (g) Subject minus controls	No. subjects/ controls
Bombay (Merchant, 1980, personal	40.0 (larger amt)	-17	(97/635)
communication)	40.0 (smaller amt)	-23	(136/635)
New York City (21,22)	34.0	-32	(263/272)
San Francisco(23)	34.0	-45	(36/43)
Philadelphia(27)	26.0	-113	(122/118)
Toronto(25,26)	21.4	-85	(90/120)
Cardiff (Elwood, personal communication)	21.2	55*	(510/441)
Aberdeen(24)	20.5–23.8	37	(90/90)
Taiwan(35)	20.0	51	(81/87)
Taiwan(36)	20.0	16	(108/105)
Bogotá(37,38)	17.9	51	(200/207)
Hyderabad(34)	16.0	540	(39/37)
New York City(21,22)	7.5	41	(263/272)
San Francisco(23)	7.5	92	(36/23)
Bombay (Merchant 1980, personal	6.7 (larger amt)	83	(122/635)
communication)	6.7 (smaller amt)	36	(157/635)

*Controlling (approximately) for disparity in frequency of smoking.

Two of the four large studies between 1982 and 1984 that comprised the NWE are relevant to this review. One was a retrospective study which related WIC benefits to perinatal outcome in 1322 counties in 19 states over the first decade of the programme's existence;[43] the other was a prospective controlled study of over 7000 births to income-eligible women, done in 58 randomly selected areas in the continental US, performed at 174 randomly chosen WIC clinics and 55 public or hospital prenatal clinics without WIC programmes.[50-52] Some of the results are presented in Tables 8 and 9.

In the birth certificate study we found statistically significant positive correlations between the volume of WIC service and early registration for prenatal care, more frequent prenatal visits, duration of gestation, mean birthweight, and most importantly, a reduction in late fetal death. The magnitude of reduction in neonatal death rate was somewhat less than that of fetal death rate, and the result was not statistically significant.

In order to study issues other than those included on birth certificates, we also executed an extensive prospective study on a large nationwide representative sample of low income pregnant women, some of the results of which are presented in Table 9.[42] Diets were increased in energy and in nutrient density; weight gain was accelerated and late pregnancy fat deposition lowered. Further, while birthweight and duration of gestation were not different the head circumferences of infants of mothers who participated in WIC were statistically significantly larger than those of controls (0.21 cms, $p>0.01$). This has been an infrequently studied outcome, but it is likely that it was a real rather than a chance finding as we found a similar, although not statistically significant, relationship among preschool children whose mothers had been enrolled in the WIC programme during pregnancy, that was not present among children enrolled after birth. This association with accelerated head and presumably brain growth is potentially of great importance, and would require follow-up in early childhood to test its constancy over time and whether it reflects changes in cognition and behaviour. Unfortunately, the US government would not support such a follow-up effort.

We found significant relationships between the quality of the individual WIC programme, as judged by each state WIC administrator and rate of fetal growth. Further, we found no relationship between the response to WIC programme benefits as seen in perinatal outcome with maternal skinfold thickness at the onset of programme participation. Skinfold thickness in early pregnancy was not an index of responsiveness to the programme.

The overall pattern of results suggested strongly that the predominant effects of WIC benefits during pregnancy were on maternal physiology, and not primarily mediated by better obstetrical care. In our contemporary study there were major effects of WIC on the woman's diet, weight gain, and skinfold thickness.[51] Also while there were marked changes over time in the background population in some perinatal outcomes, particularly a fall in neonatal death rate, there was no change in duration of gestation over the decade under study (Table 8). Since the affected indices all reflect change prior to the onset of labour (other than for intrapartum fetal death), they cannot be related to improvements in intrapartum or neonatal care.

Table 7. Studies in which the decision to supplement and the level of supplementation were not under the subjects'

Study	Population	Assignment method/ Research design	Study no.	Group treatment	Control no.
Iyengar, 1967[33]	Indian women, age 25–40 in manual labour; monthly income "rarely exceeded" 125 rupees	How protein assigned not'clear. Controls recruited in labour.		Hospitalised 4 wks before EDC, plus	26
			12	(A) 2450 Kcal, 95g protein/d	
			13	(B) 2450 Kcal, 60g protein/d	
Qureshi *et al*., 1973[24]	Rural Indian multiparae, age 20–35, manual labourers	Alternate for groups A and B from 20 weeks gestation; method of selection untreated controls unclear.	39	A) 500 Kcal/d, 20g protein plus iron and folate	37 50
Herriott *et al*., 1978[35] McDonald *et al*., 1981[36]	Taiwan, rural villages, analysis of studies initiated by Bacon Chow	Randomised, controlled, double-blind trial	81 108	40g protein 800 Kcal/d	88 105
Mora *et al*., 1979[37] Waber *et al*., 1981[38]	Bogota, Colombia; women with at least half their children under 5 years malnourished	Prospective intervention, random assignment. Postnatal feeding and stimulation, with crossover design	200	(A) 38.4g protein/d and 856 Kcal/d supplied, third trimester only	207
Merchant & Sheth, 1980 (personal communication)	Bombay, working class women registered for prenatal care	Random		Protein g/d Kcal/d	
			97	A 45* 450	501
			136	B 30* 300	134
			122	C 7.5 450	
			157	D 5.0 300	
				*25% as animal protein	

control in developing countries.

Group treatment	Results				Comments
(C) Women presenting in labour		A	B	C	Not controlled for duration of gestation; comparison of groups A or B with C likely a function of shorter duration of gestation.
	4 wk weight gain (kg)	1.25	1.27	unknown	
	Birthweight (g)	3029	3029	2704	
	Cord plasma protein (g%)	6.09	6.11	5.34	
(B) Iron and folate		A	B	C	Duration of gestation not reported; outcome not controlled for gestation, but infants premature by dates excluded from analysis.
	Weight gain from 20th wk (kg)	3.9	2.9	unknown	
	Birthweight (g)	3320	2780	5.34	
(C) Untreated					
80/Kcal/d		Birthweight (g)			
	Herriott *et al.*	Supplement	Controls	A-B	
	First (untreated) preg.	3064	3021		Supplementation began just after previous pregnancy. Analysis of Herriott *et al.* limited to those taking >50% prescribed supplements; ingestion observed.
	Second (treated) preg.	3188	3094		
	Differences 2nd–1st preg:				
	total group	124	73	51	
	Males	196	117	79	
	Females	50	16	34	
	McDonald *et al.*				
	First (untreated) preg.	3062	3033		
	Second (treated) preg.	3118	3073		
	Differences, 2nd–1st preg:				
	total group	56	40	16	
	Males	162	73	90	
	Females	-59	2	-61	
	No difference in maternal weight gain, or infant head circumference				
(B) Health care only.		Birthweight (g)			Birthweight difference not significant on 2 tailed test.
		Supplemented	Controls	A-B	
	Total	2978	2927	51	
	Males	3040	2951	89	
	Females	2911	2905	6	
	% < 2500g	11.0	8.7	2.3	
	Group	Birthweight (g)	bw (vs gps E and F combined)		All received iron, folate, B_{12}, except group F. Half also received lysine and methionine, which were unrelated to outcome. Amount of supplementation raised halfway through study (i.e. groups B and D preceded groups A and C)
E	A	2926	-17		
F (No Supplements	B	2663	-23		
	C	2769	+83 $p<0.05$		
	D	2722	+36		
	E	2695			
	F	2650			

Table 7. (continued)

Study	Population	Assignment method/ Research design	Study No.	Group treatment	Control no.
Prentice *et al.*, 1983[39]	All births in one Gambian village during 2 years of supplementation compared to outcome during prior 4 years. On average women were attending by the 16th week of pregnancy		51 42	Wet season 110 Kcal/d, Dry season 950 Kcal/d, 6d/w	95 86 6d/w
			Actual increments (Kcal/d) Wet season 430 Dry season 433		
Prentice *et al.*, 1987[40]	Expanded report of preceding study in the Gambia, two additional years of supplementation		116 81	Wet season Dry season	95 87
			Actual increments (Kcal/d) Wet season 435 Dry season 426		Energy intake (Kcal/d) West season 1462 Dry season 1475
Girija *et al.*, 1984[41]	Low SES multip. women (<$100/m family income) in third trimester	Random assignment	10	30g protein 417 Kcals/d	10
			Intake shown by semi-quantitative bar graphs; no apparent differences between supplemented and control groups		
Ross *et al.*, 1985[42]	Consecutive births among Zulus in clinic near Durban, South Africa, with expected original vaginal delivery 1977	Randomised allocation Observed supplementation from 20 wks gestation	31	773 cals/d, high bulk 5d/w	33
			31	697 cals/d, low bulk 5d/w	
			32	30 to 90 mg Zn gluconate/d	
			1403 to 1537 avg Kcal/d prior to supplementation; No data on intake during supplementation period.		

Group treatment	Results	Comments
Wet Season Dry season Energy intake (Kcal/d) West season 1464 Dry season 1468	Supplemented / Control / Difference Wet season Mean birthweight (g): 3030 / 2844 / 186 % <2500g: 4.7 / 28.2 / -23.5 Dry season Mean birthweight (g): 2892 / 2889 / 3 % <2500g: 11.7 / 8.0 / 3.7 Results adjusted for sex, parity and month of birth	Magnitude of interaction with season uncertain because of small sample Patterns of outcome do not conform to authors' interpretation
Wet season Dry season	Mean birthweight (g) Supplemented / Control / Difference Wet season: 3010 / 2810 / 200*** Dry season: 2972 / 2959 / 13 Results adjusted for sex, parity and month of birth ***p<0.001	No explanation of additional dry season control, nor of different presupplementation energy intakes, nor of different presupplementation birthweights between publications. Wet season defined as July to October (p912,915) and July to January (p914), latter chosen post hoc, after reviewing results to maximise birthweight effect, although hunger season ends in September (p912).
Not specified	Supplemented / Controls 3rd trimester Wt gain: 3.90 / 3.95 Hgb increase (g%): 1.97 / 0.17 Birthweight (g): 2939 / 2676 Length (cm): 47.7 / 45.9	Primary goal of research was to assess effect of supplementation on lactational performance and infant growth
Placebo	Low bulk / High bulk / Zn / Controls Wt gain to 20 wks (kg): 8.1 / 8.3 / 7.2 / 8.8 Dur gest (wks): 38.6 / 39.2 / 39.4 / 38.9 Birthweight (g): 3376* / 3082 / 3088 / 3171 (diff from controls (g): 205 / -89 / -83 / -) *p<0.05	Numbers of subjects too small to test hypothesis

Table 8. National evaluation of the Special Supplemental Food Program for Women, Infants and Children (WIC): Historical study of pregnancy outcome[42]

Study design	Outcome measure	Mean	Change/yr	Difference associated with WIC participation	Comment
Relationship of perinatal outcome, from fetal death certificates and linked birth (n = 13,434,000) and infant death certificates, to rate of WIC benefits to income eligible pregnant women, within at least 100 births at midpoint of time series (1975) and with all data elements necessary to specific analysis	First trimester registration for prenatal care (%)	73.9	0.9**	4.1***	Comparison of time trends with WIC effects on duration of gestation, fetal and neonatal death rates, and birth weight strongly suggests nutritional effect rather than mediation by improved medical care
	Inadequate no. of prenatal visits (%)	6.3	-2.4***	-5.0***	
	Preterm delivery (<37w; %)	6.6	-0.1	-0.7	
	Duration of gestation (wks)	39.1	0.0	0.2*	
	Mean birthweight (g)	3335	0.7***	23.9**	
	Fetal deaths, 28+ wks gest/1000	6.2	-0.3***	-2.3*	
	Neonatal deaths/1000	10.6	-0.7**	1.5	

*p<0.05
**p<0.01
***p<0.001

In the past, work on the effect of nutritional supplementation during pregnancy has focussed almost exclusively on birthweight. Studies of effects on mortality have rarely been undertaken because of the much larger study population needed. On the other hand, the NWE was a reasonably secure demonstration of a direct relationship between a feeding programme in pregnancy and lowered fetal mortality rates.

Implications for care

We can draw two main conclusions from the studies reviewed. Firstly, dietary restriction can cause markedly decreased birthweight. During famine mean birthweight can be depressed by as much as 550 g, and iatrogenic dietary manipulation and restriction can have almost as serious an effect. Although the extent to which such decrements in birthweight are associated with perinatal mortality and morbidity is unknown, there can be no rational justification either for allowing pregnant women with access to modern obstetric care to go hungry or for imposing either dietary restriction or marked manipulation of the dietary constituents upon them.

Secondly, attempts at nutritional supplementation, while well intentioned, have not always had the desired effect. It is clear that high density protein supplements are consistently associated with depression rather than increase in mean birthweight. Also, although consistent increments (on average, about 30 to 50 g) in mean birthweight have been found in association with programmes of aggressive nutritional counselling and/or supplementation with preparations of lower protein density, the magnitude of these increments is nevertheless lower than had been hoped.

Implications for research

Since the increase in mean birthweight associated with nutritional counselling and supplementation has been relatively small, further trials of these interventions must concentrate on the subsets of women in which a beneficial effect is most likely to be demonstrated. This notion is supported by the fact that in our New York study, nutritional intervention matched our expectations only among those women who were heavy smokers.(21,22) Women who are likely to benefit most from dietary supplementation might be identified in a number of ways. Reliance on dietary history alone has been unrewarding. Possibly biochemical assessment or anthropometric measurements may prove more useful.

Further research is also urgently needed to determine whether the observed range of increments in birthweight are consistently associated with decreased perinatal morbidity and mortality, and with improved long term growth and development of the infant and child. New studies with new research designs are needed. Much larger populations are required to study effects on mortality, and careful longitudinal research is essential to understand long term development. It is essential that subsequent research assesses indices of development other than weight, particularly head circumferential growth. In addition, since there is some evidence that prenatal feeding may beneficially influence subsequent psychological development independent of changes in birthweight, the possibility of such effects must not be neglected.(21,22)

REFERENCES

1. Campbell DM, Gillmer MDG. *Nutrition in Pregnancy.* Proceedings of the Tenth Study Group of the Royal College of Obstetricians and Gynaecologists. London: RCOG, 1983.
2. Rush D. Erfects of changes in protein and calorie intake during pregnancy on the growth of the human fetus. In: *Effective Care in Pregnancy and Childbirth.* Eds. M Enkin, M Keirse, I Chalmers. London: Oxford University Press, 1989.
3. Antonov AN. Children born during the seige of Leningrad in 1942. *J Pediatr* 1947; **30**: 250–259.
4. Stein Z, Susser M, Saenger G, Marolla F. *Famine and Human Development: The Dutch Hunger Winter of 1944/45.* New York: Oxford University Press, 1975.
5. Smith CA. The effect of wartime starvation in Holland upon pregnancy and its product. *Am J Obstet Gynecol* 1947; **53**: 599–608.
6. Dean RFA. The size of the baby at birth and the yield of breast milk. In: *Studies of under-nutrition. Wuppertal 1946–9.* Medical Research Council Special Report Series, No. 275. London: HMSO; pp.346–378.

Table 9. The Special Supplemental Food Program for Women, Infants and Children (WIC): Longitudinal study[49,50]

Population	Assignment method/ Research design	Study no.	Group treatment	Control no.
First time registrants for WIC, or prenatal care, first two trimesters, in 58 randomly selected areas in US, 1983.	WIC patients from 174 of 185 randomly selected WIC sites; controls were income eligible women from 55 of 80 prenatal clinics without WIC programs and in areas of low WIC penetration.	5205	Standard WIC benefits.	1358

All results adjusted for race, age, income, education, welfare status, etc.
(1) Includes those enrolled in WIC after registration.

7. Rush D. Effects of changes and calorie intake during pregnancy on the growth of the human fetus. In: *Effectiveness and Satisfaction in Antenatal Care*. Clinics in Developmental Medicine Series. Eds. M Enkin, I Chalmers. London: Spastics International Medical Publications, 1982: pp.92–113.
8. Campbell DM, MacGillivray I. The effect of a low calorie diet or a thiazide diuretic on the incidence of pre-eclampsia and on birthweight. *Br J Obstet Gynaecol* 1975; **82**: 572–577.
9. Campbell DM. Dietary restriction and its effect on neonatal outcome. In: *Nutrition in Pregnancy*. Eds. DM Campbell, MDG Gillmer. Proceedings of the Tenth Study Group of the Royal College of Obstetricians and Gynaecologists. London: RCOG 1983: pp.243–250.
10. Blumenthal I. Diet and diuretics in pregnancy and subsequent growth of off-spring. *Br Med J* 1976; **2**: 733.
11. Grieve JFK, Campbell-Brown BM, Johnstone FD. Dieting in pregnancy: a study of the effect of a high protein low carbohydrate diet on birthweight in an obstetric population. In: *Carbohydrate Metabolism in Pregnancy and the Newborn*. Eds. MW Sutherland, JM Stowers. Berlin: Springer Verlag, 1978: pp.518–533.
12. Barsa Gregory P, Rush D. Iatrogenic caloric restriction in pregnancy and birthweight. *Am J Perinatol*; In press.
13. Naeye RL, Blanc W, Paul C. Effects of maternal nutrition on the human fetus. *Pediatrics* 1973; **52**: 494–503.
14. Cameron CS, Graham S. Antenatal diet and its influences on still births and prematurity. *Glasgow Med J* 1944; **142**: 1–7.
15. Berry K, Wiehl DG. An experiment in education during pregnancy. *Milbank Memorial Fund Quarterly* 1952; **30**: 119–151.

Group treatment	Results			Comments
Routine prenatal care		WIC	Control(1)	One-quarter of controls enrolled in WIC program by 36–38th week gestation. Control group had higher incomes, educati and social status.
	Duration gestation (d)	-0.1	276.0	
	<37 wks gest (%)	-1.2	15.1	
	Mean birthweight (g)	-9	3258	
	<2500g (%)	+0.5	7.4	
	Length (cm)	-0.2	50.3	
	Head circ (cm)	+0.2**	33.8	
	Fetal\ mort (/1000)	-5.5	15.1	
	(n	2536–3192	693–813)	

16. Sweney C, Smith H, Foster JC, Place JC, Specht J, Kochenour NK, Prater BM. Effects of a nutrition intervention program during pregnancy. *J Nurse Midwifery* 1985; **3**: 149–158.
17. Habicht JP, Lechtig A, Yarbrough C, Klein RE. Maternal nutrition, birthweight and infant mortality. In: *Size at Birth.* Eds. K Elliott, J Knight. Ciba Foundation Symposium 27. Amsterdam: Elsevier, 1974: pp.353–377.
18. Dieckmann WJ, Adair FL, Michael H, Kramer S, Dunkle F, Arthur B, Costin M, Campbell A, Wensley AC, Lorang E. Calcium, phosphorous, iron and nitrogen balances in pregnant women. *Am J Obstet Gynecol* 1944; **47**: 357–368.
19. Higgins AC. Nutritional status and the outcome of pregnancy. *J Can Dietetic Assoc* 1976; **37**: 17–36.
20. Rush D. Nutritional services during pregnancy and birthweight: a retrospective matched pair analysis. *Can Med Assoc J.* 1981; **125**: 567–576.
21. Rush D, Stein Z, Susser M. A randomized controlled trial of prenatal nutritional supplementation in New York City. *Pediatrics* 1980; **65**: 683–697.
22. Rush D, Stein Z, Susser M. *A Randomized Controlled Trial of Prenatal Nutritional Supplements.* March of Dimes Birth Defects Foundation, Vol XVI, no. 3. New York: Alan R, Liss Inc, 1980.
23. Adams SO, Barr GD, Huenemann RL. Effect of nutritional supplementation in pregnancy. I: Outcome of pregnancy. *J Am Diet Assoc* 1978; **72**: 144–147.
24. Campbell–Brown M. Protein energy supplements in primigravid women at risk of low birthweight. In: *Nutrition in Pregnancy.* Proceedings of the Tenth Study Group of the Royal College of Obstetricians and Gynaecologists. Eds. DM Campbell, MDG Gillmer. London: RCOG, 1983; pp.85–98.
25. Ebbs JH, Tisdall FF, Scott WA. The influences of prenatal diet on the mother

and child. *J Nutr* 1941; **22**: 515–526.
26. Ebbs JH, Brown A, Tisdall FF, Moyle WJ, Bell M. The influence of improved nutrition upon the infant. *Can Med Assoc J* 1942; **46**: 6–8.
27. Osofsky JH. Relationships between prenatal medical and nutritional measures, pregnancy outcome, and early infant development in an urban poverty setting. I. The role of nutritional intake. *Am J Obstet Gynecol* 1975; **123**: 682–690.
28. Viegas OA, Scott PH, Cole TJ, Eaton P, Needham PG, Wharton BA. Dietary protein energy supplementation of pregnant Asian mothers at Sorrento, Birmingham. I. Unselective during second and third trimesters. *Br Med J* 1982; **285**: 589–592.
29. Watney PJM, Atton C. Dietary supplementation in pregnancy. (Letter) *Br Med J* 1986; **293**: 1102.
30. Tompkins WT, Mitchell RM, Wiehl DG. Maternal nutrition studies at Philadelphia Lying-in Hospital, 2. Prematurity and maternal nutrition. In: *The Promotion of Maternal and Newborn Health*. New York: Milbank Memorial Fund, 1955: pp.25–50.
31. Balfour MI. Supplementary feeding in pregnancy. *Lancet* 1944; **i**: 208–221.
32. Viegas OAC, Scott PH, Cole TJ, Needham PG, Wharton BA. Dietary protein energy supplementation of pregnant Asian mothers at Sorrento, Birmingham. II: Selective during the third trimester only. *Br Med J* 1982; **285**: 592–595.
33. Iyengar L. Effects of dietary supplements late in pregnancy on the expectant mother and her newborn. *Indian J Med Res* 1967; **55**: 85–89.
34. Qureshi S, Rao NP, Madhavi V, Mathur YC, Reddi YR. Effect of maternal nutrition supplementation on the birthweight of the newborn. *Indian Pediatr* 1973; **10**: 541–544.
35. Herriott RM, Hsueh AM, Aitchison R. Influence of maternal diet on offspring: growth, behaviour, feed efficiency and susceptibility (human); a study in Suilin, Taiwan, initiated by Chow BF. *Final report on AID/SCD 2944*. Baltimore: Johns Hopkins University, 1978.
36. McDonald EC, Pollitt E, Mueller W, Hsueh AM, Sherwin R. The Bacon Chow study: maternal nutrition supplementation and birth weight of offspring. *Am J Clin Nutr* 1981; **34**: 2133–2144.
37. Mora JO, de Paredes B, Wagner M, de Navarro L, Suescun J, Christiansen N, Herrera MG. Nutritional supplementation and the outcome of pregnancy. I. Birthweight. *Am J Clin Nutr* 1979; **32**: 455–462.
38. Waber DP, Vuori-Christiansen L, Ortiz N, Clement JR, Christiansen NE, Mora JO, Reed RB, Herrera MG. Nutritional supplementation, maternal education, and cognitive development of infants at risk of malnutrition. *Am J Clin Nutr* 1981; **34**: 807–813.
39. Prentice AM, Watkinson M, Whitehead RG, Lamb WH. Prenatal dietary supplementation of African women and birth weight. *Lancet* 1983; **i**: 489–491.
40. Prentice AM, Cole TJ, Foord FA, Lamb WH, Whitehead RG. Increased birthweight after prenatal dietary supplementation of rural African women. *Am J Clin Nutr* 1987; **46**: 912–925.
41. Girija A, Geervani P, Rao GN. Influence of dietary supplementation during

pregnancy on lactation performance. *J Trop Pediatr* 1984; **30**: 79–83.
42. Ross SM, Nel E, Naeye R. Differing effects of low and high bulk maternal dietary supplements during pregnancy. *Early Hum Dev* 1985; **10**: 295–302.
43. Rush D, Alvir JM, Kenny DA, Johnson SS, Horvitz DG. The National WIC Evaluation. III. Historical study of pregnancy outcomes. *Am J Clin Nutr* (Suppl) 1988; **48**: 412–428.
44. Rush D, Leighton J, Sloan NL, Alvir JM, Garbowski GC. The National WIC Evaluation. II. Review of past studies of WIC. *Am J Clin Nutr* (Suppl) 1988; **48**: 394–411.
45. Stockbauer J, Blount CR. *Evaluation of the Prenatal Participation Component of the Missouri WIC Program.* Jefferson City, MO: Missouri Department of Social Services Division of Health, 1983.
46. Stockbauer JW. Evaluation of the Missouri WIC program: prenatal components. *J Am Diet Assoc* 1986; **86**: 61–67.
47. Schramm WF. *WIC Prenatal Participation and its Relationship to Newborn Medicaid Costs in Missouri: a Cost/benefit Analysis.* Jefferson City, MO: Missouri Center for Health Statistics, 1983.
48. Schramm WF. WIC prenatal participation and its relationship to newborn Medicaid costs in Missouri – a cost/benefit analysis. *Am J Public Health* 1985; **75**: 851–857.
49. Rush D, Horvitz DG, Seaver WB et al. *Evaluation of the Special Supplemental Food Program for Infants, Women and Children.* 5 vols. Washington, DC: US Department of Agriculture, 1986. (Available from the National Technical Information Service, Springfield, VA).
50. Rush D, Horvitz DG, Seaver WB, Leighton J, Sloan NL, Johnson SS, Kulka RA, Devore JW, Holt M, Lynch JT, Virag TG, Woodside MB, Shanklin DS. The National WIC Evaluation. IV. Study methodology and sample characteristics in the longitudinal study of pregnant women, the study of children, and the food expenditures study. *Am J Clin Nutr* (Suppl) 1988; **48**: 429–438.
51. Rush D, Sloan NL, Leighton J, Alvir JM, Horvitz DG, Seaver WB, Garbowski GC, Johnson SS, Kulka RA, Holt M, Devore JW, Lynch JT, Woodside MB, Shanklin DS. The National WIC Evaluation. V. Longitudinal study of pregnant women. *Am J Clin Nutr* (Suppl) 1988; **48**: 439–483.
52. Rush D, Leighton J, Sloan NL, Alvir JM, Horvitz DG, Seaver WB, Garbowski GC, Johnson SS, Kulka RA, Devore JW, Holt M, Lynch JT, Virag TG, Woodside MB, Shanklin DS. The National WIC Evaluation: VI. Study of infants and children. *Am J Clin Nutr* (Suppl) 1988; **48**: 484–511.

Discussion

Chairman: Dr M.J. Whittle

STEER: Given the fact that we know that, as we have heard from Professor Alberman, a lot of dietary manipulations can take two or three generations to work; given that we know that prepregnancy weight is the major influence and that in women who are underweight, even if they gain 20 kg in pregnancy they will make up less than half in terms of the underweight of the babies, why is it that people are so concerned about supplementation in the indexed pregnancy? You would not expect it to have very much effect.

RUSH: I would have to disagree with both of the premises. I think that the effects of prepregnant weight and weight gain are additive and independent. Both operate until one gets into very high prepregnant weights. It is not a two or three generational change. The Japanese data are very indicative of that. One sees effects in the starvation studies. There was complete rehabilitation with third trimester feeding in Holland. There may well be cohort effects over generations, but the major effects appear to be those events immediately going on during pregnancy.

STEER: But the refeeding in Holland is refeeding after a short term stress. We are talking about long term stress over perhaps two or three generations; that is why it takes a long time to reverse. Short term starvation can be reversed very quickly, and I am not surprised that it does not have much effect on birthweight because the intrinsic stores that the woman has in terms of her body mass are much greater than in the group of women who have been deprived for generations.

RUSH: Of course there is an animal model. Stuart had studied multigenerational mouse or rat data, but what you are suggesting is almost impossible to specify in the human. Certainly there are short term effects and I tried to review what some of these were. I cannot speak to the intergenerational issue; I do not think that anyone knows.

LEVENE: This is obviously an extremely important area. I do not know enough about the methodology of your study, but one must very carefully evaluate whether these changes are actual changes or maybe influenced by other factors. I was not clear what your control group was. This clearly was not a randomised study of one group, with intervention in the other group. You are not just intervening by giving them calories. You are intervening in other more subtle ways as well. Bearing in mind those potential criticisms do you think that this study actually answers any questions at all?

RUSH: It was only in doing this work that I gained any insight into the difference between programme evaluation and doing a randomised trial. They are very different exercises. It is obvious that this is not a randomised group. A small study is done and then it is generalised to the population. We then have to know whether the programme works. I think that a great deal can be learned from this because I do not think that there are unobserved factors accounting for the outcomes. I think that the likelihood of distortion is directional; it is not random, since I know a great deal about the control group, and these are poor women. By definition they are at the same economic level as those who were included in the programme. So the directional bias is towards underestimating the programme effect because the controls are in general better off. The numbers are very large, so I think that what we have seen is almost surely real and probably an underestimate of actual programme effect. You cannot address the mortality issue in a clean and elegant and neat study because the numbers will never be large enough. Many of the studies of birthweight and nutrition are pitifully small. If one does a fairly simple straightforward power analysis to address how large a study should be in order to address a question, I think that you would need sample sizes of controls and subject to address this issue of nutritional supplementation in pregnancy of at least 250 per cell. And yet the Birmingham study said 15. That is a non study. To address problems of mortality, it is not 250; it is probably 5000. Once you need a study of that size you have to think about other strategies. I think that there is a great deal to be learned from this and I think that we could have learned an enormous amount with a follow-up about the long term consequences of the feeding programme in pregnancy.

LEVENE: Clearly this is very important. In Britain there are easily identifiable groups of women who might be benefited by a programme like this. But 2 billion dollars in 1982 is a phenomenal amount of money. Are you convinced that the data that you have would support the introduction of such a programme in a developed country?

RUSH: Without the follow-up I would not even attempt to do a cost benefit analysis. The only thing that I could say is the 2 billion dollars is one Trident submarine. We can talk in terms of certain kinds of semi-quantitative or qualitative allocations of public expenditure, but I cannot say that this money invested in this way would be better than providing more neonatal intensive care units. It cannot be done because it is enormously incomplete until one really knows the functional consequences of the intervention.

FRASER: Regarding the skin fold changes in supplemented women, does your questionnaire allow you to identify any important qualitative differences in maternal diet introduced by the programme?

RUSH: We could specify with some precision the various nutrient differences because the nature of the foods that are supplied by the programme are quite specific. It is not like foodstamps. American foodstamps are cashable vouchers with which you can buy anything short of cigarettes or alcohol. The WICK vouchers are not cash denominated. They are denominated by foods. You get so much milk and so much high Vitamin C content juice and so much cereal, and we could say specifically how their diets had changed and how they were different from the controls. But that really does not answer the question of what was going on.

STEWART: If these are deprived families, did the ladies actually eat the food?

Were they giving it to their other children?

RUSH: The answer is "yes and no." It is a large supplemental package. In fact, it comes to about 800 calories of high quality food which is just about the nature of the package that was given in the public health study, so it is a large amount of food. Nobody in the world could increase their diet by more than 800 calories for more than 2 days. But the actual diet histories which I showed you, suggested that the actual increment was about 100 calories. So what we have to suppose is that with this much food introduced into the house, 7/8 of it either went to replace other food that they no longer had to purchase, but some of it got there. The fact that we got the skin fold changes, the weight gain changes, the head circumference changes says that something was going on here. This was not a pure random mix. If one only had random answers one would not expect to get differences.

Utero–placental blood flow and fetal growth

Professor J.F. Clapp III

INTRODUCTION

This chapter will address the interaction between utero–placental blood flow and fetal growth from three perspectives. Experimental data dealing with the impact of both acute and chronic reductions in utero–placental blood flow on parameters of feto–placental growth will be reviewed. These data will then be used to support the premise that growth *in utero* is flow limited. Finally, a potential mechanism which may regulate the interaction between utero–placental blood flow and feto–placental growth will be discussed.

ANIMAL EXPERIMENTAL DATA

Methods of reducing utero–placental blood flow

Three basic approaches are used to reduce utero–placental blood flow during pregnancy. The first is to reduce by manipulating maternal factors to initiate a redistribution of maternal cardiac output away from the uterine vascular bed. These perturbations include heat stress,[1] drug administration,[2,3] nutritional deprivation[4] and probably hypoxia.[5] All appear to act via adrenergic mechanisms. The second approach is mechanically to reduce flow by either ligation,[6,7] constriction[8,9] or occlusion[10-11] of the uterine vasculature. The third approach is to reduce the cross-sectional area of the caruncular vascular bed by ablating a large fraction of the implantation area prior to pregnancy.[12]

Acute reduction of utero–placental blood flow

Data obtained in the pregnant ewe suggest that both the uterine and umbilical circulations are hyperperfused relative to the metabolic needs of the tissues at normal rates of flow.[13] Thus when uterine blood flow is reduced by 30–50% for upwards of an hour, tissue oxygen uptake is maintained due to a simple reciprocal relationship between the rate of blood flow and the amount of oxygen extracted from it.[3,9] These observations indicate that fairly large, short-term, decremental changes in uterine blood flow probably have little impact on fetal growth. They also suggest that chronic, minor decremental changes in utero–placental blood flow should not compromise either substrate availability or fetal growth.

When utero–placental blood flow is acutely reduced by more than 50% there is clear evidence of progressive fetal compromise. Fetal oxygen consumption falls precipitously, and evidence of fetal excess lactate production rapidly appears.

Despite these findings, fetal pH and utero–placental oxygen consumption are maintained unless the flow reduction exceeds 70%.[11,14,15] Similar metabolic changes are seen transiently during fetal adaptation to chronic reductions in fetal oxygen availability.[5]

Chronic reduction of utero–placental blood flow

Morphometric correlates. As noted earlier, the onset of both heat stress and nutritional deprivation are accompanied by a redistribution of maternal blood flow away from the utero–placental circulation.[1,4] Chronic exposure to both stimuli has a dramatic effect on placental and fetal growth, producing the characteristic morphometric profile of asymmetrical intrauterine growth retardation.[16–19] In the heat stress model there is a direct linear correlation between the reduction in both uterine and umbilical flow and the reduction in placental weight. In turn placental weight correlates directly with the rate of utero–placental oxygen consumption and selected measures of placental transfer capacity.[18] As might be expected, there is a direct curvilinear relationship between the reduction in placental weight and the reduction in fetal weight with an increase in the fetal weight/placental weight ratio in the animals with the smallest placentas. Although correlative flow measurements are not available in the chronic nutritionally deprived model the feto-placental morphometric interrelationships are similar, with the reduction in placental weight explaining upwards of 91% of the variance in fetal weight under the condition of chronic deprivation.[19,20]

Chronic reduction of utero–placental blood flow by vascular ligation or constriction with an externally adjustable mechanical occluder also produces the classical morphometric profile of asymmetrical fetal growth retardation in a variety of species.[6–8] In all species there is a reduction in both placental and fetal weight. However in contrast to other flow reduction models their growth appears to be affected equally, as there is no consistent directional change in the fetal weight/placental weight ratio. Serial measurements of utero–placental blood flow are available in the mechanical occluder model utilising the pregnant ewe.[8] When the rate of utero–placental flow is chronically reduced by 20% and 40%, there is a tight direct linear correlation between the rate of mean utero–placental blood flow and placental weight. A similar correlation is present between flow and fetal weight as well as several indices of the asymmetry of fetal growth. It is of note that these observations do not support the conclusion drawn earlier from the acute flow reduction data, in that a relatively minor chronic reduction in utero–placental flow clearly does restrict growth of both the fetus and placenta.

Embolisation of the uterine circulation produces a similar fetal morphometric picture.[10,11,21] Serial measurements of utero–placental blood flow demonstrate that there is a direct relationship between the rate of utero–placental blood flow and the weight of the uterus and its tissue contents as well as growth of the fetus *per se*.[11] As progressive embolic placental damage is characteristic of this flow reduction model, a detailed histological study of the placenta was necessary to establish the interrelationship between fetal and placental morphometry.[22] Surprisingly, the data indicate that there is no consistent relationship between either the degree of placental embolic damage or the density of emboli within the placenta, and the degree of fetal growth restriction assessed using one or more morphometric parameters. Rather, as shown in Figure I, the amount of remaining undamaged placenta, expressed as a functional volume, is directly related to gross fetal weight over more than a 3 kg weight range, and inversely related to the

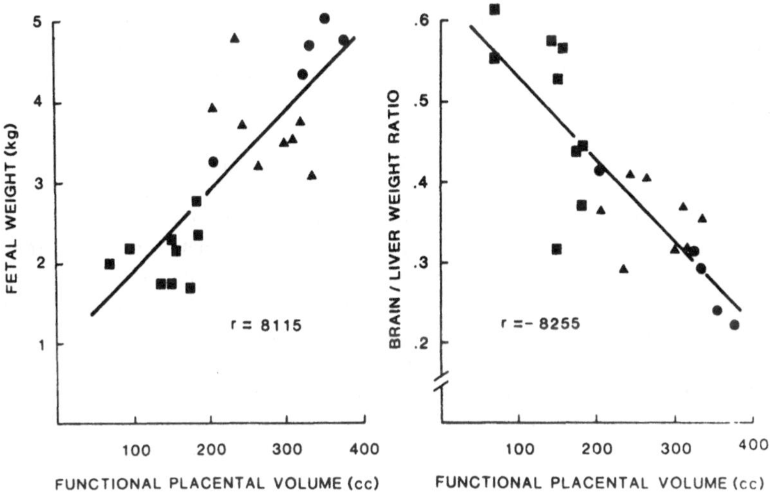

Figure I
The relationship between morphometrically quantitated functional placental volume and both fetal weight at term and the fetal brain weight/liver weight ratio in three groups of animals. All fetuses were singletons. The filled circles (●) represent fully instrumented controls, the squares (■) the fetuses with clear-cut morphometric evidence of asymmetrical growth retardation following embolisation of the uterine circulation, and the triangles (▲) the fetuses who were exposed to repetitive embolisation without clear-cut morphometric evidence of asymmetrical growth retardation. Note that only functional placental volumes under 200 cc are associated with clearly defined morphometric evidence of growth retardation.

degree of growth asymmetry, quantitated by the brain weight/liver weight ratio. This indicates that each kilogram of fetal weight in excess of 2 kg requires approximately an additional 100 gm of functional placental tissue and that, in this model, functional placental volume must be reduced below 200 cc to produce definitive morphometric evidence of fetal growth retardation. These observations, made following progressive vascular compromise, suggest that the initial development of the placenta is quite variable and may be a critical determinant of both the rate of utero–placental perfusion and the rate of feto–placental growth under normal circumstances. This speculation fits nicely with the changes in morphometric outcome observed by Alexander and Williams when the timing of heat stress was varied in relation to placental growth,[16] as well as those observed by Mellor when the timing of nutritional deprivation was varied in a similar fashion.[19]

If successful, carunculectomy prior to conception has a profound effect on placental weight, reducing it to a value between 30 and 50% of control.[12,23,24] The associated fetal morphometric profile is clearly that of asymmetrical intrauterine growth retardation and the fetal weight/placental weight ratio is increased as the placental weights decline, reaching a volume as much as 60% above that observed in controls at placental weights below 200 gm. As in other models near-term microsphere measurements of both utero–placental and umbilical flow demonstrate a direct linear relationship between absolute flow rates in the two circulations and both placental and fetal weight.[12]

Functional correlates. Longitudinal measurements of flow, substrate levels and uptakes are available in both the embolisation and mechanical occluder flow reduction models (Clark, personal communication).[21,26,27] In both models, the partial pressure of oxygen, as well as oxygen, glucose and lactate contents, remain normal until late in the course, long after there is evidence of a reduction in feto–placental growth and fetal substrate uptake. Thus, the data indicate that growth rate, blood flow, substrate availability and uptake are closely matched throughout the course of flow retardation.

Late in the course, when growth retardation is fully developed, all metabolic parameters are consistent with a restriction of substrate availability reflecting the reduction or cessation of growth. This is true in all models in which measurements have been obtained. These changes include a decrease in oxygen content, glucose content, and insulin concentration with an increase in haemoglobin, lactate and alanine concentrations, and a hormonal profile characteristic of suppressed growth.[25] Although placental transfer and substrate uptakes are markedly reduced at this point, they remain closely matched to fetal weight.[18,23,26,27] The fact that metabolic balance is maintained this late in the course suggests that continued growth under these circumstances may be externally regulated by the availability of substrate. This would have distinct survival value as it would provide a certain metabolic margin of safety for the fetus *in utero.*

In the embolisation model there is also evidence that flow distribution within the two placental circulations is altered in a fashion which improves perfusion balance between the two circulations. Functionally, this acts to minimise shunting and maximise transfer capability. The data from several initial flow studies [11,26] suggested that embolisation initiated an abrupt shift in flow in both circulations away from damaged placental tissue and a concomitant relative hyperfusion of the undamaged placental tissue. This led to a series of experiments in which perfusion balance between the uterine and umbilical placental circulations was directly assessed at a cotyledonary level by simultaneously injecting microspheres with different labels into the maternal left ventricle and fetal inferior *vena cava.*[28] Perfusion balance was expressed as the ratio of the fraction of total umbilical spheres lodged in a given cotyledon to the fraction of total uterine spheres in the same cotyledon. With this approach, a cotyledonary umbilical flow/uterine flow ratio of 1.0 represents perfect perfusion balance between the two circulations, while a ratio less than 0.75 or greater than 1.25 indicates that a fair degree of perfusion imbalance is present. The results shown in Figure II indicate that placental perfusion balance is markedly improved following progressive embolisation of the uterine side of the placental circulation with concomitant placental damage. When compared to the cotyledons obtained from the non-embolised controls, the cotyledons from the embolised animals demonstrate more than a 40% increase in the weight of cotyledonary tissue with an umbilical flow/uterine flow ratio between 0.9 and 1.1, and more than a 50% decrease in the weight of cotyledonary tissue with an umbilical flow/uterine flow ratio either less than 0.75 or greater than 1.25.

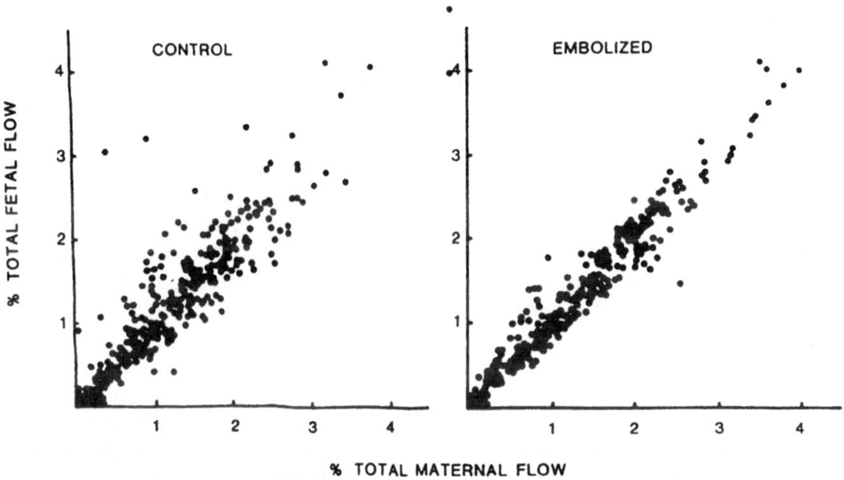

Figure II
Placental perfusion balance between the umbilical and uterine cotyledonary circulations in 4 control and 4 embolised singleton sheep placentas at 139 days gestation. Each data point represents the perfusion balance between the two circulations in a single cotyledon. A total of 320 control and 316 embolised cotyledons were examined with total weights of 980 grams and 920 grams respectively. Ideal perfusion balance is an umbilical flow/uterine flow ratio of 1.0 which is the diagonal of each graph. Note the dramatic improvement in placental perfusion balance in the embolised cotyledonary tissues.

FLOW LIMITATIONS TO FETO–PLACENTAL GROWTH

Unfortunately, correlative data between tissue weight and utero–placental blood flow is not available in all the chronic flow reduction models of intrauterine growth retardation. However, the morphometric similarities observed suggest that the correlative data from the heat stress, caruncullectomy and embolisation models are applicable to the nutritional deprivation model and those from the mechanical occluder model are applicable to the various ligation models used in rodents. In each of these flow reduction models there is a direct correlation over a wide range between the rate of utero–placental blood flow and the weight of the placenta at term. In the sheep placental weight peaks at 90–100 days gestation and the reduction in blood flow in the embolisation and mechanical occluder models does not begin until 15–20 days later. Given this time frame it is clear that both perturbations must initiate a flow dependent reduction in placental weight. Likewise, when heat stress is begun at the time of peak placental weight there is a reduction in placental weight 20 days later.[1] In the carunculectomy, nutritional deprivation and early heat stress models, the perturbation either precedes or is concurrent with the timing of placental growth and appears to restrict its growth rate and/or ultimate size. Thus in all cases it appears that a decremental change in utero–placental flow is accompanied by a reduction in placental weight, providing strong evidence that placental size is flow limited.

As noted earlier, the functional morphometric, metabolic and transfer data suggest that fetal growth is matched closely to placental functional capacity as well as size throughout the course of flow reduction. The absence of evidence of fetal substrate deprivation until late in the course indicates that fetal growth must either slow or cease very early in the course of utero–placental flow reduction in response to one or more stimuli that do not appear to require the presence of an alteration in fetal blood gas tensions for activation. The increase seen in the fetal weight/placental weight ratio at the low extremes of placental size indicates that additional adaptations such as improved perfusion balance probably act to optimise transfer function in the face of progressive morphometric restriction. These functional data, along with their morphological correlates, support the premise that the observed limitation of fetal growth following a chronic reduction in utero–placental blood flow is clearly secondary to its placental effects which are morphometrically manifested by a reduction in placental size. Nonetheless, although the effect on fetal growth appears to be secondary and mediated via the placenta, the primary mechanism controlling it is responsive to changes in utero–placental perfusion and, in that sense, fetal growth is ultimately flow limited.

A POSSIBLE CENTRAL REGULATORY MECHANISM

As noted above, all the methods of producing a chronic reduction in the rate of utero–placental blood flow are associated with a concomitant restriction of placental size. In turn, the reduction in fetal weight is closely correlated with both the restriction in flow rate and the reduction in placental weight. In addition, in the models in which data is available, the initial fetal functional response does not include haemodynamic or blood gas evidence of acute stress or metabolic compromise (Clark, personal communication).[21,26,27] Rather, there is maintenance of normal substrate levels, gradients and venoarterial differences across the umbilical circulation with a reduction in flow rate and uptake of oxygen and glucose. These findings can only be explained by an early sustained reduction in fetal growth rate that occurs long before transfer function becomes a limiting factor.

The fact that similar morphometric and functional responses to a reduction in utero–placental blood flow are seen in all the animal models suggests the presence of a common regulatory mechanism, and the early functional responses suggest that the placenta mediates the interaction. A very simple potential placental regulatory mechanism would be initiated by placental tissues sensing a reduction in utero–placental blood flow and/or substrate delivery, followed by production and release of a biochemical signal which suppresses growth long before transfer function becomes limiting. This biological strategy for growth regulation by reducing growth rate to match substrate availability is physiologically sound, is observed in post-natal life and assures the maintenance of a wide margin of safety between substrate availability and the demands of growth.

The possibility that this type of central substrate dependent growth regulating mechanism exists in the placenta is supported by several additional lines of experimental evidence. First, in the guinea pig vascular ligation model umbilical placental venous effluent from growth retarded fetuses contains a protein moiety which suppresses hepatocyte protein synthesis in culture as assessed by thymidine incorporation.[(7)] Additional *in vitro* experiments in the same model demonstrate the existence of a plasma factor in severely growth retarded fetuses which completely inhibits sulphation activity despite a several-fold elevation of plasma IGF-2 levels. Furthermore, the degree of inhibition of sulphation correlates directly with the magnitude of the morphometric growth restriction over a wide range of less severely growth retarded fetuses.[(29)] Similar data have recently been obtained in the growth retarded fetal sheep carunculectomy model[(31)] indicating that these findings are not species specific. Hormonal profiles in the embolisation model also suggest that the pattern of placental progesterone production and release are modified and the change is temporally related to documented changes in the regional distribution of placental flows.[(31)] This group of observations is certainly consistent with a regulatory role for the placenta. Second, the variability in fetal growth rate that is superimposed on the variability in initial placental growth in control, nutritionally deprived and embolisation models,[(19,22,26)] coupled with the responses in growth factors in the fetal circulation following acute reductions of uteroplacental perfusion,[(29,30)] indicates that the placenta must have a central role in the regulatory process. Finally, the observation that the embolically induced reductions in placental and fetal weight can be entirely prevented by improving substrate availability from the fetal side intravenously but not intragastrically,[(20,21)] argues that a deficiency in placental substrate availability may well be the initiator of the process.

Thus a large body of evidence supports the concept that the initial process of placentation itself, coupled with a primary placental response to superimposed chronic reductions in utero–placental blood flow, regulates fetal growth rate. In addition, its own morphometric response to a diminution in utero–placental blood flow indicates that the same mechanism also autoregulates its own size.

SUMMARY

The experimental data currently available in a variety of flow reduction animal models indicates that both placental and fetal size are limited by the rate of utero–placental blood flow. Furthermore growth rate appears to be quite sensitive to this stimulus, as minor reductions in flow restrict growth with no evidence of metabolic compromise. This sensitivity of growth to the substrate supply available has obvious survival value. The similarity of the morphometric response and its timing across models, coupled with a commonality in time-linked functional responses, point to the placenta as the likely site of growth regulation. A probable mechanism, supported by a wide variety of data, is that a decrease in placental perfusion and/or substrate delivery induces the placental release of one or more peptide moieties which inhibit the effect of multiple growth factors and thereby suppress the rate of fetal and placental growth.

ACKNOWLEDGEMENTS

Portions of this work were supported by United States Public Health Service grants RO1 11122 and K04 00213.

REFERENCES

1. Alexander G, Hales JRS, Stevens D, Donnelly JB. Effects of acute and prolonged exposure to heat on regional blood flows in pregnant sheep. *J Dev Physiol* 1987; **9**: 1–15.
2. Rosenfeld CR, Barton MD, Meschia G. Effects of epinephrine on distribution of uterine blood flow in the pregnant ewe. *Am J Obstet Gynecol* 1976; **124**: 156–163.
3. Clapp JF. Effect of epinephrine infusion on maternal and uterine oxygen uptake in the pregnant ewe. *Am J Obstet Gynecol* 1979; **133**: 208–212.
4. Morriss FH, Rosenfeld CR, Crandell SS, Adcock EW. Effects of fasting on uterine blood flow and substrate uptake in sheep. *J Nutr* 1980; **110**: 2433–2443.
5. Jacobs R, Robinson JS, Owens JA, Falconer J, Webster MED. The effect of prolonged hypobaric hypoxia on growth of fetal sheep. *J Dev Physiol* 1988; **10**: 97–112.
6. Wigglesworth JS. Experimental growth retardation in the foetal rat. *J Pathol Bacteriol* 1964; **88**: 1–13.
7. Jones CT. Reprogramming of metabolic development by restriction of fetal growth. *Biochem Soc Trans* 1985; **13**: 89–91.
8. Clark KE, Mack CE. A new model of growth retardation – fetal growth is blood flow dependent. *Proc Soc Gynecol Invest* 1986; Abst No. 137.
9. Gu W, Jones CT, Parer JT. Metabolic and cardiovascular effects on fetal sheep of sustained reduction of uterine blood flow. *J Physiol* 1985; **368**: 109–129.
10. Creasy RK, Barrett CK, De Swiet M, Kahanpaa KV, Rudolph AM. Experimental intrauterine growth retardation in the sheep. *Am J Obstet Gynecol* 1972; **112**: 566–573.
11. Clapp JF, McLaughlin MK, Larrow R, Farnham J, Mann LI. The uterine hemodynamic response to repetitive unilateral vascular embolization in the pregnant ewe. *Am J Obstet Gynecol* 1982; **82**: 309–318.

12. Owens JA, Falconer J, Robinson JS. Effect of restriction of placental growth on umbilical and uterine blood flows. *Am J Physiol* 1986; **250**: R427–R434.
13. Clapp JF. The relationship between blood flow and oxygen uptake in the uterine and umbilical circulations. *Am J Obstet Gynecol* 1978; **132**: 410–413.
14. Clapp JF. Placental bed blood flow in the pregnant ewe. In: *Placental Transfer*. Eds: GVP Chamberlain, AW Wilkenson. London: Pitman Medical, 1979; pp.60–75.
15. Skillman CA, Clarke KE. Fetal beta-endorphin levels in response to reductions in uterine blood flow. *Biol Neonate* 1987; **51**: 217–223.
16. Alexander G, Williams D. Heat stress and the development of the conceptus in domestic sheep. *J Agric Sci Camb* 1971; **76**: 53–72.
17. Reynolds LP, Ferrell CL, Nienaber JA. Effects of chronic environmental heat stress on blood flow and nutrient uptake of the gravid bovine uterus and foetus. *J Agric Sci Camb* 1985; **104**: 289–297.
18. Bell AW, Wilkening RB, Meschia G. Some aspects of placental function in chronically heat-stressed ewes. *J Dev Physiol* 1987; **9**: 17–29.
19. Mellor D. Nutritional and placental determinants of foetal growth rate in sheep and consequences for the newborn lamb. *Br Vet J* 1983; **139**: 307–324.
20. Charlton V, Johengen M. Effect of intrauterine nutritional supplementation on fetal growth retardation. *Biol Neonate* 1985; **48**: 125–142.
21. Charlton V, Johengen M. Fetal intravenous nutritional supplementation ameliorates the development of embolization-induced growth retardation in sheep. *Pediatr Res* 1987; **22**: 55–61.
22. Clapp JF, Larrow R, Hewitt J, Mann LI. Fetoplacental morphometric correlates in intrauterine growth retardation. *Proc Soc Gynecol Invest* 1982; Abst No. 159.
23. Harding JE, Jones CT, Robinson JS. Studies on experimental growth retardation in sheep. The effects of a small placenta in restricting transport to and growth of the fetus. *J Dev Physiol* 1985; **7**: 427–442.
24. Robinson JS, Kingston JE, Jones CT, Thorburn GD. Studies on experimental growth retardation in sheep. The effect of removal of endometrial caruncles on fetal size and metabolism. *J Dev Physiol* 1979; **1**: 379–398.
25. Robinson JS, Falconer J, Owens JA. Intrauterine growth retardation: clinical and experimental. *Acta Paediatr Scand* (suppl) 1985; **319**: 135–142.
26. Clapp JF, Szeto HH, Larrow R, Hewitt J, Mann LI. Umbilical blood flow response to embolization of the uterine circulation. *Am J Obstet Gynecol* 1980; **138**: 60–67.
27. Clapp JF, Szeto HH, Larrow R, Hewitt J, Mann LI. Fetal metabolic response to experimental placental vascular damage. *Am J Obstet Gynecol* 1981; **140**: 446–451.
28. Clapp JF, McLaughlin MK, Larrow R, Farnham J, Mann LI. Perfusion balance in the ovine placenta following embolic damage. *Proc Soc Gynecol Invest* 1982; Abst No. 305.
29. Jones CT, Lafeber HN, Price DA, Parer JT. Studies on the growth of the fetal guinea pig. Effects of reduction in uterine blood flow on plasma sulphation-

promoting activity and on the concentration of insulin-like growth factors-I and-II. *J Dev Physiol* 1987; **9**: 181–201.

30. Jones CT, Gu W, Harding JE, Price DA, Parer JT. Studies on the growth of the fetal sheep. Effects of surgical reduction in placental size, or experimental manipulation of uterine blood flow on plasma sulphation activity and on the concentration of insulin–like growth factors-I and-II. *J Dev Physiol* 1988; **10**: 179–189.
31. Clapp JF, Auletta FJ, Farnham J, Larrow R, Mann LI. The ovine fetoplacental endocrine response to placental damage. *Am J Obstet Gynecol* 1982; **144**: 47–54.

Discussion

Chairman: Dr M.J. Whittle

HAY: I must take issue with the point that you made about fetal growth being flow limited. I do not think that you have shown that at all. The model that you used is one that reduces the size of the placenta. You lose the functioning surface area, and that is quite different from reducing blood flow. While blood flow is reduced at the same time it is quite a different thing to restricting blood flow to a fully functioning organ across which substances are transported either by flow limited clearance, diffusional processes or by diffusion limited processes. My understanding of reducing blood flow with a fully functioning placenta, whether this is done acutely or chronically in the instrumented animal at least, is that you need sustained reductions of over 50% from control before you see any reduction in a flow limited substance, and even further in diffusion limited substances. That is quite different from restricting the size of the placenta where you could imagine a reduction in diffusional limited substances that is proportional to the loss of placenta. That is why you might see these differences in substrate versus oxygen.

CLAPP: You are certainly right in terms of the embolisation model. However, Ken Clark (personal communication) in the vascular occlusion model where he reduces uterine blood flow chronically over time by both 20% and 40%, has virtually identical findings to ours in the embolisation model. He has small placentas, small fetuses, no change in blood gases and reduced substrate uptakes that are very equivalent. That is the only other model that has been studied longitudinally; all the other models have been studied long after the growth retardation has been well established, at near term, at a time when the pO_2 is down. I think that his group of animals really makes the case strongly for the cascade of flow or substrate delivery at the placental side being an initial stimulus that triggers the placental response that then inhibits growth very early on. I cannot give you any other data because there are no other longitudinal data dealing with the issue. The relationship between flow and placental size is inescapable, and the symmetry of growth reduction between the placenta and fetus is the same until one gets to extremes of growth as one does especially in heat stress models. My second point is about pulling out the stops in terms of reserve functional capacity in the placenta in a variety of ways whether it be lipolysis, steroidogenesis or others.

HAY: What you have said confirms my point that a small placenta, regardless of how it is produced, transports less nutrients. That is different from saying that a flow reduction has selected properties....

CLAPP: What I said was that a flow reduction has a primary effect on placental growth and that placental growth change is signalled rapidly by the placenta to cause an equal reduction in growth of the fetus very early on in the process. So the balance between profusion of supply/delivery is a demand-regulated system as opposed to a supply-regulated system much like you would see after birth with nutritional deprivation.

CAMPBELL: I was trying to work out why a fall of pO_2 is a relatively late phenomenon in your model in the fetus. I wondered whether you could replicate the kind of changes that occur in the placental villi in human pregnancy. For instance, when there is impaired uterine perfusion of the intervillous space there is perivillous fibrin deposition, loss of villi, failure of tertiary stem villus formation and loss of small arterioles in the tertiary stem villi.

CLAPP: As far as I know that has only been shown in one study.(1) Two other people have been unable to confirm that (unpublished data).

CAMPBELL: No, these are well defined, well described changes in the villi.

CLAPP: But in terms of actually looking at flow Doppler-derived information versus actual morphometric study, as far as I know, the only group has been Truninger's group.(1)

CAMPBELL: I am not talking about Doppler. These are well described changes in the villi described by Fox(2) along with several other people. These are changes in the villi in response to poor perfusion on the maternal side. Am I saying something heretical?

CLAPP: When this data has been examined critically it is clear that the morphometric studies show a defined relationship between a variety of placental morphometric parameters and fetal growth, that is true. But the issue has always been that those things are there in placentae anyway. Perhaps as with the sheep, with the human there is a critical volume of functional placental tissue that is necessary to sustain adequate growth. You have to have enough damage to get beyond that point before you see much of anything.

CAMPBELL: Do you get infarctions?

CLAPP: Oh yes.

HAY: Perhaps you could tell us from Dr Clark's work where the sheep's placenta is actually decreasing in weight during the period of study? It is certainly not growing all that much.

CLAPP: That is right.

HAY: If Clark sees a change it must be degenerative rather than a restriction in growth. I am wondering if that ties in with what Professor Campbell is trying to get at, that is that we see a comparable picture in the human. He is making the inference that this is a degenerative change that is a result of poor flow.

CLAPP: I see in the heat stress model, in the vascular reduction model that Clark used and in the nutritional stress model, the evidence is very strong. When one looks at these placentae versus the placentae of simultaneously studied control animals there is no escaping the conclusion that there is degeneration. The stimuli are all adminstered after the time of peak growth and the placental weights at term parallel the reduction in flow at term.

CAMPBELL: Why does the trophoblast produce more progesterone? Is this not compensatory?

CLAPP: I think that this is a flow regulatory associated phenomenon that we are looking into, but I do not know why. I look at that as one of many signals, many of which are unidentified to date. Probably that is a very unimportant one; I am just using it as an example of a concept of placental signalling being the primary regulator of the slowing or the suppression or down-regulation of fetal growth processes in a way that allows fetal survival.

SNOW: In rodents there has been a longstanding association between placental and fetal growth. That has been correlated in the mouse with blood flow through the uterus. The story in rodents does not really seem to hold up because if you look at the fetal weight distribution which is characteristic in the rat, it does not mimic that in the mouse. Yet the blood flow through the uterus is the same. If the fetal weights in those two species were related to blood flow characteristics, then you have to assume that there are other factors involved. As I recall Bob Brent and colleagues did vascular clamping experiments in the rat in an attempt to dissect out this haemodynamic theory of fetal growth, without a great deal of success. He found that in order to get an effect on fetal growth he had to restrict blood flow very significantly and for very long periods of time.

WIGGLESWORTH: I thought they originally used very short periods of clamping. They found that they got an excessive retardation over any other effect.

SNOW: That was the inital study, but there have been two follow up studies in the late seventies which monitored the rate of flow over much longer periods than 20 minutes to try and see where the cut off levels of impact on fetal growth actually came in. The restriction that was required was very significant and I do not know whether they got data which would allow them to say whether there was a proportional decrease in fetal weight once one had passed a critical flow restriction.

CLAPP: I think that Professor Wigglesworth's initial work showed the same relationship between fetal weight and placental weight. I know in species like the pig that this is very well defined. There is a very tight relationship between placenta size and fetal weight. If you look at the position in the horn and at the localised placental perfusion issue I think that holds up. There is data in the guinea pig from Colorado which says the same thing; the big placenta gets the big blood flow and grows the big fetus.

HAY: Yes, but what came first?

CLAPP: That is why a longitudinal study is important and looking at it on a daily basis is important. Unfortunately, there is not enough of that information in other models.

SNOW: Let us go back to the rodent for a minute, which I know is far removed from humans, and look at the tight correlation between fetal weight and placental weight which exists in the mouse. In experiments which we have done in the lab to try and push up early fetal weight by reducing litter size we cannot make any impact at all on fetal weight up to about 15 or 16 days. In the rodent system the fetal overgrowth that you get which is associated with placental size and reduced litter size is a late phenomenon.

MILNER: What we have just heard helps to reconcile the experimental observation that was made by de Prins(3) in collaboration with us, and which has only very recently been published although the experiments were carried out some three years ago. De Prins was interested in using a rat model to study the effects of maternal hyperalimentation to correct fetal undergrowth. He then went on to use the Wigglesworth classical model to produce fetal undergrowth and hyperalimented the test mothers by gavage. He did not improve the growth of the growth retarded fetuses in the ligated horn, but he significantly reduced fetal mortality in that horn. In light of what we have heard this morning, what previously had been a total puzzle to me might have some functional significance.

CAMPBELL: You measured both volume flow and vascular resistance. What was the relationship between these two parameters?

CLAPP: Resistance is a calculated number from pressure gradient and flow, and the pressure gradient did not change. As flow fell resistance went up. We also looked at the systolic/diastolic (S/D) ratios on the umbilical circulations both with the Doppler and with the flow probe, and we see absolutely no change in S/D ratio in these animals. If we embolise the umbilical side of the circulation and give an excess of 120 million spheres acutely we can produce a change in the S/D ratio, but that is only when resistance is so high that it is unbelievable. I think part of the difference may be whether or not one has diffuse versus non-diffuse placental damage. When you get up around 100 million spheres you can see a transient change in the S/D ratio, then everything goes back to normal. But we have not been able to see a change in the S/D ratio even late in the process of growth retardation in the embolisation model, even when the pO_2 is down.

WHITTLE: We have heard a wealth of information from some reknowned experts and talked about the environmental factors that are involved in growth. It occurs to me that it might be the ability of the baby, and perhaps the placenta, to adjust its growth potential to what is available in terms of substrate supply and indeed oxygen. It may be that which tells us whether it is going to survive or not.

REFERENCES

1. Trudinger BJ, Giles WB, Cook CM. Fetoplacental blood flow resistance and placental microvascular anatomy: a Doppler ultrasound – pathological correlation. *J Ultrasound Med* 1983; **2:** 59–78.
2. Fox H. *Pathology of the Placenta*. London, Philadelphia: EB Saunders, 1978.
3. De Prins F, Hill DJ, Milner RDG, Van Assche A. Effect of maternal hyperalimentation on intrauterine growth retardation. *Arch Dis Child* 1988; **63**: 733–736.

SECTION 5

CLINICAL IMPLICATIONS OF FETAL UNDERGROWTH

The detection of intrauterine growth retardation

Professor S. Campbell

The terms "small for gestational age" (SGA) and "intrauterine growth retardation" (IUGR) are firmly fixed in the vocabulary of perinatal medicine. Both are ill-defined and are often used as synonymous terms.[1,2] This should not be so. SGA merely indicates that a fetus or neonate is below a defined reference range of size or weight for a gestational age; IUGR indicates that a pathological process is operating to modify the growth potential of the fetus by reducing its growth rate.

This is an important distinction for two reasons: i) many SGA fetuses do not suffer from IUGR, but are small because of perfectly normal genetic influences; ii) many IUGR fetuses are not SGA e.g. a fetus with a growth potential that will result in a birthweight of 4 kg at term could receive less than the optimal growth support from the mother and be only 3 kg. This birthweight would fall outside any definition of SGA but the fetus would be more at risk than most SGA fetuses.

DETECTION OF THE SGA FETUS

On the premise that most IUGR fetuses are SGA, most antenatal screening programmes for IUGR judge their efficacy on the ability to predict the birthweight of an infant which is on or below the 5th centile birthweight for gestation or, alternatively, below 2 standard deviations (SD) (approximately 3rd centile) of the mean birthweight for gestation. The 10th centile limit is also commonly used but it is likely that with this definition the growth retarded population is being diluted by a large number of normally nourished babies.[3]

The detection of an SGA infant contains two elements: firstly, the accurate assessment of gestational age and secondly the recognition of fetal smallness. Any method of detection must apply to the whole obstetric population for it would be impossible to identify the majority of SGA infants on the basis of risk factors.[4]

Gestational age

Routine ultrasound dating is now widely regarded as a prerequisite for optimal detection of the SGA fetus. Predictions are made by comparing an ultrasound fetal measurement with the mean growth line for the appropriate reference range, reading off a gestational age and calculating an ultrasound expected date for delivery (EDD). The ultrasound prediction will be more accurate than an optimal last menstrual period as long as the scatter about the mean caused by the variation in fetal growth rate is less than that caused by variations in the length of the follicular phase of the menstrual cycle.[5] Thus, the earlier in gestation the measurement is made the better should be the prediction of gestational age. The fetal measurement has also to be highly reproducible and before 20 weeks; reproducibility appears to be more important than timing in terms of reliable predictions. For example, the biparietal diameter (BPD) between 12–18 weeks has been shown to be a better predictor than the crown-rump length measurement taken between 6 and 12 weeks.[6] Originally, predictions were made from the biparietal diameter,[7] but a wide variety of parameters have been used such as the head circumference, femur length, abdominal circumference, the inter-orbital diameter, the foot length and the first trimester crown-rump length.[8–13] The biparietal diameter is still the most commonly used parameter, probably because it is the most easily obtained and reproducible measurement. Two studies have demonstrated the superiority of early BPD dating when compared to predictions made from an optimal last menstrual period. The first[6] compared the predictions of an expected date of confinement (EDC) from Naegele's formula, based on a certain LMP against those based on BPD measurements made after 12 weeks' gestation. Only pregnancies that ended in spontaneous labour with the delivery of a mature infant were considered. The measurement of the BPD between 12 and 18 weeks was superior to an optimal menstrual cycle in predicting the date of delivery ($p < 0.001$); 89.4% delivered within 2 weeks of the BPD prediction; the figure for certain dates was 85%. The second study[14] compared several ultrasound measurements and also a certain LMP as a means of predicting a Dubowitz score shortly after delivery. Between 18 and 23 weeks (the earliest time at which measurements were made) the biparietal diameter was the single most accurate ultrasound parameter and both the mean and random errors were significantly less than those associated with last menstrual period (LMP) predictions.

There is thus good evidence to indicate that routine ultrasound dating between 12 and 23 weeks' gestation is more effective than gestational age assessment based on the last menstrual period and thus should be part of an SGA screening programme.

Size

Obstetricians and midwives screen patients for the SGA fetus at each antenatal visit by palpation of the uterine size. This method is known to be inaccurate[15] and results in detection of only approximately one-third of cases[16] with a 60% false positive rate. For this reason, ultrasound measurements have been investigated extensively as a means of improving the detection rate for the SGA fetus. The most commonly measured fetal dimensions are the BPD, head circumference, abdomen circumference and femur length. All studies show that the abdominal circumference is the single most effective parameter for predicting fetal weight, for it is reduced in both symmetrical and asymmetrical types of IUGR. Head measurements and femur length are often unaffected in asymmetric IUGR.[17,18] Campbell and Wilkin[19] demonstrated that there was a constant percentage error in predictions made from the abdominal circumference throughout the birthweight range, the 95% confidence limits being ± 16% of the actual birthweight. Subsequent studies[20,21] showed that formulae incorporating the abdominal circumference with other parameters, such as the biparietal diameter, reduce the random variation of the predictions. One of the most elegant studies was that of Hadlock *et al.*[22] who used several regression models incorporating all the commonly used fetal measurement parameters. As can be seen from Table 1, with the addition of biparietal

Table 1. Mean and random errors in the estimation of fetal weight by regression models incorporating the abdominal circumference alone and in combination with other fetal parameters.

Parameter	Mean Deviation	± SD%
AC	0.6	± 11.1
AC : BPD	0.4	± 9.1
AC : HC	0.4	± 9.1
AC : FL	0.3	± 8.2
AC: BPD : FL	0.3	± 7.7
AC : HC : FL	0.3	± 7.6
AC: BPD : HC: FL	0.3	±7.5

AC = abdominal circumference.
BPD = biparietal diameter.
HC = head circumference.
FL = femur length.
(Reference 22, with permission)

Table 2. Comparison between Serial Symphysis – fundal weight measurements and a single ultrasound measurement of the fetal abdominal circumference at 34 or 36 weeks' gestation in the detection of the SGA infant.

Measurement	Sensitivity %	Specificity %	Predictive value positive %	Predictive value negative %
SFH	76	79	36	95
AC	83	79	39	87

SFH = symphysis fundal height measurement
AC = abdominal circumference measurement
(Reference 26, with permission)

diameter, head circumference, femur length and combinations of these parameters to the abdominal circumference (AC) measurement, the mean deviation was reduced from 0.6% to 0.3% and the random variation from 11.1% to 7.5% per standard deviation of the actual birthweight.

There is a large number of publications(23-25) designed to test the effectiveness of these measuring techniques in screening out the SGA fetus in unselected populations. Comparison is difficult due to the large number of variables that can affect the result. For example, the sensitivity, specificity and predictive value can be affected by the gestation at assessment, the prevalence of SGA in the population, the cut-off point for a positive diagnosis and other more subtle variables such as the experience of the operators and the quality of the equipment. However, the following overall conclusions can be drawn: i) abdomen circumference is the best predictor, and the addition of other measurement variables does not seem to improve significantly the sensitivity; ii) even with a cut-off point as high as the 25th centile, sensitivities are disappointingly low, in the region of 60% to 85%; iii) the closer the measurement is made to the time of delivery, the better the detection rate for the SGA fetus; iv) due to the low prevelance of the condition, predictive values are low, in the region of 20% to 40%.

In the light of these generally poor results for the ultrasound detection of the SGA fetus, Pearce and Campbell(26) carried out a comparison between the clinical efficacy of a single AC measurement made at either 34 or 36 weeks with serial measurements of the symphysis fundal height (SFH) for the detection of the SGA infant. To make the tests comparable, the lower cut-off point of the AC measurement was altered until the specificity matched that of the SFH. All patients had early ultrasound confirmation of the gestational age. The results are summarised in Table 2.

Although the sensitivity of the AC measurement was slightly better than that of the SFH measurement, this was not statistically significant. Each test had a high false positive rate and a low predictive value. Screening with both tests improved the sensitivity to 93% but as expected decreased the specificity to 67% and the positive predictive value to 32%.

In summary, both ultrasound and clinical methods of screening for the SGA fetus are far from ideal. However, the combination of a single third trimester AC measurement and serial SFH measurements would seem to be the best option. For a screening test, a high sensitivity is essential and subsequent detailed diagnostic tests for IUGR (*vide infra*) will hopefully identify the small group of pregnancies that are at risk.

DETECTION OF IUGR: REDUCED GROWTH POTENTIAL

Altered genetic potential

When an SGA fetus is suspected it is important to know whether there is a structural abnormality or karyotypic defect, both of which can cause IUGR. A detailed ultrasound scan at 18 weeks should be performed on all pregnancies(27) and should recognise the majority of structural abnormalities. Cordocentesis or late placental biopsy and rapid karotyping will reveal if there is a chromosomal abnormality.

In a series of 263 severely SGA fetuses (i.e. fetal abdominal circumference below the 3rd centile for gestation) where karotyping was performed in our unit, chromosomal abnormalities were found in 42 (16%). These included triploidy (19 cases), trisomies (11 cases), and deletions or translocations (12 cases). The triploidies were most commonly encountered in the second trimester while the aneuploidies, deletions and translocations were found in the third trimester group of fetuses. These findings suggest that triploidy is associated with the most severe form of early onset growth retardation and that the majority of affected fetuses die before the third trimester of pregnancy. Sixteen of the triploid fetuses were found to have severe asymmetrical IUGR with a very high head to abdomen circumference ratio, and although most of the fetuses were hypoxic the degree of asymmetry was significantly greater than that expected from the degree of hypoxia.

Uteroplacental insufficiency

Placental failure to support fetal growth results in reduced placental transfer of oxygen leading to reduced pO_2 levels in the fetus.[28,29] Subsequently, there is failure to excrete CO_2 and lactate, resulting in progressive respiratory and metabolic acidosis. A fall in fetal pO_2 is almost certainly an early event and if this diagnosis is made antenatally, it is useful to call such a situation hypoxic intrauterine growth retardation. There are now a large number of antenatal investigations designed to recognise these events.

Serial measurements

Serial measurements, if they show severe reduction or cessation of growth, are diagnostic of IUGR. For example, the late flattening growth retardation pattern[30] is clearly diagnostic of a pathological process. However, even in the most obsessional hands, the reproducibility of head circumference and abdomen circumference measurements would not allow a definitive diagnosis of cessation of growth in less than two weeks and a more realistic time span would be four weeks.[3] This limits the usefulness of serial measurements in severe cases of IUGR where early diagnosis is required.

Head/abdomen ratio and ponderal index

Placental failure results in asymmetrical growth retardation due to the preferential redistribution of blood to the fetal brain at the expense of the liver, kidneys and other abdominal viscera as a response to hypoxia. This occurs even before there is a demonstrable fall in fetal pO_2 in the umbilical venous blood. The head/abdomen circumference ratio[17] was introduced to try to distinguish the wasted hypoxic IUGR fetus from the fetus which is symmetrically small but normally nourished. This ratio has proved to be a useful but not infallible method of identifying the wasted IUGR fetus. This is especially true with early onset (second trimester) IUGR for two reasons. Firstly, it is possible to have symmetrical IUGR associated with severe uteroplacental insufficiency due possibly to delay in blood flow redistribution as a result of chemoreceptor insensitivity. Secondly, as stated above, severe asymmetrical IUGR can be associated with triploidy with or without significant fetal hypoxaemia.

The neonatal ponderal index (weight in grams divided by length in cm^3 x 100) is accepted as a reliable method of distinguishing the symmetrical from the asymmetrical growth retarded infant.(32) Vintzileos *et al.*(32) have found that there is a good correlation between the fetal femur length and the neonatal crown/heel (fetal length = 6.18 + 5.9 x the femur length) and have thus calculated an intrauterine fetal ponderal index. The sensitivity of this index for predicting an abnormal neonatal ponderal index was 77% with a specificity of 87%. It is possible that a combination of the head/abdomen circumference ratio and the fetal ponderal index may be more useful in identifying asymmetrical growth retardation.

Amniotic fluid volume

Reduction in amniotic fluid volume is widely recognised to be associated with asymmetric IUGR. This is almost certainly due to a reduction in renal blood flow as part of the circulatory redistribution with fetal hypoxia. Accurate quantification by ultrasound is clearly difficult as amniotic fluid is collected in a multitude of pockets surrounding the fetal shape. Manning *et al*(33) describe a "qualitative technique" in which oligohydramnios is diagnosed when the maximal amniotic fluid pool is less than 1 cm in its broadest diameter (subsequently amended to vertical diameter). They found a high association between this qualitative definition of oligohydramnios and IUGR, fetal distress in labour and perinatal death.(34) These findings prompted their inclusion of amniotic fluid measurement in the biophysical profile.(36) Others(37) have not been able to substantiate these findings and Hoddick *et al.* have found "the 1 cm sign" was present in only 4% of SGA pregnancies.(35) While many of these pregnancies were probably not associated with IUGR, this does seem a rather low sensitivity and suggests that methodological problems might be at the root of these disparate results. Many workers recognise that isolated pockets of greater than 1 cm or even 2 cm exist when there is a generalised reduction of amniotic fluid. Furthermore, sometimes a "pool" greater than 2 cm can be occupied by loops of cord which in the obese patient are difficult to see. We have not been able to identify a correlation between qualitative measurements of amniotic fluid volume and fetal hypoxia as diagnosed by cordocentesis (Nicolaides, personal communication). Thus, oligohydramnios as diagnosed by the Manning method should not be taken seriously.

Fetal urinary production rate

Measurement of the fetal bladder in three dimensions allows its volume to be calculated.(36) Fetal urinary production rates are calculated by taking serial bladder volume measurements during the filling phase and calculating the hourly rate of increase (HFUPR).(37) The original normal values for HFUPR during gestation have now been revised upwards (Rabinowitz, personal communication) using real-time ultrasound to obtain measurements at 2–5 minute intervals. There is a strong correlation between HFUPR rates and fetal pO_2 levels in umbilical venous blood obtained by cordocentesis (Nicolaides, personal communication). Thus, HFUPR measurements appear to be a more sensitive indicator of hypoxic IUGR than amniotic fluid volume measurements. Although previously regarded as being impractical, HFUPR measurements should be re-evaluated in view of the ease with which such measurements can be made with real-time ultrasound and the newly recognised shorter bladder cycle which makes a diagnosis possible in 15 minutes.

Biophysical profile

This is now the most commonly used test for the antenatal detection of fetal hypoxia in the USA and is fully discussed elsewhere in this volume. There is little doubt that the test is excellent in identifying the non-hypoxic SGA fetus, but when the test is equivocal or abnormal it can be a time consuming exercise making a definitive diagnosis of hypoxic IUGR.(38) For this reason, in the UK the test is usually condensed to an assessment of two variables: amniotic fluid volume and antepartum cardiotocograph (CTG).

We have looked at the ability of the antepartum CTG (performed immediately before cordocentesis) to predict the blood pO_2 and pH in SGA fetuses at 27–38 weeks' gestation. Preliminary results indicate that moderate to severe fetal hypoxia or acidosis are associated with changes in fetal heart rate patterns, but in milder degrees of hypoxia the fetal heart rate pattern is normal.

Doppler studies

The principles and clinical application of Doppler examination in pregnancy is described elsewhere in this volume. Simple continuous wave Doppler equipment can be used to measure flow impedence in the uterine(39) and umbilical arteries.(40) The test has several advantages: it uses inexpensive mobile equipment, the technique is quickly learned and the examination time for this technique is usually less than 15 minutes. Failure of trophoblast invasion will result in high impedence waveforms in the uterine artery as early as 16–18 weeks' gestation and studies at this time have been used to predict intrauterine growth retardation and pregnancy-induced hypertension.(41) Absence of end-diastolic velocities in the umbilical artery correlate well with fetal hypoxaemia and acidaemia in umbilical venous blood samples obtained by cordocentesis.(42) We have previously described the biometric changes in asymmetrical IUGR which are due to a redistribution of the fetal circulation in response to hypoxia. It is now possible to measure this redistribution by pulsed Doppler examination of the fetal circulation by comparing the blood velocity and flow impedence in the common carotid artery supplying the brain with the same parameters in the thoracic aorta supplying the abdominal viscera and placenta. We have carried out a Doppler study of the fetal and uteroplacental circulations in 41 pregnant women with SGA fetuses and 10 with appropriate for gestational age (AGA) fetuses between 19 and 37 weeks' gestation. Blood gases and pH measured in umbilical venous samples within one hour of the Doppler examination were correlated individually and as an "asphyxia index" to the Doppler and ultrasound biometric measurements. The ranking order of these variables in their ability to predict the asphyxia index is shown in Table 3. The best predictor of asphyxia was an index comprising the aortic mean velocity and the common carotid artery pulsatility index. When this index was abnormal, 89% of fetuses had an asphyxia index one standard deviation above the mean and 60% two standard deviations above the mean. A normal index was always associated with normal blood gases. Thus, Doppler examination of the fetal circulation appears to be a sensitive indicator of the chemoreceptor response to falling pO_2 values and probably gives the earliest warning of hypoxic intrauterine growth retardation. It also suggests that alterations in the fetal circulation probably occur before there are gross changes in fetal pO_2, thus explaining why asymmetric IUGR can exist in the presence of apparently normal pO_2 values.

Table 3. Prediction of asphyxia index from individual variables (n = 50).

	Res SD	R
Carotid PI/aortic V Mean Score	18.66	0.67
Carotid/aortic Δ V Mean	19.03	0.68
Carotid/aortic Δ PI	19.35	0.66
Aortic Δ V Mean	19.74	0.62
Aortic Δ PI	19.98	−0.61
Carotid Δ PI	20.20	0.60
Aortic EDF (absent)	20.22	−0.60
Umbilical artery Δ PI	21.07	0.54
Umbilical artery EDF (absent)	21.26	0.54
Δ Abdominal circumference	22.12	0.48
Utero-placental RI	22.36	−0.48
Δ Head circumference	22.85	0.44
Δ Carotid V Mean	22.96	0.43
Head/abdomen circumference ratio	23.64	−0.36

Res SD= Residual standard deviation
R= Correlation coefficient
PI = pulsatility index
V Mean = Time averaged mean blood velocity
Δ = Corrected for gestational age
EDI = end-diastolic frequencies
Asphyxia index = $\Delta pO_2 + 1.43 (\Delta pCO_2) - 180.2 (\Delta pH)$

Cordocentesis

This test provides samples of umbilical venous or arterial blood for detailed analysis and thus permits the most precise diagnosis of hypoxic IUGR. It is also the least expensive method, requiring only a 20 gauge spinal needle in addition to the standard ultrasound equipment. The procedure requires great skill and expertise, and has a small procedure-related mortality (less than 1%), so should only be used when there is a substantial risk of karyotype abnormality or when precise knowledge of blood gases and acid-base states is necessary to determine management of the pregnancy.[28,29]

CONCLUSION

Identification of IUGR at the present time is an inexact science. It involves fetal biometry to determine whether the fetus is SGA and then a series of biophysical tests to identify those fetuses which are growth retarded. Although it is an invasive procedure, cordocentesis and fetal blood analysis has emerged as a very important step in the diagnostic process. Firstly, it is justified when severe SGA is diagnosed to identify a possible karyotypic cause for IUGR. Secondly, by permitting measurement of blood gases and acid-base status, it provides the gold standard against which to assess the statistical and clinical effectiveness of the large range of second line diagnostic tests. Most of these tests assess the effects of hypoxia on fetal behavioural states and cardiovascular system. In the future, it is likely that IUGR will be diagnosed directly by investigations targeted to identify the pathophysiological processes involved in IUGR. The early identification of resistance to flow in the uterine artery is a promising example of this new approach. It is on this basis that therapeutic regimes can be properly established.

REFERENCES

1. Johnson MP, Evans MI. Intra-uterine growth retardation; pathophysiology and possibilities for intra-uterine treatment. *Fetal Therapy* 1987; 2:109-122.
2. Mintz MC, Landon MB. Sonographic diagnosis of fetal growth disorders. *Clin Obstet Gynecol* 1988; **31:** 44-52.
3. Campbell S. Fetal growth. In: *Fetal Growth in Fetal Physiology and Medicine*. Eds. RW Beard, PW Nathanielsz. London: Saunders, 1976: pp.271-301.
4. Rosenberg K, Grant JM, Hepburn M. Antenatal detection of growth retardation: actual practice in a large maternity hospital. *Br J Obstet Gynaecol* 1982; **89**: 12-15.
5. Persson PH, Grennert L, Gennser G, Gullberg B. Normal range curves for the intrauterine growth of the biparietal diameter. *Acta Obstet Gynecol Scand, Supplement* 1978; **78:** 15-20.
6. Campbell S, Warsof SL, Little D, Cooper D. Routine ultrasound screening for the prediction of gestational age. *Obstet Gynecol* 1985; **65**:613-620.
7. Campbell S. The prediction of fetal maturity by ultrasonic measurement of the biparietal diameter. *J Obstet Gynaecol Br Commonw* 1969; **76**: 603-609.
8. Hadlock FB, Deter RL. Harrist RB, Park SK. Fetal head circumference: relation to menstrual age. *AJR* 1982; **138**: 649-653.
9. O'Brien GD, Queenan JT, Campbell S. Assessment of gestational age in the second trimester by real-time ultrasound measurement of the femur length. *Am J Obstet Gynecol* 1981; **139**: 540-545.
10. Hadlock FB, Deter RL, Harrist RB, Park SK. Fetal abdominal circumference

as a predictor of menstrual age. *AJR* 1982; **139**: 367-370.

11. Mayden K, Tortora M, Berkowitz RL, Bracken M, Hobbins JC. Orbital diameters: a new parameter for prenatal diagnosis and dating. *Am J Obstet Gynecol* 1982; **144**: 289-297.
12. Mercer BM, Sklar S, Shariatmadar A, Gillieson MS, D'Alton ME. Fetal foot length as a predictor of gestational age. *Am J Obstet Gynecol* 1987; **156**: 350-355.
13. Robinson HP, Fleming JE. A critical evaluation of sonar crown-rump length measurements. *Br J Obstet Gynaecol* 1975; **82**: 702-710.
14. Ott WJ. Accurate gestational dating. *Obstet Gynecol* 1985; **66**: 311-315.
15. Beazley JM, Underhill RA. Fallacy of the fundal height. *Br Med J* 1970; **4**: 404-406.
16. Hall MH, Chng PK, MacGillivray I. Is routine antenatal care worthwhile? *Lancet* 1980; **ii**: 78-80.
17. Campbell S, Thoms A. Ultrasound measurement of the fetal head to abdominal circumference ratio in the assessment of growth retardation. *Br J Obstet Gynaecol* 1977; **84**: 165-174.
18. Yagel S, Zacut D, Igelstein S, Palti Z, Hurwitz A, Rosenn B. In utero ponderal index as a prognostic factor in the evaluation of intrauterine growth retardation. *Am J Obstet Gynecol* 1987; **157**: 415-419.
19. Campbell S, Wilkin D. Ultrasonic measurement of fetal abdomen circumference in the estimation of fetal weight. *Br J Obstet Gynaecol* 1975; **82**: 689-697.
20. Warsof SL, Gohari P, Berkowitz RL, Hobbins JC. The estimation of fetal weight by computer assisted analysis. *Am J Obstet Gynecol* 1977; **128**: 881-892.
21. Shepard MJ, Richards VA, Berkowitz RL, Warsof SL, Hobbins JC. An evaluation of two equations for predicting fetal weight by ultrasound. *Am J Obstet Gynecol* 1982; **142**: 47-54.
22. Hadlock FP, Harrist RB, Carpenter RJ, Deter RL, Park SK. Sonographic estimation of fetal weight. The value of femur length in addition to head and abdomen measurements. *Radiology* 1984; **150**: 535-540.
23. Nielson JP, Whitfield CR, Aitcheson TC. Screening for the small for dates fetus: a two-stage ultrasound examination schedule. *Br Med* J 1980; **1**: 1203-1206.
24. Warsof SL, Cooper DJ, Little E, Campbell S. Routine ultrasound screening for antenatal detection of intrauterine growth retardation. *Obstet Gynecol* 1986; **67**: 33-39.
25. Ferrazzi E, Nicolini U, Kustermann A, Pardi G. Routine obstetric ultrasound: effectiveness of cross-sectional screening for fetal growth retardation. *JCU* 1986; **14**: 17-22.
26. Pearce MJ, Campbell S. A comparison of symphysis fundal height and ultrasound as screening tests for light for gestational age infants. *Br J Obstet Gynaecol* 1987; **94**: 100-104.
27. Campbell S, Smith P. Routine screening for congenital anomalies by ultra-

sound. In: *Prenatal Diagnosis*. Eds. CH Rodeck, KH Nicolaides. London: Royal College of Obstetricians and Gynaecologists, 1984: pp.325-330.

28. Soothill PW, Nicolaides KH, Rodeck CH, Campbell S. The effect of gestational age on fetal and intervillous blood gas and acid-base values in human pregnancy. *Fetal Therapy* 1986; **1**: 166-173.
29. Nicolaides KH, Economides DL, Soothill PW. Blood gases and pH in appropriate and small for gestational age fetuses. *Am J Obstet Gynecol* 1989; In press.
30. Campbell S. The assessment of fetal development by diagnostic ultrasound. *Clin Perinatol* 1974; **1**: 507.
31. Miller HC, Hassanein K. Diagnosis of impaired fetal growth in newborn infants. *Pediatrics* 1971; **48**: 511.
32. Vintzileos AM, Lodeiro JG, Feinstein SJ, Campbell WA, Weinbaum PJ, Nochimson DJ. The value of fetal ponderal index in predicting growth retardation. *Obstet Gynecol* 1986; **67**: 584-588.
33. Manning FA, Hill LM, Platt LD. Qualitative amniotic fluid determination by ultrasound: antepartum detection of intra-uterine growth retardation. *Am J Obstet Gynecol* 1981; **139**: 254-258.
34. Manning FA, Platt LD, Sipos L. Antepartum fetal evaluation: development of a fetal biophysical profile. *Am J Obstet Gynecol* 1980; **136**: 787-795.
35. Hoddick WK, Callen PW, Filly RA, Creasy RK. Ultrasonographic determination of qualitative amniotic fluid volume in intrauterine growth retardation: reassessment of the 1 cm rule. *Am J Obstet Gynecol* 1984; **149**: 758-762.
36. Campbell S, Wladimiroff JW, Dewhurst CJ. The antenatal measurement of fetal urine production. *J Obstet Gynaecol Br Commonw* 1973; **80**: 680-686.
37. Wladimiroff JW, Campbell S. Fetal urine production rates in normal and complicated pregnancy. *Lancet* 1974; **i**: 151-154.
38. Vintzileos AM, Campbell WA, Nochimson DJ, Weinbaum PW. The use and misuse of the fetal biophysical profile. *Am J Obstet Gynecol* 1987; **156**: 527-533.
39. Campbell S, Diaz-Recasens J, Griffin DR, Cohen-Overbeck TE, Pearce JM, Willson K. New Doppler technique for assessing uteroplacental blood flow. *Lancet* 1983; **i**: 675-677.
40. Trudinger BJ, Giles WB, Cook CM, Bombardieri J, Collins L. Fetal umbilical artery flow velocity waveforms and placental resistance: pathological correlation. *Br J Obstet Gynaecol* 1985; **92**: 23-30.
41. Campbell S, Pearce JM, Hackett G, Coen-Overbeek T, Hernandez C. Qualitative assessment of uteroplacental blood flow: early screening test for high risk pregnancies. *Obstet Gynecol* 1986; **68**: 649-653.
42. Nicolaides KH, Bilardo CM, Soothill PW, Campbell S. Absence of end diastolic frequencies in the umbilical artery: a sign of fetal hypoxia and acidosis. *Br Med J* 1988; **297**: 1026-1027.

Detection of fetal growth retardation by biochemical tests

Professor T. Chard and Dr R.J.S. Howell

In the late 1970s biochemical tests of fetal wellbeing or placental function tests (PFT) were among the most widely investigative tools in clinical obstetrics. Today they have been almost entirely abandoned: totally so in the US, to a lesser extent in Europe. Why is this, and do such tests have any remaining use or potential future application?

BIOCHEMICAL DETECTION OF FETAL GROWTH RETARDATION IN THE FIRST HALF OF PREGNANCY

Only one biochemical parameter measured in the first half of pregnancy has been shown to have a clear relationship to the delivered weight of the fetus in the second half of pregnancy: maternal serum alphafetoprotein (MSAFP). The evidence that MSAFP has predictive value in respect of "low birthweight" has been reviewed in detail by Chard and colleagues.[1] Numerous studies have shown a statistical association between low birthweight and elevated MSAFP. However, the association is weak, and at a clinical level the test is almost valueless. Thus, the test would miss five out of every six cases of low birthweight and there would be nine false positives for every case correctly identified.

BIOCHEMICAL DETECTION OF FETAL GROWTH RETARDATION IN THE SECOND HALF OF PREGNANCY

The biochemical detection of fetal growth retaraation in the second half of pregnancy depends upon the measurement in the mother of a range of fetoplacental materials which are either quantitatively or qualitatively specific to pregnancy. These materials have been classified into three groups according to a variety of clinical and biological criteria (Tables 1 and 2).

Table 1. A classification of placental products.

Group 1	Group 2	Group 3
Enzymes Steroids hCG, SP1	PP5 PAPP-A	PP12, PP14

N.B. PP12 and PP14 are products of the endometrium/decidua (i.e. maternal tissue) rather than the placenta (fetal tissue). Because these proteins were identified simultaneously by different groups, they also have a number of synonyms.

Table 2. Biological features of the three groups of placental and pregnancy-associated products

	Group 1	Group 2	Group 3
Source	Trophoblast	Trophoblast	Endometrium/decidua
Control mechanisms	Trophoblast mass and uteroplacental bloodflow	Trophoblast mass and uteroplacental bloodflow plus other factors	Placenta or ovarian steroids
Postulated functions	Hormone/enzymatic	Local (immune and coagulation systems)	Maternal response to pregnancy

GROUP 1 PRODUCTS

Group 1 includes most of the better known products of the human placenta (Tables 1 and 2). These materials serve no very obvious function in the pregnant woman;[2] indeed, a pregnancy can be entirely normal in those rare cases in which one or the other of these products is totally absent. The only exception would seem to be the luteotrophic action of hCG in early pregnancy, which is probably essential to the maintenance of the corpus luteum.

There are also no obvious feedback control mechanisms for Group 1 products. Indeed, it is likely that placental protein production is simply a function of the total mass of the trophoblast so that in the short term the main controlling factor is the rate of uteroplacental blood flow.[3] The reduction of fetoplacental products in the mother in complicated pregnancies could thus be the result of either changes in blood flow or damage to the trophoblast.

Clinical applications of Group 1 products

In the 1970s much of the literature on PFT consisted of argument as to the relative merits of one or the other of the Group 1 compounds. However, one hypothesis proposed that all tests were identical.[2] This was based on the fact that all products used as PFT are produced by the same tissue (the trophoblast), and all are apparently the subject of the same rather non-specific control mechanisms (trophoblast mass and uteroplacental blood flow). There is no subsequent evidence which would negate this hypothesis, particularly if a further caveat is added: 'providing the systems of measurement have similar analytical precision'.

Clinical practice now focuses on just two blood tests: human placental lactogen (hPL) and oestriol (E_3). The distinction between these at a clinical level is very marginal when they are compared by an appropriate study design.[4] There is no current evidence which suggests that any of the more recently discovered Group 1 products such as Schwangerschaftsprotein 1 (SP1) will show any advantage over the "classical" tests.[5]

There was at one time a belief that E_3 was the best test because its synthesis depends on fetal precursors; and that the best fluid in which to measure it should be urine because the latter integrates and thereby eliminates the time-to-time variation in circulating levels. The first belief is correct physiologically but irrelevant to clinical practice. Most of the pathology which underlies "fetal deprivation" originates in the placenta and not the fetus itself. Since the placental trophoblast carries out the final and rate-limiting step in oestriol synthesis, and also all steps of hPL synthesis, it is not surprising that the two compounds vary in parallel in the presence of fetal pathology.[4, 6] The second belief, that the variability can be reduced by a 24 h urine collection, is not supported by the only published investigation of this topic.[7] The argument that variability can be attributed to problems of sample collection simply reinforces the reasons why measurement of E_3 in urine has long since been rejected.

What does a Group 1 PFT predict?

PFT are still used in a fairly non-specific manner for the detection of "fetal deprivation". This condition has a number of different manifestations: growth failure,

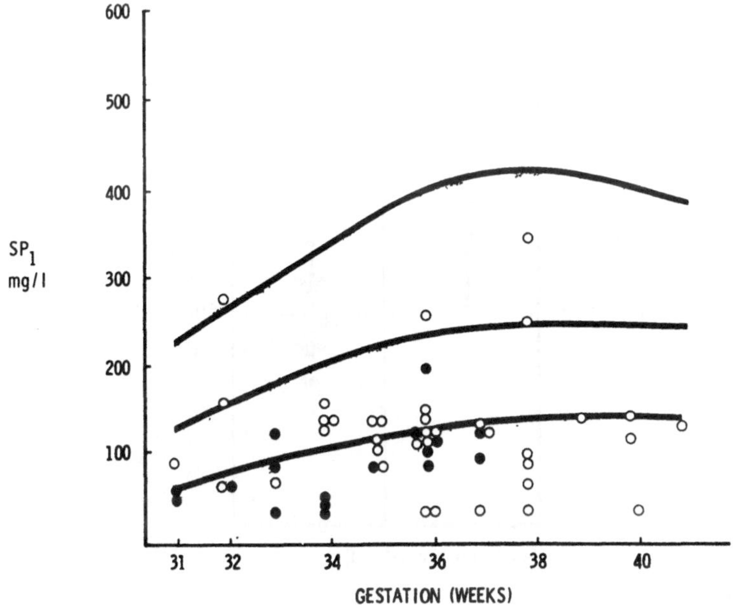

Figure I
Maternal serum SP1 levels in patients with (●) and without (○) hypertension in whom there was growth retardation of the fetus. The solid lines show the median and 10th and 90th centiles of the normal range.

fetal distress, brain damage and fetal death. All studies on PFT agree that low levels of Group 1 products are associated with fetal growth retardation (Figure I), and that abnormal results often precede fetal death.[8] What is less clear is whether PFT can predict acute events such as fetal distress during labour. The only study on PFT in which this point was specifically examined showed that the greatest predictive value of hPL was in respect of growth failure; there was a smaller and much less obvious association with acute fetal distress.[9] The general conclusion is that abnormal results of a PFT predict a high risk of growth retardation and a much lower but not insignificant risk of fetal distress, brain damage and fetal death.

Another important question is whether a PFT reflects 'growth retardation', which is the result of a pathological process, or merely small babies in general. This distinction is clearly made by biophysical procedures which can distinguish "symmetrical" from "asymmetrical" growth retardation. The only detailed investigation on this point suggested that pathological growth retardation ("dysmaturity") was associated with lower hPL levels than were cases with small but normal babies (Figure II). [10]

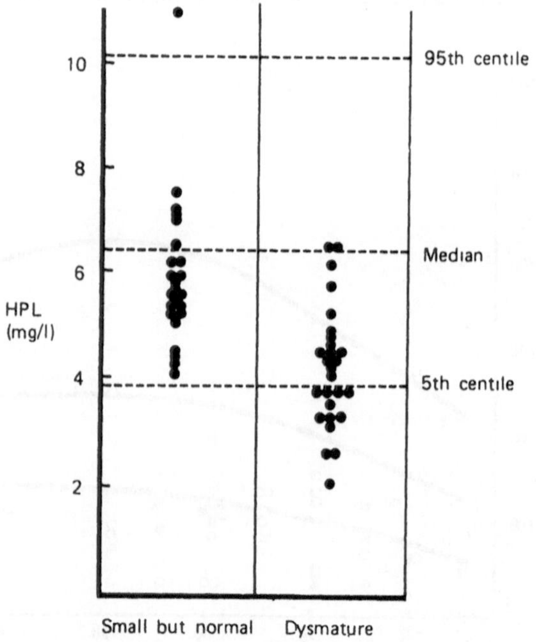

Figure II
Maternal blood hPL in 51 women who delivered a child with birthweight below the 10th centile of the population. In the left column 24 subjects with a small but normal infant; in the right column 27 women whose infants showed clinical evidence of dysmaturity. The interrupted lines show the median, 5th and 95th centiles of hPL for a normal population.

The clinical efficiency of PFT

Much of the literature on PFT was published at a time when the concept of clinical efficiency of test results was at a rudimentary stage. The criteria which are now routinely applied to evaluation of biophysical tests (indices such as sensitivity, specificity, predictive valve, and relative risk) were rarely quoted. Even now they are often misused. For example, it is possible to generate a high "sensitivity" merely by shifting the cut-off point between normal and abnormal. The apparent sensitivity of any test can be greatly increased by using the 20th centile of the normal range instead of the 10th centile.(11)

Current knowledge of PFT can be summarised by the statement that both the sensitivity and predictive value of these tests in respect of intrauterine growth retardation are of the order of 30–50% with rather less efficiency in prediction of fetal distress. The main reason for the decline in the use of PTF is not that they are ineffective, but that the alternative biophysical technology is a more efficient predictor of these risks.(12) For example measurement of multiple sections through the fetus has a sensitivity and predictive value of the order of 50–80% in respect of both absolute fetal weight and of its distribution. When PFT were widely used there was a myth that only serial levels were of any value, because serial levels showed falling concentrations in those cases at greatest risk. In reality, a true and rapid decrease is rare, occurring only in the most extreme and clinically obvious circumstances such as abruption of half or more of the placenta. Most so-called falls are the result of normal, random time-to-time fluctuations which, if not correctly interpreted, can be misleading and dangerous.(13) The real value of serial levels of PFT is the same as that for any other numerical parameter in diagnostic medicine: the fact that the mean of a series of values gives a far better estimate than does a single value of the relationship of the individual patient to the population of which she is part.(14)

Some general problems of tests of fetal wellbeing

The only fetal outcomes which are truly significant are death and long term neurological damage to the child. But both of these are rare, especially after exclusion of cases due to prematurity or congenital abnormality. Most investigations on tests of fetal wellbeing use commoner but intermediate endpoints which on their own are not necessarily of great significance. Most severely anoxic babies do not suffer any intellectual or neurological sequelae.(15) The "small-for-dates" child may just as often be the lower end of a statistically normal range as the result of specific pathology; even in the latter case the long term prognosis is usually favourable.(16) Furthermore, no study on growth retardation has addressed the child with a 4000 g genetic potential which, as a result of placental insufficiency, has a birthweight of 3000 g.(17)

Another problem of both biochemical and biophysical tests is that the only specific therapy for the fetus identified as being "at risk" is to remove the child from its unsatisfactory environment: elective early delivery by artificial induction of labour or Caesarean section. This will avoid acute events such as fetal distress or fetal death which might occur a week or more later but has no effect on the growth retardation itself. Indeed, there is no direct therapy for this condition.[18] Furthermore, it is difficult to prove that intervention has any positive therapeutic effect. For example, the Caesarean section rate has little or no relationship to measures of fetal outcome.[19]

GROUP 2 PRODUCTS

The products of Group 2 are placental protein 5 (PP5) and pregnancy-associated plasma protein A (PAPP-A) (Table 1). The common features of these are that their proposed activities (anti-complementary, anticoagulant and anti-proteolytic[20–22]) would be exerted locally at the trophoblast surface. Whether or not these functions are essential is uncertain. A specific deficiency of PAPP-A has been reported: this was associated with a normal pregnancy and a child with the Cornelia de Lange syndrome.[23]

The main controlling factors of Group 2 products would appear to be trophoblast mass and uteroplacental blood flow. However, it has been shown that injection of heparin in sub-therapeutic doses can produce a massive rise in PP5 levels, an effect not found with PAPP-A or any other placental product.[24] It is possible that this phenomenon might be related to the close analogy between PP5 and anti-thrombin 3.[21]

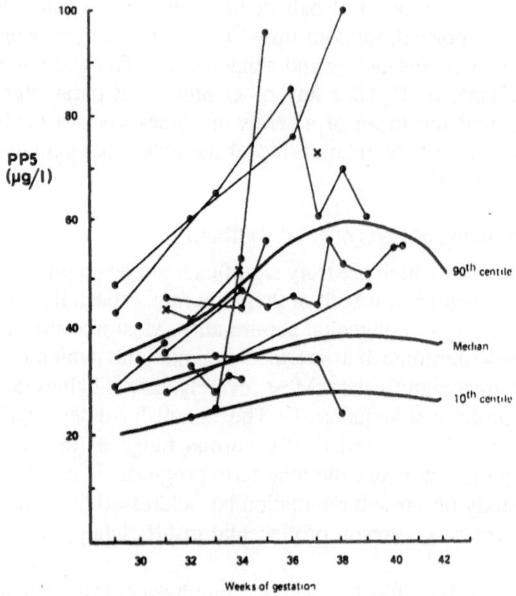

Figure III
Circulating PP5 levels in serial samples from 12 patients with placental abruption. The solid lines show the median, 10th, and 90th centiles of the normal range.

Clinical applications of Group 2 products

The levels of both PP5 and PAPP-A show a weak relationship to the size of the fetus. A much more striking phenomenon is the association of PP5 with coagulation processes at the placental site: elevated levels of PP5 have been shown in cases of placental abruption (Figure III),[25] and in some cases of pre-eclampsia and eclampsia. [26, 27] Furthermore, there is a substantial differentation between cases of growth retardation in hypertensive and non-hypertensive pregnancies.[26] The common thread in these observations could be placental damage leading to release of PP5 as a defence mechanism against further coagulation in the intervillous space.

GROUP 3 PRODUCTS

Much current interest centres around the Group 3 products (PP12 and PP14; Tables 1 and 2).[28] These are not specific to pregnancy but show a very striking rise at that time. They are produced by various maternal tissues including the endometrium/decidua.[29] It has been shown by amino acid analysis that PP12 is identified with the small IGF-1 binding protein, [29] and that PP14 is analogous to beta-lactoglobulin.[30] The demonstration that PP12 can act as a binding protein for

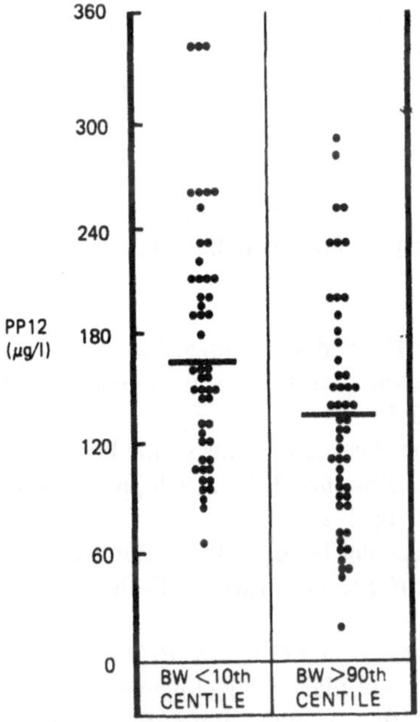

Figure IV
Circulating PP12 levels at 36 weeks in women delivering infants below the 10th centile and above the 90th centile of birthweight.

growth factors suggests that it might have a *negative* effect on fetal and placental growth. This hypothesis has been clearly confirmed with the demonstration of an *inverse* correlation with the weight of the fetus at term (Figure IV).[31] There is a relationship between PP14 and progesterone levels in the luteal phase of the menstrual cycle, but no relationship to fetal weight at term. [32]

Clinical application of Group 3 products

The site of production of Group 3 products suggests that their secretion might reflect the maternal response to a pregnancy. Measurement of PP12 and PP14 might therefore prove to be an important clinical parameter of the wellbeing of early or late pregnancy. The inverse relationship between PP12 and birthweight has some predictive value, similar or even slightly superior to that of hPL.[31] However, the main value of this test will arise if PP12 levels prove to relate to some fundamental aspect of the control of fetal growth, rather than simply a somewhat crude and indirect means of weighing the fetus *in utero*.

CONCLUSIONS

The classical placental functions tests — measurement of hPL or oestriol in the mother — have now been substantially replaced by biophysical tests which have greater diagnostic efficiency in respect of fetal risk, especially growth retardation and fetal distress. Biochemical tests are now of value only in those units (still very numerous) which do not have access to a full range of state-of-the art biophysical technology.

A new generation of materials—the Group 2 and 3 products—offer some exciting new possibilities for the diagnosis of complications such as placental abruption and fetal growth failure. Thus, levels of PP5 and PP12 may directly reflect some of the fundamental aspects of the pathology which underlie these fetal risks.

REFERENCES

1. Chard T, Rice A, Kitau MJ, Hird V, Grudzinskas JG, Nysenbaum AM. Midtrimester levels of alphafetoprotein in the screening of low birthweight. *Brit J Obstet Gynaecol* 1986; **93**:36-38.
2. Gordon YB, Chard T. The specific proteins of the human placenta: some new hypotheses. In: *Placental Proteins*. Eds. A Klopper and T Chard. Springer-Verlag, Heidelberg; 1979. pp.1-22.
3. Chard T. Synthesis of placental lactogen by human placentae. In: *Hormones in Normal and Abnormal Tissues*. Eds. K Fotherby, SB Pal. Berlin: de Gruyter, 1981: pp.409-428.
4. Chard T, Sturdee J, Cockrill B and Obiekwe BC. Which is the best placental function test? A comparison of placental lactogen and unconjugated oestriol in the prediction of intrauterine growth retardation. *Eur J Obstet Gynecol Reprod Biol* 1985; **9**:13-17.
5. Westergaard JG, Teisner B, Grudzinskas JG. Biochemical assessment of placental function — late pregnancy. In: *Clinics in Obstetrics and Gynaecology. The Placenta*. Ed. T Chard. London: Saunders, 1986; pp. 571-591.

6. Perry L, Hickson R, Obiekwe BC, Chard T. Maternal oestriol levels reflect placental function rather than foetal function. *Acta Endocrinol (Copenh)*1986; **111:** 563-566.
7. Klopper A, Wilson G, Cooke I. Studies on the variability of urinary oestriol and pregnanediol output during pregnancy. *J Endocrinol* 1969; **43**: 295-300.
8. Spellacy WN, Buhi WC and Birk SA. The effectiveness of human placental lactogen measurements as an adjunct in decreasing perinatal deaths. *Am J Obstet Gynecol* 1975; **121**: 835-844.
9. Obiekwe BC, Chard T. What do placental functions tests predict? Observations on placental lactogen levels in growth retardation and fetal distress. *Eur J Obstet Gynecol Reprod Biol* 1982; **14**: 69-73.
10. Westergaard JG, Teisner B, Hau J, Grudzinskas JG, Chard T. Placement function studies in low birth weight infants with and without dysmaturity. *Obstet Gynecol* 1985; **65**: 316-318.
11. Lilford RJ, Obiekwe BC, Chard T. Maternal blood levels of human placental lactogen in the prediction of fetal growth retardation: choosing a cut-off point between normal and abnormal. *Br J Obstet Gynaecol* 1983; **90**: 511-515.
12. Chard T. What is happening to placental function tests? *Ann Clin Biochem* 1987; **24**: 435-439.
13. Chard T. Normality and abnormality. In: *Plasma Hormone Assays in Evaluation of Foetal Well-being*. Ed. A Klopper. Edinburgh: Churchill Livingstone, 1976: pp.1–19.
14. Obiekwe BC, Chard T, Sturdee DW, Cockrill BL. The value of serial estimations of placental lactogen for fetoplacental function testing in the diagnosis of intrauterine growth retardation. *J Obstet Gynaecol* 1984; **4**: 157-160.
15. Paneth N, Stark R. Cerebral palsy and mental retardation in relation to indicators of perinatal asphyxia. An epidemiological overview. *Am J Obstet Gynecol* 1983; **147**: 960-966.
16. Hepburn M, Rosenberg K. An audit of the detection and management of small-for-gestational age babies. *Br J Obstet Gynaecol* 1986; **93**: 212-216.
17. Chard T. Placental functions tests. In: *Antenatal and Neonatal Screening*. Ed. NJH Wald. Oxford: Oxford University Press, 1984: pp.510-522.
18. Neilson JP Munjanja SP, Whitfield CR. Screening for small for dates fetuses: a controlled trial. *Br Med J* 1984; **289**: 1179-1182.
19. Porreco RP. High Cesarean section rate: a new perspective. *Obstet Gynecol* 1985; **65**: 307-311.
20. Bischof P. Purification and characterization of pregnancy associated plasma protein A (PAPP-A). *Arch Gynecol* 1979; **227**: 315-326.
21. Salem HT, Seppälä M, Chard T. The effect of thrombin on serum placental proteins (PP5): Is PP5 the naturally occuring antithrombin III of the human placenta? *Placenta* 1981; **2**: 205-209.
22. Sinosich MJ, Davey MW, Ghosh P, Grudzinskas J G. Specific inhibition of human granulocyte elastase by human pregnancy-associated plasma protein A. *Biochem Internat* 1982; **56**: 777-786.
23. Westergaard JG, Chemnitz J, Teisner B, Poulsen HK, Ipsen L, Beck B,

Grudzinskas JK. Pregnancy-associated plasma protein A: a possible mårker in the classification and prenatal diagnosis of Cornelia de Lange syndrome. *Prenat Diagn* 1983; **3**: 225-232.

24. Menabawey M, Silman R, Rice A, Chard T. Dramatic increase of placental protein 5 levels following injection of small doses of heparin. *Br J Obstet Gynaecol* 1985; **92**: 207-210.
25. Salem HT, Westergaard JG, Hindersson P, Seppälä M, Chard T. Placental protein 5 (PP5) in placental abruption. *Br J Obstet Gynaecol* 1981; **88**: 500-503.
26. Salem HT, Westergaard JG, Hindersson P, Lee JN, Grudzinskas JG and Chard T. Maternal serum levels of placental protein 5 in complications of late pregnancy. *Obstet Gynecol* 1982; **59**: 467-471.
27. Takayama M, Soma H, Isaka K, Okudera K, Ogawa T, Ueda A. Serum concentrations of placental proteins (PP5 and PP10) in toxemia of pregnancy as related to intrauterine growth retardation. *Gynecol Obstet Invest* 1987; **23**: 89-96.
28. Seppälä M, Ruttinen L, Julkunen M, Kostinen R, Wahlstrom T, Lino MK, Alfthan H, Stenman UH and Huhtala ML. Structural studies, localization in tissue and clinical aspects of human endometrial proteins. *J Reprod Fert* (Suppl) 1988; **36**: 127-145.
29. Koistinen R, Kalkkinen N, Huhtala, ML Seppälä, Bohn H, Rutanen M. Placental protein 12 is a decidual protein that binds somatomedin and has an identical N-terminal amino acid sequence with somatomedin-binding protein from human aminotic fluid. *Endocrinology* 1986; **118**: 1375-1378.
30. Huhtala, ML, Seppälä M, Narvanen A, Palomaki P, Julkunen M, Bohn H. Amino acid sequence homology between human placental protein 14 and beta-lactoglobulins from various species. *Endocrinology* 1987; **120**: 2620-2622.
31. Howell RJ, Perry LA, Choglay NS, Bohn H, Chard T. Placental protein 12 (PP12): a new test for the prediction of the small-for-gestational-age infant. *Br J Obstet Gynaecol* 1985; **92**: 1141-1144.
32. Howell RJ, Bolton AE and Chard T. Placental protein 14 (PP14) in late pregnancy. *Arch Gynecol* 1986; **239**: 27-29.

Discussion

Chairman: Dr N. Patel

LEVENE: Could I ask Professor Campbell to define intrauterine growth retardation?

CAMPBELL: I am not interested in definitions because I do not think that we know. We think that not all small-for-dates fetuses are IUGR. What we are trying to do is to discover the basic fundamental problem. This is why using Doppler we are groping towards understanding what the basic mechanism of the growth problem, if there is one, might be. Forty-five percent of small babies as diagnosed by ultrasound have perfectly normal Doppler and usually deliver at term without any trouble. Therefore, we are by this means getting to know which small babies are perhaps growth retarded or in trouble. If it is physically normal, if there is no chromosome abnormality, if there is no Doppler abnormality, no fetal/placental perfusion problem and the fetal circulation is normal, then that small baby is small for innocent reasons, possibly genetic or other. That is why I kept using the words "hypoxic IUGR". If it is normal and not hypoxic or in danger of being hypoxic as shown by a normal uterine circulation, then you do not need to worry.

LEVENE: You seem to have created a circular argument and you are only able to prove what you want to prove. You need a "gold standard". We need to know what you mean by intrauterine growth retardation. What are you trying to prevent? If you are preventing it in your belief, then you are not going to see it in any case. It is the same with the concept of asphyxia. What you mean by asphyxia is not necessarily what I mean by asphyxia. Until you can tell us your definition of growth retardation, which must have something to do with growth, it is very difficult to evaluate the techniques that you are currently using.

CAMPBELL: We are trying to detect placental insufficiency of some kind, whether it is feto-placental or utero-placental. Usually utero-placental is the first problem. That is what we are trying to predict and that is why I am fairly careless about the words "IUGR" or "small-for-dates". It is merely a manifestation of a disease process and I am trying to diagnose the disease process. If it is a small baby because of chromosome abnormality it is intrauterine growth retardation. If it is a small baby where all the parameters that we use are normal, then it is not.

HALL: If it is a normal weight baby that is in trouble is it growth retardation?

CAMPBELL: Yes.

HALL: Why are we using the word "growth" and why are we using the word "retardation"?

CAMPBELL: The simple matter is if the baby is programmed to be 4 kg and ends up at 3 kg but has abnormal Doppler and is hypoxic, that is intrauterine growth retardation.

PATEL: Professor Campbell is not interested in weight at all as long as it is Doppler normal. "Normal Doppler" is the new criterion for a normal baby!

CAMPBELL: It is "Doppler and cordocentesis normal".

GILLMER: There is good animal data to support what Professor Campbell is saying, I believe. The work done by Jeff Robinson originally in Oxford and carried on in Australia admittedly using the carunculectomy model does show that you can modify the ultimate outcome of the pregnancy by reducing the available placental reserve to that fetus. Logically it would be possible to have a fetus for whom the potential growth could be 4.5 kg, but as a result of whatever constraint is applied (and it is those constraints that we do not fully understand) ends up at 3 kg. That baby, as we well know, could be the one that dies suddenly. We think it is suddenly but it has probably been asphyxiated for a long time. We have had a number of cases in Oxford where we have followed up babies that are seemingly of normal size, but who clearly are suffering chronic asphyxial stress. I do not think that it is that important to have definitions either of macrosomia or of intrauterine growth retardation.

LEVENE: I accept that that is true, but if those assumptions are made implicitly, then you are never going to answer the question. As I said, it becomes a self-fulfilling prophecy. Professor Campbell spoke of differential growth between head and body. There I am with you because you are obviously measuring a real difference which we as neonatologists can measure. I think that we are very bad at measuring lengths and perhaps we should be looking at ratios of length and weight or head circumference, or whatever. Then we will be able to agree as to what we mean by differential growth. However, if you take that one step further with your Doppler studies, I am beginning to get uneasy that you are making measurements and then you are intervening. We are never going to know whether those interventions are valid or not.

STEWART: I think that we have got a terminology problem. You are not talking about whether the baby is small or heavy or fat or thin. You are talking about what you believe to be a disease process of which one of the symptoms may be deviations in measurements. We have actually got to say that we are either talking about a disease process or a condition, or not. Retardation is one thing, but if you are going to be abnormal the fact that your birthweight is, for example, under 1500 g at term, that is not just retardation, that is an absolute abnormality as defined. We have an enormous mix up of terminology, mixing symptoms and conditions. Until we manage to clarify it all and accept the fact that we have got to be a bit disciplined it is going to be impossible to make sense out of the literature.

CAMPBELL: What we have got are small-for-gestational-age fetuses. Some of them are perfectly normal and are just programmed to be small; some of them are small because they are abnormal. What we are trying to do is make that diagnosis. If we find a small fetus with abnormal uteroplacental flow and fetoplacental flow, I would call that IUGR. If it is small because of a chromosome abnormality, I would call that IUGR. It is small for gestational age, but it is also IUGR. If we can find no cause we cannot possibly call it IUGR, because we have not been able to identify an aetiological mechanism. Therefore it is just small for gestational age.

HOWIE: What you are postulating is that the disease process that you are measuring may have a better relationship either to death, immediate morbidity or possibly to long term morbidity. I think that, before you can really establish whether your way of defining abnormality by disease process is true or not, you will have to relate what you measure or you define as a disease process by Doppler, or whatever, to these measures of death, immediate or long term morbidity. That really is the bottom line. One point that David Taylor picked up in the Dundee study(1) is that he started with the babies that had long term morbidity and then went back, and babies who were morbid were more likely to have been small. So there is a relationship between size and morbidity.

CAMPBELL: But I have shown that. We looked at small-for-dates fetuses below 2 kg and they were all below the 10th centile. So it was a very severe group. They were fairly similar in the gestational age at which they were born. We divided them into those who had severe abnonnalities in the fetal thoracic aorta, and those who did not. There was a mean of 10 days between the two. The neonatal mortality and morbidity was much higher in those with abnormal Doppler. This is borne out by the randomised study where we revealed Doppler and did not reveal Doppler results. When it was revealed doctors tended to intervene a bit earlier before the antenatal heart traces became abnormal. These babies had a lower neonatal morbidity. The morbid features were necrotising enterocolitis, renal failure and coagulation problems due to the redistribution affecting the liver.

PATEL: How close to delivery were these abnormal measurements?

CAMPBELL: Because these patients were in the hospital they were done very frequently right up to the time of delivery. Indeed we showed a correlation between the duration of the abnormal Doppler findings and the incidence of morbidity. In other words, when they had no end-diastolic flow for around four or five weeks they had a much higher incidence of morbidity. We can demonstrate the centralisation of fetal flow sometimes for weeks before the fetus is delivered. This is a response to chronically low pO_2 values; therefore we believe that the human fetus must be different from the animal model.

WHITTLE: One of the other important issues is the difference between screening and diagnostic tests. In that particular study, Professor Campbell, you were looking at a very selected population. I think that many of us would agree that you are going to find abnormalities in that group. If that was a screening test then I do not think that it was very good because the positive predictive valve was very low. Most clinical studies have suggested that you can pick up between 30-40%. I realise that your tests were done at a very early stage, but applying that as a screening test those figures are fairly meaningless.

CAMPBELL: I have another study now which shows that 60% of abnormalities which you can relate to uterine flow were detected by the early screening tests. But I do think that picking up a third of all the severe IUGR fetuses by a test at 20 weeks plus a third of all the severe fulminating pre-eclampsias plus a half of the abruptios, etc., plus a third of the intrauterine deaths is not too bad for a screening test.

WHITTLE: Yes, but there is high incidence of false positives.

REFERENCES

1. Taylor DJ, Howie PW, Davidson J, Davidson D, Drillien CH. Do pregnancy complications contribute to neurodevelopmental disability? *Lancet* 1985; i: 713–716.

Technical basis for Doppler blood flow measurement

Professor S. H. Eik-Nes

INTRODUCTION

The ultrasound technique has been extensively used in imaging. Especially in the field of obstetrics and gynaecology where traditional techniques have had limitations because of their invasive ionising nature, ultrasound has had a great impact on diagnosis and clinical management. In the imaging mode ultrasound is flooded into a field of tissue and the backscattered sound is used to generate an image as in radar and sonar.

Parallel to the development of imaging techniques using ultrasound, the first experiment utilising the same basic principle to measure velocity began.(1) By emitting sound towards a vessel and utilising the Doppler principle, it is possible to elicit information concerning the velocity distribution. The first crude blood velocity results were obtained using Doppler instruments in the continuous mode.(1-3) Later, Peronneau and Baker introduced the pulsed ultrasonic Doppler mode.(4,5) In the pulsed mode, the blood velocities in a small range cell can be studied separately and thus produce information necessary for the quantification of blood flow.(6,7)

In cardiology there is a need for the assessment of detailed spatial flow information in small areas as well as for measuring very high velocities in specific areas. Because of the general limitation in measuring high velocities in the pulsed mode, instruments that combined pulsed and continuous mode were made to overcome these problems(8) and such instruments have been widely used in cardiology.(9,10)

In peripheral vascular work and in cardiology it has been of interest to combine imaging ultrasound with measurement of velocity, and to direct the velocity displaying beam to a certain location in the imaged area. These requirements were fulfilled with the introduction of the duplex scanners.(11) The latest innovation in ultrasound is the simultaneous two dimensional tissue and velocity imaging, the so-called colour flow mapping technique.(12)

Present research work is aimed towards the combined use of computer technology and digital storage for advanced analysis of the information obtained from the imaging and Doppler ultrasound signals.

DOPPLER EFFECT

The Doppler effect is named after its first describer, an Austrian physicist, Christian Johann Doppler (1803 – 1853). In 1842, he explained how the colour of the light emitted from a star changes according to the direction and the velocity of the movement of the star in relation to the observer on earth.(13)

The Doppler effect is found in all kinds of waves where there is movement between the observer and the wave emitting source. When the receiver is stationary, and the wave emitting source is moving towards the receiver, the wavelength is compressed and thus the frequency received is higher than the emitted frequency. If the wave source is moving away from the receiver, the waves are elongated and the received frequency is decreased (Figure I). This can be observed every day by listening to the pitch of a siren on an ambulance passing by. The Doppler principle is widely used in, for example, radar, sonar, security systems, etc.

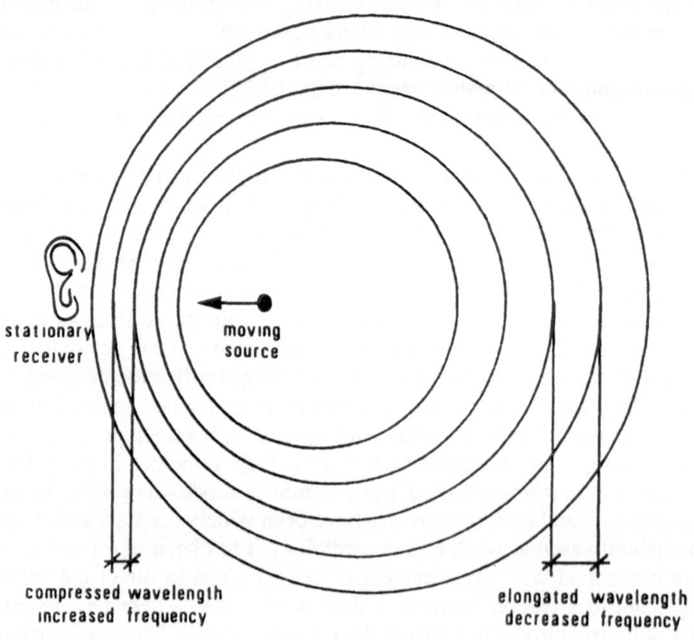

Figure I
Illustration of the Doppler effect.
(Reprinted with permission from Angelsen and Hatle: *Doppler Ultrasound in Cardiology*, 1982).

DOPPLER ULTRASOUND IN CLINICAL PRACTICE

The Doppler principle can also be utilised to measure the velocity of moving blood. The moving red blood cells act as scatterers and reflect the sound emitted towards them. The change in frequency between the emitted and received sound is called the Doppler shift. The Doppler shift, f_d, is described by the equation

$$f_d = 2 f_0 \frac{v \cos \alpha}{c}$$

where f_0 is the transmitted frequency, c, the velocity of sound in the tissue, α the angle between the direction of the sound beam and the velocity direction of the moving blood, and v the velocity of blood. In clinical Doppler ultrasound, the emitted frequency is usually 2 MHz. For typical blood velocities the Doppler shift is in the audible range for the human ear (16 000 – 20 000 Hz) and pulsatile and venous blood flow can be evaluated by its typical sound during the examination.

The decomposition of a velocity vector in a blood vessel is shown in Figure II. Using the Doppler principle, one measures the velocity vector in the direction of the beam. The velocity vector in the direction of the vessel must be calculated as shown. Cos 90^0 is 0 and cos 0^0 is 1. Thus one can never pick up the Doppler shift if the sound beam is approaching the vessel at a 90° angle. Errors of the estimate of flow are more likely to occur when the angle is near 90°. Optimum results are obtained with an angle ranging from 0° to 60°.

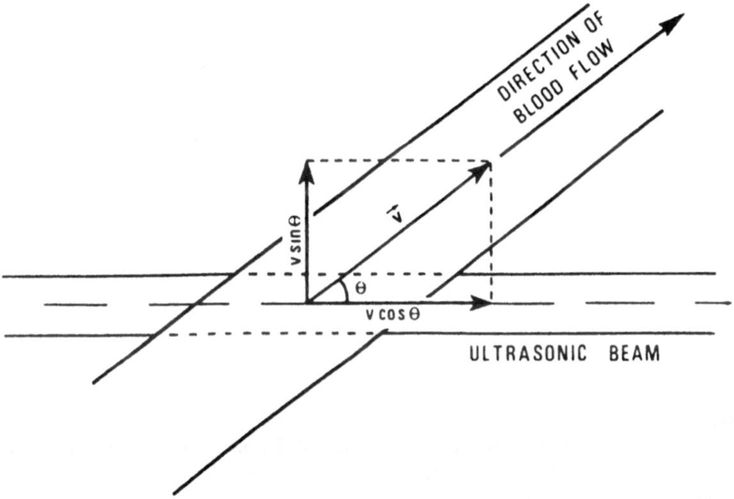

Figure II
Decomposition of a velocity vector into a component parallel to the beam and at an angle of 90° to the beam.
(Reprinted with permission from Angelsen and Hatle: *Doppler Ultrasound in Cardiology*, 1982).

The frequency spectrum (corresponding to the velocity) is usually recorded along the y-axis and the time along the x-axis.

Continuous wave

The first Doppler instruments operated in the continuous mode, i.e. emitting and receiving sound at the same time utilising two different transducers or one split transducer as illustrated in Figure III. Various reflectors, for example vessels at different depth in the path of the beam could thus cause a Doppler shift. Such a system has therefore no range resolution. In some circumstances this can be a disadvantage. On the other hand, there is no limit on the maximum velocity to be measured in the continuous mode. Especially in cardiology, this can be an advantage. The sensitivity of a continuous wave Doppler system is usually poórer than for a pulsed one.

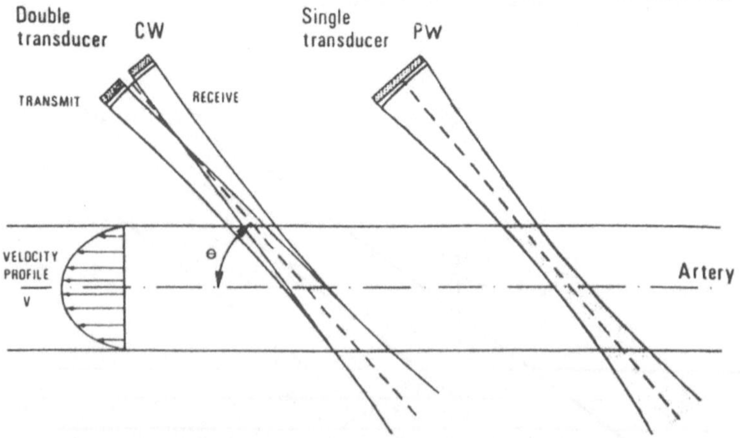

Figure III
Principles of ultrasonic Doppler velocity measurement. In the continuous mode a double transducer, and in the pulsed mode a single transducer is used.

Doppler shift: $f_d = 2f_0 \frac{v \cos \alpha}{c}$
Transmitted frequency: f_0
Velocity of sound: c
(Reprinted with permission from Angelsen and Hatle: *Doppler Ultrasound in Cardiology*, 1982).

The application of continuous Doppler ultrasound is established in peripheral vascular work, in cardiology and in monitoring the fetal condition antenatally, especially during labour (cardiotocography). On a research basis, the technique is used in obstetrics to obtain information about various velocity patterns in the umbilical artery and in the maternal arteries branching off towards the base of the placenta. The changes in the velocity pattern observed here during various clinical conditions might be of prognostic importance.

Pulsed wave

In a pulsed Doppler ultrasound system, a short burst of sound is emitted at a specified repetition frequency. Because the sound is first transmitted from, then received by the transducer, the sound is sampled with a time delay after the pulse transmission. Thus only scatterers from a small area are sampled in the received signal. This area is usually referred to as a sample volume (diameter given by the transducer diameter, and length by the length of the transmitted pulse). The boundaries of the sample volume are diffuse. The basic concept is illustrated in Figure III.

The major advantage of the pulsed Doppler system is its range resolution. In the pulsed mode, a relatively high power output is used compared to that used in continuous mode, a fact which must be considered in fetal use. Pulsed Doppler instruments are more complex than the continuous, and thus more expensive.

Frequency aliasing

The major disadvantage of the pulsed Doppler system is its limitation in measuring relatively high velocities at relatively great depth. This is due to the fact that an emitted soundburst must be allowed to travel back to the receiver before the next one is submitted to avoid ambiguity in depth.

As seen in Figure IV, there is a relationship between the maximum velocity detectable at a certain depth and the specified emitted frequency. Violation of this relationship will cause frequency aliasing. Frequency aliasing is the inability of the Doppler instrument to present a true description of the frequency distribution. Frequency aliasing can easily be recognized on a spectrum analysis of the Doppler shift.

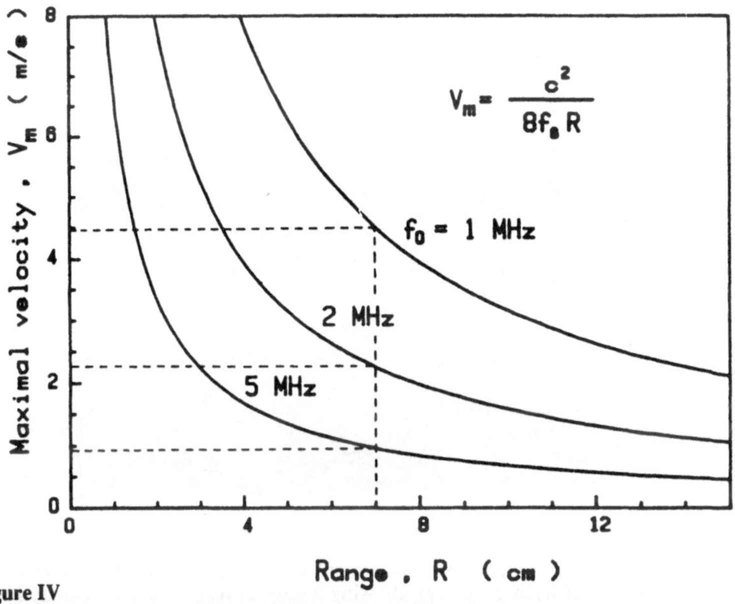

Figure IV
Range velocity product. With a 2MHz probe at 7 cm depth one can measure a velocity of approximately 4.5 m/s without running into aliasing problems. With a 5 MHz probe, the maximum detectable velocity would be approximately 2.25 m/s.
(Reprinted with permission from Angelsen and Hatle: *Doppler Ultrasound in Cardiology*, 1982).

DOPPLER INSTRUMENTS

Doppler instruments are produced in a variety of models from small portable units that give audible demonstration of pulsation in peripheral vessels or heart activity in early pregnancy, to complicated instruments with continuous and pulsed modes. The latter are capable of producing several useful output signals, like the maximum and mean velocity, the integral and derivative of the velocity and various indices describing the velocity pattern. In addition, they can perform sophisticated analysis of the Doppler spectrum.

Stand alone instruments

In obstetrics, small Doppler instruments operating in the continuous mode for registration of fetal heart activity in early pregnancy are widely used. Most pregnancies today are monitored by cardiotocography, which includes a Doppler-unit for the detailed registration of a tracing of fetal heart activity. For research purposes, continuous wave and pulsed wave evaluation of the pattern of the velocity in the fetal umbilical artery and in the branches of the uterine artery are being made. A typical printout from such an instrument (Vingmed Goldline Doppler, Vingmed Sound A/S, Horten, Norway) is shown in Figure V. Similar instruments have been used to measure blood flow in the fetus.[14,15]

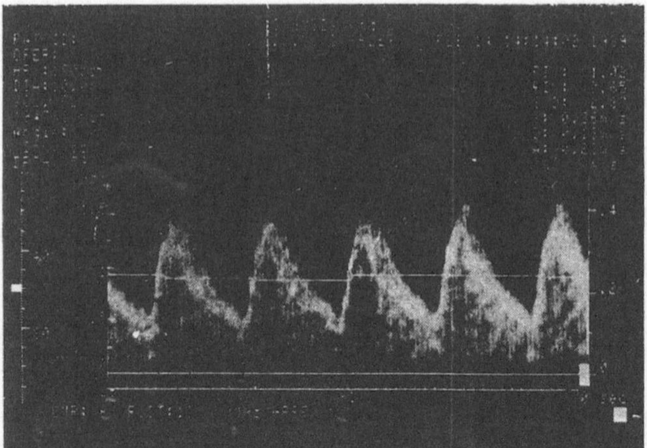

Figure V
Printout from a stand alone Doppler instrument (Vingmed Sound Goldline Doppler, Vingmed Sound A/S, Horten, Norway), showing a normal tracing of the velocity in the umbilical artery. Calculation of PI, RI, A/B-ratio, maximum, mean and average velocity and heart rate are done automatically. Volume flow is calculated when the diameter of the vessel and the angle between the vessel and the Doppler beam are given.

Duplex scanners

To obtain adequate information concerning blood flow it is important to aim the positioning of a Doppler sample volume to a certain area, or to look for vessels in a certain field of interest. This has been made possible by instruments combining two dimensional imaging of tissue with the Doppler measurement of velocity. The first instrument produced[11] did not allow a simultaneous real-time display of tissue and velocity, but on a frozen image the sample volume could be guided to the area of interest in the vessel. Later developments allowed a frequent update of the tissue image, and by using modern time-sharing techniques it is now possible to have a simultaneous imaging of the velocity pattern in a vessel and the tissue.[16] Most of the available instruments use a phased or an annular array system. The image and the blood flow information are then created by the same transducer. In obstetrics it then may be problematic to access the vessel at a small angle. Doppler measurements of the fetal heart usually do not present a problem with this approach, but tracing other fetal vessels which are often found parallel to the surface, and thus at an unfortunate angle (close to 90°), might prove difficult. New instruments using two transducers with the Doppler transducer at an offset are being developed.

Colour Doppler

Traditionally, blood velocity measurement is acquired with the Doppler sample volume put in an area with flow and the frequency spectrum displayed. Interest has been shown in developing a Doppler scanner which, in addition to a traditional two-dimensional tissue image, produces a two-dimensional image of the velocity distribution in an area, so-called colour flow mapping. This can be done by scanning an area in the tissue image with Doppler and looking at the velocity in several small sample volumes covering this area. Blood flow away from the transducer is coded in blue and towards the transducer in red. The various velocities are illustrated in shades of the respective colour. Aliasing can be displayed in a diverging colour (green) and thus areas of high velocities can be detected easily. For detailed information, a single sample volume can be isolated and the Doppler signal displayed in the ordinary way. In addition to obtaining the spatial distribution of flow, such an instrument also has the advantage of locating the flow in small vessels which cannot be resolved on regular 2D images, for example, small branches of the uterine arteries approaching the placenta or small fetal vessels such as the renal or cerebral arteries.

The use of a colour flow instrument has found its place in adult and paediatric cardiology, as well as in peripheral vascular work, and is presently being evaluated in fetal cardiology. Its place in the monitoring of fetal–maternal vessels remains to be seen.

CONCLUSION

There has been a constant development of new Doppler techniques for application in clinical medicine as a result of the fruitful cooperation between clinicians and technicians. Presently interesting possibilities for the clinician are arising as a result of technical research on advanced use of digital storage and computer processing of Doppler data. This is an important field in obstetrics, since there are reasons to believe that Doppler monitoring of fetal vascular parameters can be of clinical importance in future surveillance of the pregnancy at risk.

REFERENCES

1. Satumora S. Ultrasonic Doppler method for the inspection of cardiac functions. *J Acoust Soc Am* 1957; **29:** 1181-1185.
2. Franklin DL, Schlegal WA, Rushmer RF. Blood flow measured by Doppler frequency shift of backscattered ultrasound. *Science* 1961; **134:** 564-565.
3. Edler I, Lindström K. Ultrasonic Doppler technique used in heart disease. II. Clinical application. In: *Ultrasonographica Medica.* Eds J Bock, K Ossoing. Vienna: Verlag Wiener Med Akad, 1969.
4. Peronneau P, Deloche A, Bui-Mong-Hugn, Hinglais J. Debimetrie ultrasonore: Dévelopments et applications expérimentales. *Eur Surg Res* 1969; **1:** 147-156.
5. Baker DW. Pulsed ultrasonic Doppler blood-flow sensing. *IEEE Trans on S and US.* 1970; **SU-17:** 170-185
6. Eik-Nes SH, Brubakk AO, Ulstein M. Measurement of human fetal blood flow. *Br Med J* 1980; **1:** 283-84.
7. Eik-Nes SH, Maršál K, Brubakk AO, Ulstein M. Ultrasonic measurement of human fetal blood flow. *J Biomed Eng* 1982; **4:** 28-236.
8. Angelsen BAJ. *Transcutaneous measurement of blood velocity and flow in the thorax by ultrasound and the Doppler effect.* Trondheim: Inst Eng Cyb. Norwegian Institute of Technology, 1974; Report 75-78-W.
9. Hatle L, Brubakk AO, Tromsdal A, Angelsen B. Noninvasive assessment of pressure drop in mitral stenosis by Doppler ultrasound. *Br Heart J* 1978; **40:** 131-140.
10. Hatle L Angelsen BA, Tromsdal A. Non-invasive assessment of aortic stenosis by Doppler ultrasound. *Br Heart J* 1980; **43:** 284-292.
11. Phillips DJ, Powers JE, Eyer MK, Blackshear WM Jr, Bodily KC, Strandness DE Jr, Baker DW. Detection of peripheral vascular disease using the Duplex scanner III. *Ultrasound Med Biol* 1980; **205:** 28.
12. Omoto R. In: *Color Atlas of Real-time Two-Dimensional Doppler Echocardiography.* Ed. R Omoto. Tokyo: Shinidan-To-Chiryo Co, Ltd, 1984; p.11.
13. Doppler C. Über das farbige Licht der Doppelsterne und einiger anderer Gestirne des Himmels. Sectionssitzung 25 Königl böhm. Prague: Gesellschaft der Wissenschaften zu Prag, 1842; pp.467-482.
14. Eik-Nes SH, Maršál K, Kristoffersen K. Methology and basic problems related to blood flow studies in the human fetus. *Ultrasound Med Biol* 1984; **10:** 329-337.
15. Maršál K, Lindblad A, Lingman G. Eik-Nes SH. Blood flow in the fetal descending aorta; intrinsic factors affecting fetal blood flow, i.e.fetal breathing

movements and cardiac arrhythmia. *Ultrasound Med Biol* 1984; **3:** 339-348.
16. Angelsen BAJ, Kristoffersen K. Combination of 2D-echo amplitude imaging and Doppler measurements. In: *Cardiac Doppler Diagnosis*. Ed. MP Spencer. Boston: Martinus Nijhoff, 1984.

Volume flow calculation in the human fetus using pulsed Doppler ultrasound: basic problems

Professor S. H. Eik-Nes

INTRODUCTION

Parallel with the development of ultrasound imaging techniques, instruments facilitating blood velocity measurements based on the Doppler principle have been developed and continuously improved.[1-3] The combined use of such instruments made it possible for the first time to obtain quantitative information on blood flow in the human fetus in a non-invasive way.[4,5] The ultrasound techniques have thus opened a new era in the physiological assessment of human fetal haemodynamics. In addition to establishing previously unknown information about the human fetus, the various techniques have been used clinically in order to find and evaluate possible new methods for the assessment of fetal wellbeing.[6-8] During the early years, the main interest focussed on the quantification of blood flow. As this turned out to be too inaccurate for clinical use, the major interest diverged towards qualitative assessment of flow.

History

The first attempts to analyse human fetal blood flow by non-invasive ultrasound methods were made in 1977 by Fitzgerald and Drumm.[9] They used a 5 MHz system combined with a two-dimensional B-mode imaging device, and presented spectral analysis from the blood velocity in the umbilical artery and vein. A year later McCallum *et al.* used a similar technique and indicated that the flow pattern in the umbilical artery of fetuses in normal pregnancies differed from the flow pattern in the fetuses of pre-eclamptic mothers.[10] In 1979 Gill and Kossoff managed to quantify blood flow in the umbilical vein using a B-mode scanner (Octoson).[4] Their system did not allow measurement of the high velocities in the fetal arterial system due to the limited range velocity product of the Octoson. In 1980 Eik-Nes *et al.*[5] published a method which used a 3.5 MHz linear B-mode scanner in combination with a 2 MHz pulsed Doppler fixed to the linear transducer at an offset. This set-up made it possible to quantify flow in both the umbilical vein and the fetal aorta.

DOPPLER METHOD

The original method for blood flow measurement in the human fetus is shown in Figure 1.[5,11] Later methods developed for blood flow measurement use the same

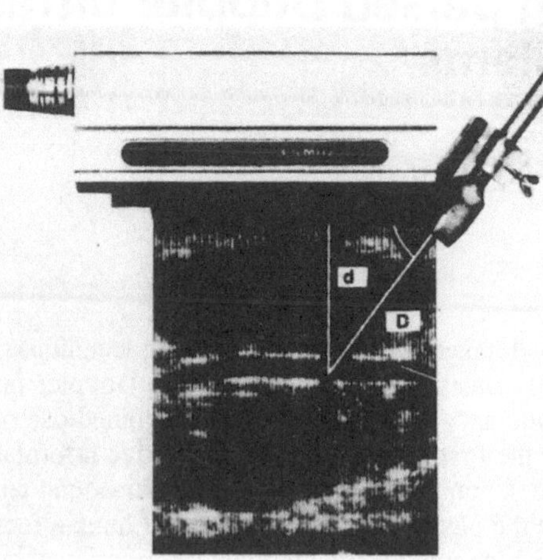

Figure I
Principle of the method for transcutaneous measurements of fetal blood flow. The unit includes a real-time transducer (left) and a 2MHz Doppler transducer (right).

basic set-up.[8] In order to quantitate blood flow in a fetal vessel, four problems must be solved: location of the vessel, angle between the vessel and the Doppler beam, measurement of the blood velocities, and diameter of the vessel.

Location of the vessel

With the transducer combination illustrated in Figure I, the fetal vessel was located and the real-time transducer put parallel to the vessel of interest. Thus, the angle between the vessel and the Doppler beam was known because it corresponded to the angle between the two transducers. Along a line drawn on the screen or electronically generated, the distance of the vessel from the Doppler transducer could be measured and the sample volume put in the correct position, spanning the vessel.

Measurement of blood velocity

The blood velocity was measured with a 2 MHz pulsed Doppler instrument (ALFRED,Vingmed A/S, Oslo, Norway). The instrument can produce multiple frequencies, but was used in the 2 MHz mode. To eliminate low frequencies from the vessel wall and tissue movements a pulsed Doppler system always uses a high-pass filter. This was set to 100 Hz, thus minimising the influence on the calculation of flow values. The pulse repetition frequency of the instrument was automatically changed from 9.5 to 5.2 kHz depending on the depth range. The size of the sample volume was determined by the diameter of the transducer (10 mm) and its length could be set at either 5 or 10 mm. When the sample volume was positioned at the correct depth, the fine tuning of the location of the sample volume was done by audible guidance, by visual analysis of the Doppler spectrum on an oscilloscope, or both. The Doppler signals were processed in several ways. On-line, an analogue tracing of the maximum and mean velocity, as well as the integral of the mean velocity was given. On a separate screen, the spectral analysis was given (DAISY, Vingmed, A/S, Oslo, Norway). In addition the Doppler signal was modulated, then stored on a standard tape recorder for later off-line analysis.

Measurement of the vessel diameter

Two methods for measurement of the vessel diameter were used. [12] One method involved measuring the diameter from the outer to the inner outline of the vessel wall on a frozen static image of the B-mode scanner. The calliper operated in 0.4 mm steps. This procedure was repeated 10 times, then the average was calculated as the vessel diameter. Since the images were frozen at random, the calculated diameter then approximately represented the time-average diameter. This method was relatively simple, not time-consuming and could be used in clinical practice.

The other method involved the use of the time-distance recorder (TD-recorder).[13] On the B-mode image, two markers were positioned proximal to the vessel wall echoes and the TD-recorder then "locked" on the vessel walls and a detailed tracing of the wall movement could be obtained (Figure II). The results obtained with the two methods were comparable.[6]

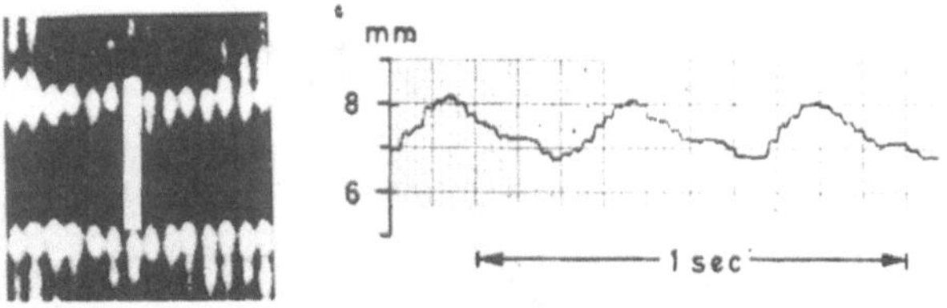

Figure II
Time-distance recording (TD-recording) of the vessel diameter. Left: real-time image of a longitudinal section of the aorta; the white line visualises the diameter measured automatically from the outer to the inner outline of the vessel wall echoes along an image line. Right: tracing by a TD-recorder of the fetal aortic diameter.

Calculation of flow

With the ultrasound Doppler technique described above it is possible to estimate blood flow quantitatively. The blood flow, Q, in a vessel is given by the equation:

$$Q = \frac{v \cdot (D/2)^2 \cdot \pi}{\cos \alpha}$$

v is the mean blood velocity over the vessel cross-sectional area, D is the diameter, and α is the angle between the vessel and the insonating Doppler ultrasound beam.

In vivo comparison

In an *in vivo* experiment the blood flow in the abdominal aorta of pigs was measured combining the described Doppler technique and an electromagnetic method (Blood flowmeter 376, Nycotron, Drammen, Norway) simultaneously.[14] An electromagnetic transducer was mounted on the aorta which was dissected free. The abdominal cavity was filled with salt water and the Doppler ultrasound transducer was applied in the waterbath for measurement of blood flow in the aorta in the same way as was done on the human fetus. The diameter of the aorta was measured with the real-time technique described above. The simultaneous recordings of the blood flow employing the two techniques is shown in Figure III. The correlation between the two techniques was, r = 0.91, and no systematic error could be demonstrated. It must be emphasised though, that the experiment was done in a highly controlled situation and might not represent results which can be obtained clinically.

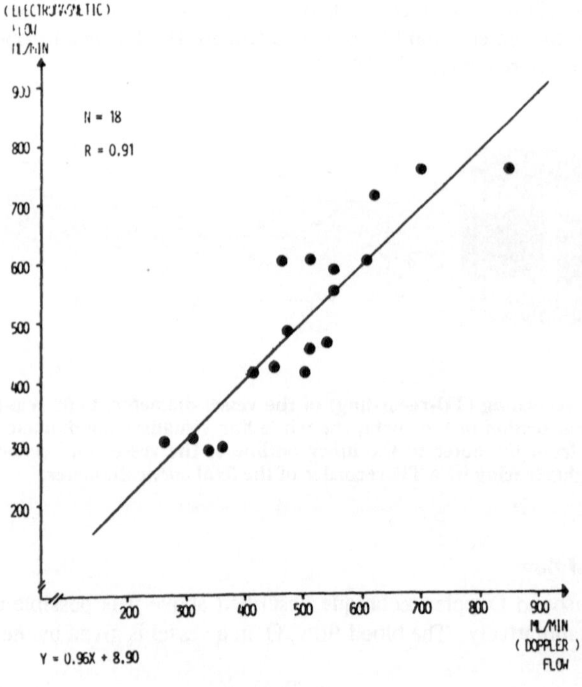

Figure III
Correlation between the simultaneous measurements of aortic blood flow in the pig with electromagnetic and Doppler method.
(Reference 14, with permission)

SOURCES OF ERROR

The quantification of blood flow is based on a number of single measurements using various technical procedures. All of them are subject to error, and a careful analysis of the possible pitfalls is therefore indicated.

Vessel diameter

The area of the vessel is calculated from the diameter, since it is not possible to measure the area directly. To calculate the area, the diameter is squared, making the calculation most sensitive to errors in measurement (Figure IV). In late pregnancy the diameter of the aorta or the umbilical vein is in the range between 6 and 8 mm and an error of 0.4 mm can then cause an error of 10% in the calculated flow. It is clearly demonstrated in Figure III that for smaller vessels the error can be easily in the range of 25–50% and one should then be most careful with blood flow quantification. The pulsatile expansion of the fetal aortic diameter is in the range of 10 – 15% of the minimum diameter (Figure II). Due to interference between the Doppler and the imaging ultrasound it is not possible to make these measurements simultaneously. At present, blood flow is calculated as the product of the time-averaged velocity. The correct procedure would be to calculate flow from the integral of the product of the two. In pulsating vessels this might lead to errors in the estimate. The solution to the latter problem is the simultaneous

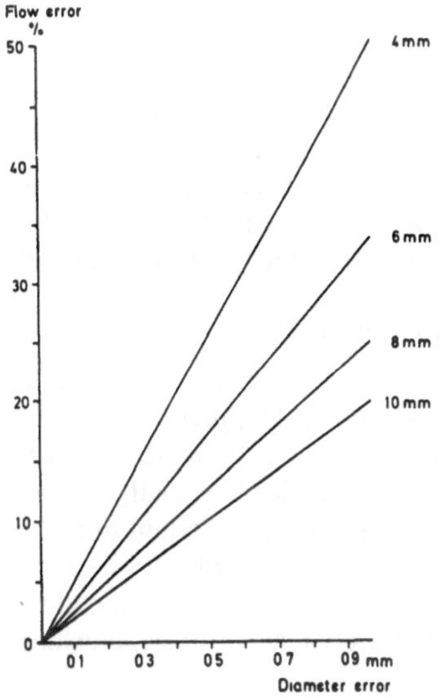

Figure IV
Error in flow measurement due to diameter error at four different vessel diameters (4, 6, 8 and 10 mm)

measurement of velocity and diameter, a procedure which is not yet possible. With advanced use of time-sharing techniques it might be possible in the near future.

High-pass filter

In order to remove signals from the slowly moving tissue in the path of the beam as well as signals from the vessel wall movement, the Doppler signal must pass through a high-pass filter. The filter also removes the low frequencies in the Doppler frequency spectrum, affecting the volume flow calculation.

Initially, the high-pass filter was set in the range of 400 Hz as is common in adult cardiology, but experience has shown that the filter can be lowered to 100 Hz in fetal use, thus having minimal influence on the volume calculation of the flow. In the umbilical vein a 100 Hz filter will cause an overestimation of 2.7 cm/s which is about 5% for a normal pregnancy at term. The maximum velocity will not be affected by the high-pass filter, as long as the maximum frequency exceeds the cut-off frequency of the high-pass filter. The flow profile in the aorta is flat in systole and the volume flow will therefore not be affected significantly by the high-pass filter. In qualitative evaluation of the flow in the umbilical artery, where the amount of diastolic blood flow is important, the high-pass filter can be a source of significant misinterpretation.

Sample of the Doppler instrument

Over the vessel cross-sectional area, the flow in a vessel is proportional to the mean blood flow velocity. This assumes that the sound beam has a uniform intensity across the blood vessel and that the sample volume covers the whole vessel cross-section. Too large a sample volume might include signals from nearby vessels and cause errors. If the sample volume is too small and does not cover the whole vessel cross-sectional area, it might cause both over- or underestimation, depending on where the sample volume is positioned within the vessel.

Angle between the vessel and the Doppler ultrasound beam

An error in the estimate might also occur as a result of an error in the assumed angle between the vessel and the Doppler beam. Since the relative difference between cosine to the angle is smaller for angles closer to 0° than to 90°, it is safer to operate at a relatively small angle. Especially in the qualitative assessment of flow in the umbilical artery, it is very important to be aware of the fact that when the angle approaches 90°, the high-pass filter (which has a fixed frequency level) chops off frequencies which, at that angle, correspond to a considerable amount of blood velocity. This might falsely lead to the conclusion that the flow in diastole is low or absent.

Estimation of fetal weight

When the blood flow in the human fetus is quantitatively assessed, it is expressed in ml/min/kg fetal weight. Then the result depends on our ability to estimate fetal weight. Again errors in the range of 10% must be considered common, with larger errors occurring.[15]

CLINICAL RESULTS

Initially, several groups set out to establish normal data for the blood flow in the umbilical vein and the thoracic aorta.[7,8,16,17] Most of the results obtained in the umbilical vein corresponded, while those from the aorta were more variable. As time went on, the values in the fetal aorta seemed to increase and corresponded more for the different observers, probably as a consequence of improved technique and better experience. The velocity in the descending aorta of growth retarded fetuses, has been found to be low, but the volume flow was not significantly different from the controls.[8,18] In the umbilical vein, though, the volume flow in several growth retarded fetuses has been found to be very low[19] and sometimes not detectable.[20] The reason is unclear, and may possibly result from technical problems.

Very low flow values in the umbilical vein have been found in fetuses immediately prior to development of cardiotocographic signs of compromise.[20] In these fetuses there was loss of blood velocity late in diastole.[21] These and other studies stimulated researchers to study qualitative rather than quantitative changes in the human fetal circulation as a parameter for the assessment of fetal wellbeing.[22,23]

Generally, it has not been possible to obtain results of clinical importance for the surveillance of the fetus at risk, with few exceptions. Some groups familiar with the method have found use in the monitoring of volume flow in the aorta in fetuses with arrhythmia[23,24] and during fetal digoxin treatment[25] in cases of imminent heart failure.

Volume flow is definitely of importance, but using the present methods it is not possible to measure it precisely enough for the result to be of clinical significance. There are reasons to believe that technical improvements in the near future will help overcome some of the problems and that future clinical research will come back to this field.

CONCLUSION

In obstetrics the noninvasive method for quantitative assessment of blood flow in the fetus has led to the first information of haemodynamics being obtained in human fetuses. In clinical practice the method at present probably is not precise enough to be of any value. But there is reason to believe that the Doppler blood velocity monitoring of fetal vascular parameters can be done with such a precision that it can be of clinical importance in future surveillance of the pregnancy at risk. With technical improvement it may also be possible in the future to measure blood flow quantitatively with sufficient precision that it could have clinical consequences. It is important though, that the development of new technology is followed up by well designed studies to evaluate their true benefit in perinatal medicine.

REFERENCES

1. Satumora S. Ultrasonic Doppler method for the inspection of cardiac functions. *J Acoust Soc Am* 1957; **29**:1181-1185.
2. Baker DW. Pulsed ultrasonic Doppler blood-flow sensing. *IEEE Trans on S and US* 1970; **SU-17:** 0-185.
3. Angelsen BAJ. *Transcutaneous measurement of blood velocity and flow in the thorax by ultrasound and the Doppler effect.* Trondheim: Inst Eng Cyb. Norwegian Institute of Technology, 1974; Report 75-78-W.
4. Gill RW, Kossoff G. Pulsed Doppler combined with B-mode imaging for blood flow measurement. *Contrib Gynecol Obstet* 1979; **6:** 139-141.
5. Eik-Nes SH, Brubakk AO, Ulstein M. Measurement of human fetal blood flow. *Br Med J* 1980; **280:**283– 284.
6. Maršál K, Eik-Nes SH, Lindblad A, Lingman G. Blood flow in the fetal descending aorta; intrinsic factors affecting fetal blood flow, i.e. fetal breathing movements and cardiac arrythmia. *Ultrasound Med Biol* 1984; **3:** 339-348.
7. Tonge HM, Struijk PC, Custers P, Wladimiroff JW. Vascular dynamics in the descending aorta of the human fetus in normal late pregnancy. *Early Hum Dev* 1983; **9:** 21-26.
8. Griffin D, Cohen-Overbeek T, Campbell S. Fetal and utero-placental blood flow. In: *Clinical Obstetrics and Gynaecology,* Vol 10 Ed. S Campbell. London. Philadelphia, Toronto: WB Saunders, 1983: pp.562-602.
9. Fitzgerald DE, Drumm JE. Non-invasive measurement of human fetal circulation using ultrasound: a new method. *Br Med J* 1977; **2:** 1450-1451.
10. McCallum WD, Williams CS, Napel S, Diagle RE. Fetal blood velocity waveforms. *Am J Obstet Gynecol* 1978; **132:** 425 - 429.
11. Eik-Nes SH, Maršál K, Brubakk AO, Ulstein M. Ultrasonic measurement of human fetal blood flow. *J Biomed Eng* 1982; **4:** 28-36.
12. Eik-Nes SH, Maršál K, Kristoffersen K. Methodology and basic problems related to blood flow studies in the human fetus. *Ultrasound Med Biol* 1984; **10:** 329-337.
13. Lindström K, Maršál K, Gennser G, Bengtsson L, Benthin M, Dahl P.Device for measurement of fetal breathing movements–I. The TD-recorder. A new system for recording the distance between two-echogenerating structures as a function of time. *Ultrasound Med Biol* 1977; **3:** 143-151.
14. Eik-Nes SH, Grip, A, Kristoffersen K, Lingman G, Maršál K, Vernersson E. Comparison of blood flow measurements by real-time/Doppler ultrasound and electromagnetic flowmeter. *J Clin Ultrasound* 1989;In press.
15. Eik-Nes SH, Grøttum P, Andersson NJ. Estimation of fetal weight by ultrasound measurement. II. Clinical application of a new formula. *Acta Obstet Gynecol Scand* 1982; **61:** 307-312.
16. Gill RW, Warren PS, Griffiths KA, Garrett WJ, Kossoff G. Umbilical blood flow in high risk pregnancy. In: *Recent Advances in Ultrasound Diagnosis 3.* Eds. A Kurjak, A Kratochwil. Amsterdam Oxford Princeton: Excerpta Medica, 1981:pp. 220-225.

17. Jouppila P, Kirkinen P, Eik-Nes SH, Koivula A. Fetal and intervillus blood flow measurements in late pregnancy. In: *Recent Advances in Ultrasound Diagnosis 3*. Eds. A Kurjak, A Kratochwil. Amsterdam Oxford Princeton: Excerpta Medica, 1981: pp. 226-233.
18. Laurin J, Lingman G, Maršál K,Persson PH. Fetal blood flow in pregnancies complicated by intrauterine growth retardation. *Obstet Gynecol* 1987; **69:** 895-902.
19. Gill RW. Pulsed Doppler with B-mode imaging for quantitative blood flow measurement. *Ultrasound Med Biol* 1979; **5:** 223-235.
20. Jouppila P, Kirkinen P. Umbilical vein blood flow as an indicator of fetal hypoxia. *Br J Obstet Gynaecol* 1984; **91:**107-110.
21. Jouppila P, Kirkinen P. Increased vascular resistance in the descending aorta of the human fetus in hypoxia. *Br Obstet Gynaecol* 1984; **91:** 853-856.
22. Trudinger BJ, Giles WB, Cook CM. Flow velocity waveforms in the maternal uteroplacental and fetal umbilical placental circulations. *Am J Obstet Gynecol* 1985; **152:** 155-163.
23. Tonge HM, Stewart PA, Wladimiroff JW. Fetal blood flow measurements during fetal cardiac arrhythmia. *Early Hum Dev* 1984; **10:** 23-34.
24. Lingman G, Dahlström JA, Eik-Nes SH, Maršál K, Ohlin P. Ohrlander S. Haemodynamic assessment of fetal heart arrhythmias. *Br J Obstet Gynaecol* 1984; **91:** 647-652.
25. Lingman G, Lundström NR, Maršál K. Clinical outcome and circulatory effects of fetal cardiac arrhythmia. *Acta Paediatr Scand* 1986; **Suppl 329:** 120-126.

Fetal and placental blood flow

Dr K. Marsál

INTRODUCTION

In animal experiments, uteroplacental blood flow has been shown to be one of the most important determinants of fetal growth.(1) Experimentally induced reduction of the blood flow to the uterus results in intrauterine growth retardation (IUGR).(2) Certain complications of human pregnancy, e.g. pre-eclampsia, restrict the blood flow through the placental vascular bed and predispose to IUGR.(3) In growth retarded fetal lambs the umbilical blood flow is reduced.(4) During intrauterine hypoxia, which is more likely to occur in growth retarded than in normal fetuses, fetal blood flow is redistributed to ensure preferential blood supply to vital organs.(5,6) This phenomenon has been named the brain-sparing effect.

It is obviously of great interest and of clinical importance to measure blood flow on both sides of the placenta and within the fetus itself, in human pregnancies at risk of developing IUGR. Therefore, the first reports on Doppler ultrasound estimation of fetal blood flow(7,8) aroused great interest among both clinicians and perinatal physiologists. However, numerous methodological problems and sources of error inherent in the ultrasonic volumetric estimation of fetal blood flow(9) led to moderation of the initial enthusiasm. Most of the research groups have rejected the estimation of volume blood flow in favour of analysing the waveform of the fetal and umbilical arterial blood velocity as it has been shown in a number of studies to contain information related to the outcome of pregnancy.(10–15) Nevertheless, using advanced Doppler ultrasound techniques in experienced hands it is possible reliably to estimate the blood flow.(16) As for the future, it may be surmised that it will not be long before the development of ultrasound techniques will make it possible simultaneously and accurately to measure the vessel diameter and blood velocity, thus circumventing the present methodological problems, and so the volume flow method will regain the interest of obstetricians.

In the following, some methodological considerations will be given and a short review of results obtained in growth retarded fetuses will be presented, concerning both the blood flow and blood velocity waveform.

BLOOD VELOCITY WAVEFORM ANALYSIS

Waveform analysis is performed on the envelope of the Doppler shift frequencies, i.e. on the maximum blood velocity, recorded from the fetal or uteroplacental arteries. The waveform can be characterised by various indices: those most often used are the systolic/diastolic ratio (A/B ratio),(17) resistance index(18) and pulsatility index (Figure I).(19) All three indices are said to be a measure of the peripheral vascular resistance. The first two indices have the advantage of being easily derived from the Doppler spectrum, even by manual analysis of the tracings. However,

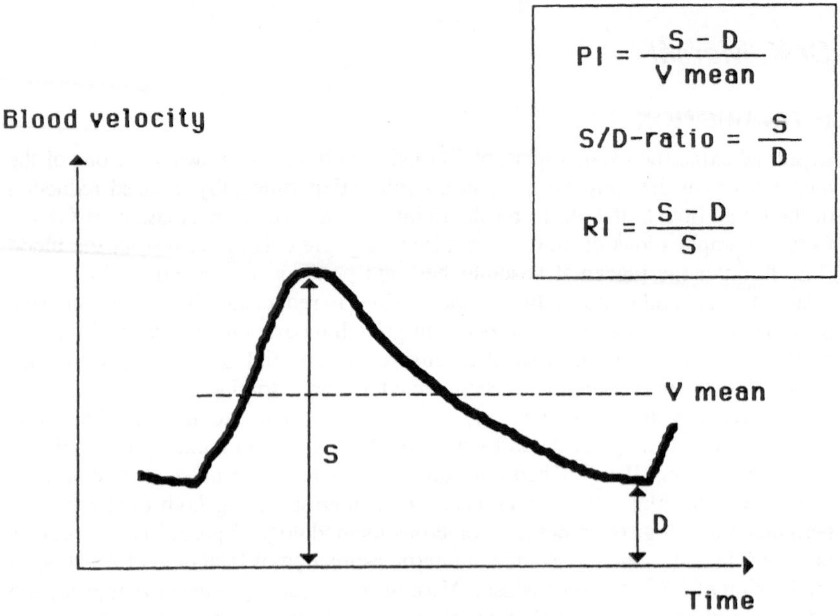

Figure I
Indices of the maximum blood velocity waveform. PI: Pulsatility index; S/D ratio: systolic to diastolic velocity ratio (A/B ratio); RI: Resistance index; S: peak velocity; D: the least diastolic velocity; V mean: average velocity over the heart cycle.

when the diastolic velocity approaches zero, both those indices lose their resolution. In this respect the pulsatility index (PI) is superior, as it increases in a linear fashion with increasing resistance.

The above statement, that the PI and other waveform indices reflect the resistance in the vascular bed peripheral to the site of measurement, should not be accepted without reservation. The indices are indeed strongly influenced by the peripheral resistance; however, they are not independent of other influences like blood pressure, preload, etc. This can be illustrated by the results from the experiments on lamb fetuses, where we have found that the rising slope of the acceleration part of the aortic velocity waveform has the best correlation to the myocardial contractility, expressed as dP/dt of the left ventricle.[20] The next best correlation was found for the PI.

In normal fetuses the diastolic flow is always present as an expression of the low-resistance feto-placental circulation (Figure II). With increasing peripheral resistance, the end-diastolic flow decreases and is eventually eliminated. In growth retarded fetuses developing cardiotocographic signs of distress, the Doppler recorded velocity in the aorta and umbilical artery is often missing in diastole (Figure III). This caused us to design a semi-quantitative evaluation of the fetal blood velocity waveform, the blood flow classes (BFC):[21] BFC 0 (normal) =

positive flow throughout the cardiac cycle + normal PI; BFC I = positive flow + PI ≥ mean + 2 SD; BFC II = end-diastolic velocity non detectable; BFC III = absence of positive flow through the major part of diastole and/or reverse flow in diastole. The concept of BFC proved to offer an efficient diagnostic tool in the case of the development of intrauterine distress.(22) This suggests that, in the future, an automated analysis of the complex waveform pattern may be preferable to simple mathematical indices.

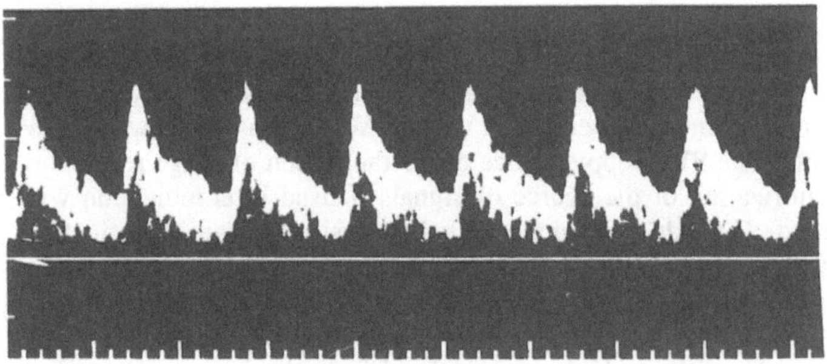

Figure II
Doppler spectrum of blood velocity signals recorded from the umbilical artery of a healthy fetus. Note the presence of a positive velocity throughout the cycle.

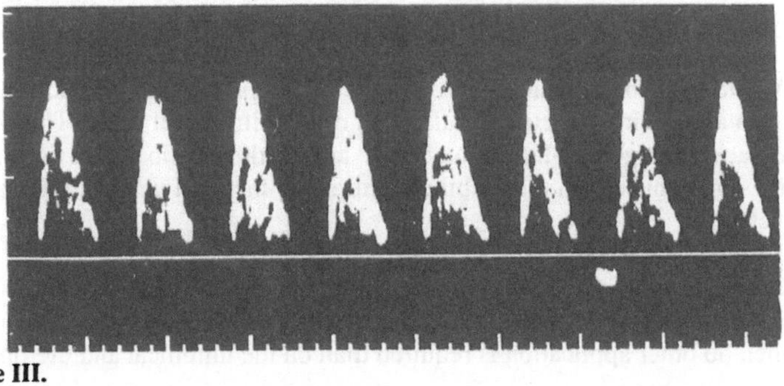

Figure III.
Doppler spectrum of blood velocity signals recorded from the umbilical artery of a fetus in distress. The diastolic velocities are missing, and, in one cycle, there is even a short-lasting reversal of flow.

It should be mentioned that the quality of the primary Doppler signals is crucial both for proper estimation of blood flow and for waveform analysis. All Doppler ultrasound systems include high pass filters for removal of low velocity signals. It has been demonstrated that the filter may profoundly affect the estimation of volume flow. However, it may also affect the appearance of the blood velocity waveform. In cases where the end-diastolic frequency shifts are below the cut-off level of the filter, the velocity will be interpreted as missing. If the insonation angle is large the velocities erroneously eliminated may be quite considerable.(22) Accordingly, the recommendation that insonation angles should not exceed 60°(7)

is also valid for Doppler recordings used in waveform analysis even when indices independent of the angle of insonation are used. There seems now to be agreement between users that a filter with low cut-off level (100 Hz) should be used. In a situation where the insonation angle cannot be controlled, e.g. in recordings of signals from the umbilical artery, the finding of the absence of end-diastolic velocities should be reproduced by insonating the cord from different angles before it is accepted as a pathological finding.

CONTINUOUS WAVE AND PULSED WAVE DOPPLER ULTRASOUND

Signals of the fetal and uteroplacental blood flow velocity can be detected and recorded by means of either pulsed wave (PW) or continuous wave (CW) Doppler ultrasound. The PW Doppler mode offers the option of range resolution and positive identification of the source of signals if used in combination with imaging ultrasound. It produces signals with better signal-to-noise ratio than the CW Doppler does, and enables estimation of the time-averaged mean velocity, which can be used for estimation of blood flow. A disadvantage of the PW-Doppler systems is that they are relatively complicated technically, and therefore are more expensive. The PW mode comprises the risk of aliasing, and the pulse repetition frequency limits the maximum velocity to be recorded. When a spectrum analysis is used on-line, possible aliasing can be easily recognised. Furthermore, the velocities to be detected from a pregnant uterus usually do not exceed the given maximum velocity, and the above limitations only seldom constitute a practical problem.

The CW Doppler systems are technically less complex and therefore cheaper than PW Doppler instruments. The output CW Doppler signals include frequency shifts from all moving structures in the path of the ultrasound beam. Thus, the CW systems lack a range resolution, and their application in obstetrics is limited to recordings of signals from the umbilical arteries in the cord and from the uteroplacental vessels.

The results obtained from the umbilical and/or uteroplacental vessels by the two Doppler modes in the same fetuses were compared in several studies and no significant differences were found.[23–26] Thus, the cheaper CW systems can be reliably used when no other application is required than on the umbilical and uteroplacental arteries.

AORTIC AND UMBILICAL VENOUS BLOOD FLOW IN GROWTH RETARDED FETUSES

In a prospective study on 159 fetuses suspected of IUGR blood flow was estimated in the descending aorta and intra-abdominal part of the umbilical vein.[21] The pregnancies were selected on the basis of routine ultrasound fetometry at 32 weeks' gestation (all pregnancies having been previously dated by an early routine ultrasound examination). At birth, 74 of the newborns were small-for-gestational age (birthweight < mean – 2 SD of the general population) and considered to be growth retarded. In these fetuses, the mean flow velocity both in the descending aorta and the umbilical vein was significantly lower than the reference values (Table 1). The blood flow per fetal weight was also lower. Previously, in normal

Table 1. Mean blood velocity in the descending aorta and umbilical vein in four groups of fetuses according to weight deviation. (Means ± SD).[21]

(n)	Group 1 (24)	Group 2 (61)	Group 3 (48)	Group 4 (26)	Reference group (21)
Descending aorta	30.9 ±4.1	28.6* ±5.4	24.8* ±5.9	20.8* ±5.3	34.6 ±5.5
Umbilical vein	12.4 ±4.1	11.6 ±4.4	9.6* ±3.4	8.6* ±2.6	12.6 ±3.1

*: significance of the difference from the reference value, $p<0.01$
Group 1: Birthweight deviation from the age-related normal mean 0 to -10%; Group 2: - 11 to -21%; Group 3: -22 to -32%: Group 4: more than -32%.

fetuses, a close correlation between the umbilical venous flow and placental weight was found; the correlation between the fetal weight and flow was less good.[27] In the group of IUGR fetuses, the relative flow to placenta was calculated and found to be 35 ml/min/100 g placenta[21] while in normal fetuses, the corresponding value was 65 ml/min/100 g placenta weight.

Concurrent reports on low umbilical flow in IUGR fetuses have been presented in the literature.[21,28,29] The results are also in accord with the experimental data.[4] When evaluated as a possible clinical test, however, the aortic and umbilical volume flow measurements showed a relatively low capacity.[22] This is probably due to the large variation of the normal results as a consequence of the methodological difficulties already discussed.

BLOOD VELOCITY WAVEFORM CHANGES IN GROWTH RETARDED FETUSES

In growth retarded fetuses, the diastolic velocity in the descending aorta and umbilical artery is often decreased or even missing.[10,11,30] The reduction of diastolic flow suggests that there is an increase in the placental vascular resistance. Giles *et al.*[31] found that in cases with umbilical artery waveform changes (i.e. with high A/B ratio), many small muscular arteries in the tertiary stem villi of the placenta have been obliterated.

The vascular bed supplied by the descending aorta of the fetus includes, in addition to the placenta, the lower part of the fetal body including kidneys, viscera and lower extremities. The waveform of the aortic velocity is influenced not only by the resistance in the different parts of the vascular bed but also by the heart's action. Therefore the recording of the aortic velocity probably does not give the same information as an examination of the umbilical artery velocities.

The waveform of the blood velocities recorded from the common carotid artery of growth retarded fetuses shows a relative increase in the diastolic velocity with a decrease in the PI as a consequence.[32] This finding, suggesting a decrease in the peripheral resistance of the cranial vascular bed — the brain-sparing phenomenon — was confirmed on recordings from the intracranial vessels.(33,34) To enhance the abnormal findings in IUGR the use of a ratio between the umbilical artery and internal carotid artery PI was suggested.(33,35)

On the maternal side of the placenta of IUGR fetuses, a decrease in the diastolic velocity and occurrence of a "notch" in the deceleration part of the waveform were found, suggesting an increase in the vascular resistance.(36) Campbell *et al.* (37) described that a finding of pathological velocity waveforms in the uteroplacental arteries before 20 weeks' gestation could give an indication of subsequent development of IUGR and pre-eclampsia.

BLOOD FLOW STUDIES AS A DIAGNOSTIC TEST IN IUGR

After experience from descriptive studies on pregnancies with IUGR had been collected, several prospective studies were performed to evaluate the predictive capacity of the blood flow studies with regard to fetal weight and outcome. These studies had to cope with the difficulty known from other perinatal studies, i.e. how to define the outcome variables, the standard against which the test was to be evaluated. In our studies, the following variables were used as end-points: age-related birthweight and weight deviation from the normal population (mean – 2 SD being the cut-off value for the definition of IUGR), Apgar scores, cord blood pH, occurence of intrauterine distress — defined as the necessity for operative delivery for fetal distress (ODFD) — and neonatal morbidity (days in the neonatal intensive care unit, days in the respirator, etc). An important feature of the studies was the fact that clinicians managing the patients were not aware of the results of the blood flow studies, which thus had no impact on the outcome of pregnancies.

The capacity of blood flow examinations as a test for predicting fetal outcome was evaluated in terms of sensitivity, specificity and predictive value. The agreement between the test results and the actual outcome was tested by calculating the Kappa index.(38) A Kappa index close to 1.0 indicates the best agreement. For comparison of the predictive capacity of various blood flow variables and for choosing suitable cut-off levels for the variables, graphic representation of the relationship between the sensitivity and the false positive rate at various cut-off levels, the so-called Receiver Operating Characteristic (ROC) curves, were used.(39)

In the previously mentioned study on aortic and umbilical venous blood flow in 159 fetuses,(22) the sensitivity in predicting IUGR was 41% for aortic PI, 57% for aortic BFC and 21% for venous blood flow. In predicting fetal distress (defined as ODFD), the corresponding values were 76, 87, and 38% respectively. The Kappa values for the prediction of IUGR were 0.36 for aortic PI, 0.48 for aortic BFC and 0.36 for venous flow. For the prediction of ODFD, the corresponding values of Kappa were 0.44, 0.64, and 0.45, respectively.

In a subsequent study performed at our laboratory in Malmö on a group of 129 patients, the predictive values of the blood velocity waveforms recorded from the umbilical and uteroplacental arteries were compared.(40) The sensitivity in predicting IUGR was 56% for the umbilical artery PI and 39% for the uteroplacental PI. In predicting fetal distress, the corresponding values were 83% for the umbilical artery and 43% for the uteroplacental artery. The Kappa values for the prediction of IUGR were 0.56 for the umbilical PI and 0.11 for the uteroplacental PI. For the prediction of ODFD, the corresponding values of Kappa were 0.63 and 0.08.

The results suggest that the Doppler studies are better indicators of fetal health than of fetal size. This is not surprising as the size of the fetus is determined by many factors. The IUGR can be of other than circulatory origin, and furthermore, some of the very small fetuses can be genetically small, but otherwise healthy with normal blood circulation. The results also showed that the waveform analysis of fetal arterial velocity signals was superior to the estimation of the volume flow in great fetal vessels. Furthermore, a significant difference was found between the predictive capacity of the umbilical and uteroplacental blood velocity waveforms, the latter being a relatively poor predictor of the current fetal condition. When the findings on both sides of placenta were evaluated in the same fetuses, only in cases of abnormal umbilical artery PI was this related to unfavourable clinical outcome.(40) The performance of various blood flow variables was demonstrated by ROC curves. An example of an ROC curve in a case of ODFD is given in Figure IV. A comparison between the fetal aortic and umbilical blood velocity waveforms gave very similar results for both vessels; the umbilical PI was the best predictor of

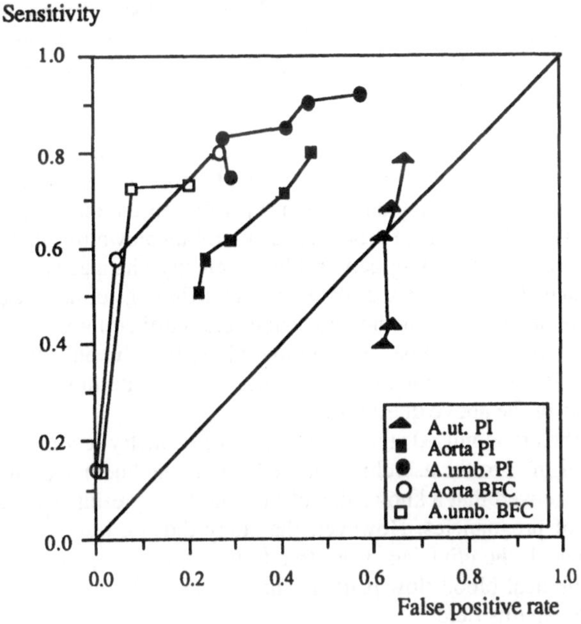

Figure IV
Receiver Operating Characteristic (ROC) curves showing the sensitivity and false positive rate for 5 blood flow variables in the prediction of operative delivery for fetal distress (ODFD). The cut-off levels are changed in steps of 0.5 SD from the mean, from right to left. PI: pulsatility index; BFC: blood flow class; A.ut.: uteroplacental arteries; Aorta: descending aorta; A.umb.: umbilical artery.

IUGR and the aortic BFC was the best predictor of ODFD.[41]

Arduini *et al.*[35] evaluated the ratio between the PI in the umbilical artery and internal carotid artery at 26–28 weeks' gestation and reported a sensitivity of 78% and a specificity of 92% with regard to the subsequent development of IUGR. The blood flow changes seem to occur earlier than any other detectable signs of IUGR.

BLOOD FLOW STUDIES IN THE CLINICAL MANAGEMENT OF IUGR

The results of the Malmö studies[22,40] and a number of studies reported from other centres[12–14,42] suggest that the blood velocity waveforms recorded from the fetal vessels (umbilical artery, descending aorta, cranial arteries) are sensitive indicators of the fetal circulatory state. Especially the absence of end-diastolic velocities in the descending aorta and/or umbilical artery of growth retarded fetuses seems to be a reliable and early indication of fetal distress. In our recent prospective study Doppler examinations of fetal circulation were used as a secondary diagnostic test on a group of fetuses preselected by routine ultrasound fetometry at 32 weeks' gestation as being at risk of IUGR.[43] The study showed the very good capacity of the Doppler examination for predicting unfavourable outcome and indicated that a combined use of the ultrasound fetometry and Doppler velocimetry would reduce the number of pregnancies suspected of IUGR requiring intensive surveillance. Similar conclusions were also arrived at by Berkowitz *et al.*[44] Gaziano *et al.*[45] and Dixon *et al.*[46]

All the evidence presented suggests that the Doppler method is a very promising clinical tool. However, there are still some important questions to be answered before recommendation can be made for use of the Doppler method in monitoring fetuses suspected of IUGR. The time relationship between the onset of the blood velocity changes and other signs of fetal distress is still unknown for the most part. The clinical importance of finding certain blood velocity changes seems to vary with gestational age. There is a risk of obtaining false findings of absent end-diastolic blood flow on the basis of methodological errors. Furthermore, suitable management protocols for various types of abnormal blood flow findings have not yet been established. Prospective randomised studies may be the most reliable and fastest way to answer the above questions.

The first published randomised study on Doppler velocimetry seems to vindicate the original optimism as to the usefulness of the Doppler method in a clinical situation.[47] The study proved that a knowledge of the blood flow results had an impact on the outcome of pregnancies. However, the study did not test a standardised management protocol; the clinicians were free to use or to disregard the information about the umbilical blood flow pattern. There is no doubt that there is a need for further research in this field.

SUMMARY AND CONCLUSIONS

Doppler ultrasound methods can be used in two ways for evaluation of the fetal uteroplacental circulation: volume flow in large fetal vessels can be estimated, or the waveform of arterial velocities can be analysed. At present, the estimation of flow is open to several possible errors and does not seem to provide reliable information on fetal circulation in cases of IUGR. The aortic and umbilical blood velocities are relatively easy to record and their waveform can be analysed and characterised by various mathematical indices. In cases of severe IUGR and in fetuses in distress, the end-diastolic velocities decrease and eventually disappear as the expression of increased peripheral vascular resistance. Similar changes are found also in the uteroplacental vessels. In the cerebral vessels of the growth retarded fetus, the diastolic flow velocities increase, probably reflecting the brain-sparing effect with redistribution of the blood flow.

Prospective studies on preselected groups of fetuses at risk of IUGR demonstrated that the blood velocity waveform changes have a very good capacity to predict IUGR and fetal distress. The umbilical and aortic flow velocity waveforms are comparable in this respect, both being superior to the uteroplacental velocity waveforms. There is little doubt that the Doppler ultrasound method has significant clinical potential as a secondary diagnostic test of IUGR and a method of fetal surveillance. However, the understanding of the pathophysiological background of the blood velocity changes in IUGR is far from complete, and this question requires further research. Also, the type of clinical management suitable in cases of IUGR fetuses with abnormal blood flow has to be established, e.g. in prospective randomised studies, before any recommendations for general clinical use can be made.

REFERENCES

1. Wootton R, McFayden IR, Cooper JE. Measurement of placental blood flow in the pig and its relation to placental and fetal weight. *Biol Neonate* 1977; **31**: 333–339.
2. Jansson T. Responsiveness to norepinephrine of the vessels supplying the placenta of growth-retarded fetuses. *Am J Obstet Gynecol* 1988; **158**: 1233–1237.
3. Brosens I, Dixon HG, Robertson WB. Fetal growth retardation and the arteries of the placental bed. *Br J Obstet Gynaecol* 1977; **84**: 656–663.
4. Clapp JF III, Szeto HH, Larrow R, Hewitt J, Mann LI. Umbilical blood flow response to embolization of the uterine circulation. *Am J Obstet Gynecol* 1980; **138**: 60–67.
5. Creasy RK, DeSwiet M, Kahanpää KV, Young WP, Rudolph AM. Pathophysiological changes in the foetal lamb with growth retardation. In: *Fetal and Neonatal Physiology*. Sir Joseph Barcroft Symposium. Eds. RS Comline, KW Cross, GS Dawes, PW Nathanielsz. Cambridge: University Press, 1973; pp.398–402.
6. Cohn HE, Sacks, EJ, Heymann MA, Rudolph AM. Cardiovascular responses to hypoxemia and acidemia in fetal lambs. *Am J Obstet Gynecol* 1974; **120**: 817–824.
7. Gill RW. Pulsed Doppler with B-mode imaging for quantitative blood flow measurements. *Ultrasound Med Biol* 1979; **5**: 223–235.
8. Eik-Nes SH, Brubakk AO, Ulstein M. Measurement of human fetal blood

flow. *Br Med J* 1980; **1**: 283–284.
9. Eik-Nes SH, Maršál K, Kristoffersen K. Methodology and basic problems related to blood flow studies in the human fetus. *Ultrasound Med Biol* 1984; **10**: 329–337.
10. Lingman G, Laurin J, Maršál K. Circulatory changes in fetuses with imminent asphyxia. *Biol Neonate* 1986; **49**: 66–73.
11. Jouppila P, Kirkinen P. Increased vascular resistance in the descending aorta of the human fetus in hypoxia. *Br J Obstet Gynaecol* 1984; **91**: 853–856.
12. Trudinger BJ, Giles WB, Cook CM. Flow velocity waveforms in the maternal uteroplacental and fetal umbilical placental circulation. *Am J Obstet Gynecol* 1985; **152**: 155–163.
13. Fleischer A, Schulman H, Farmakides G, Bracero L, Blattner P, Randolph G. Umbilical artery velocity waveforms and intrauterine growth retardation. *A m J Obstet Gynecol* 1985; **151**: 502–505.
14. Rochelson B, Schulman H, Farmakides G, Bracero L, Ducey J, Fleischer A, Penny B, Winter D. The significance of absent end-diastolic velocity in umbilical artery velocity waveform. *Am J Obstet Gynecol* 1987; **156**: 1213–1218.
15. Reuwer PJHM, Bruinse HW, Stoutenbeek P, Haspels AA. Doppler assessment of the feto-placental circulation in normal and growth-retarded fetuses. *Europ J Obstet Gynecol Reprod Biol* 1984; **18**: 199–205.
16. Eik-Nes SH, Grip A, Kristoffersen K, Lingman G, Maršál K, Vernersson E. Comparison of blood flow measurements by real-time/Doppler ultrasound and electromagnetic flowmeter. *J Clin Ultrasound* 1989; In press.
17. Fitzgerald DE, Drumm JE. Non-invasive measurements of the fetal circulation using ultrasound: a new method. *Br Med J* 1977; **2**: 1450–1451.
18. Pourcelot L. *Applications cliniques de l'examen Doppler transcutane*. Paris: INSERM 1974; **34**: 213–240.
19. Gosling RG, Dunbar G, King DH, Newman DL, Side CD, Woodcock JP, Fitzgerald DE, Keates JS, MacMillan D. The quantitative analysis of occlusive peripheral arterial disease by a non-intrusive ultrasound technique. *Angiology* 1971; **22**: 52–55.
20. Maršál K, Lingman G, Rosén KG, Kjrellmer I. Myocardial contractility and ultrasonically measured blood velocity in fetal lamb. In: *WFUMB'85*. Eds RW Gill, MJ Dadd. Sydney: Pergamon Press, 1985; p.256.
21. Laurin J, Lingman G, Maršál K, Persson PH. Fetal blood flow in pregnancies complicated by intrauterine growth retardation. *Obstet Gynecol* 1987; **69**: 895–902.
22. Laurin J, Maršál K, Persson PH, Lingman G. Ultrasound measurement of fetal blood flow in predicting fetal outcome. *Br J Obstet Gynaecol* 1987; **94**: 940–948.
23. Giles WB, Lingman G, Maršál K, Trudinger BJ. Fetal volume blood flow and umbilical artery flow velocity waveform analysis. A comparison. *Br J Obstet Gynaecol* 1986; **93**: 461–465.
24. Gudmundsson S, Fairlie F, Lingman G, Maršál K. Recording of blood flow velocity waveforms in the uteroplacental and umbilical circulation – repro-

ducibility study and comparison of pulsed and continuous wave Doppler ultrasound. *J Clin Ultrasound* 1989; In press.
25. Mehalek KE, Berkowitz GS, Chitkara U, Rosenberg J, Berkowitz RL. Comparison of continuous-wave and pulsed Doppler S/D ratios of umbilical and uterine arteries. *Obstet Gynecol* 1988; **72**: 603–606.
26. Brar HS, Medearis AL, DeVore G, Platt LD. Fetal umbilical velocimetry using continuous-wave and pulsed-wave Doppler ultrasound in high-risk pregnancies: a comparison of systolic to diastolic ratios. *Obstet Gynecol* 1988; **72**: 607–610.
27. Lingman G, Maršál K. Fetal central blood circulation in the third trimester of normal pregnancy. Longitudinal study. I. Aortic and umbilical blood flow. *Early Hum Dev* 1986; **13**: 137–150.
28. Gill RW, Kossoff G, Warren PS, Garrett WJ. Umbilical venous flow in normal and complicated pregnancy. *Ultrasound Med Biol* 1984; **10**: 349–363.
29. Jouppila P, Kirkinen P. Umbilical vein blood flow as an indicator of fetal hypoxia. *Br J Obstet Gynaecol* 1984; **91**: 107–110.
30. Erskine RLA, Ritchie JWK. Umbilical artery blood flow characteristics in normal and growth-retarded fetuses. *Br J Obstet Gynaecol* 1985; **92**: 605–610.
31. Giles WB, Trudinger BJ, Baird PJ. Fetal umbilical artery flow velocity waveforms and placental resistance: pathological correlation. *Br J Obstet Gynaecol* 1985; **92**: 31–38.
32. Maršál K, Lingman G, Giles W. Evaluation of the carotid, aortic and umbilical blood velocity waveforms in the human fetus. In: *Proceedings XI Annual Conference of the Society of Fetal Physiology*. Oxford, 1984; C33.
33. Wladimiroff JW, Wijngaard JA, Degani S. Cerebral and umbilical arterial blood flow velocity waveforms in normal and growth-retarded pregnancies. *Obstet Gynecol* 1987; **69**: 705.
34. Kirkinen P, Muller R, Huch R, Huch A. Blood flow velocity waveforms in human fetal intracranial arteries. *Obstet Gynecol* 1987; **70**: 617–621.
35. Arduini D, Rizzo G, Romanini C, Mancuso S. Fetal blood flow velocity waveforms as predictors of growth retardation. *Obstet Gynecol* 1987; **70**: 7–10.
36. Campbell S, Diaz-Recasens J, Griffin DR, Cohen-Overbeek TE, Pearce JMF, Willson K, Teague MJ. New Doppler technique for assessing uteroplacental blood flow. *Lancet* 1983; **i**: 675–677.
37. Campbell S, Pearce JMF, Hackett G, Cohen-Overbeek TE, Hernandez C. Qualitative assessment of uteroplacental blood flow: early screening test for high-risk pregnancies. *Obstet Gynecol* 1986; **68**: 649–653.
38. Fleiss JL. *Statistical Methods for Rates and Proportions*. New York: John Wiley & Sons, 1973.
39. Richardson DK, Schwartz JS, Weinbaum PJ, Gabbe SG. Diagnostic tests in obstetrics: A method for improved evaluation. *Am J Obstet Gynecol* 1985; **152**: 613–618.
40. Gudmundsson S, Maršäl K. Umbilical and uteroplacental blood flow velocity waveforms in pregnancies with intrauterine growth retardation. *Europ J Obstet Gynecol Reprod Biol* 1988; **27**: 187–196.

41. Gudmundsson S, Maršál K. Fetal aortic and umbilical artery blood velocity waveforms in predicting fetal outcome. A comparison. *Am J Perinatology* 1989; In press.
42. Reuwer PJHM, Sijmons EA, Rietman GW, van Tiel MWM, Bruinse HW. Intrauterine growth retardation: prediction of perinatal distress by Doppler ultrasound. *Lancet* 1987; **ii**: 415–418.
43. Maršál K, Persson PH. Ultrasonic measurement of fetal blood velocity wave form as a secondary diagnostic test in screening for intrauterine growth retardation. *J Clin Ultrasound* 1988; **16**: 239–244.
44. Berkowitz GS, Chitkara U, Rosenberg J, Cogswell C, Walker B, Lahman EA, Mehalek KE, Berkowitz RL. Sonographic estimation of fetal weight and Doppler analysis of umbilical artery velocimetry in the prediction of intrauterine growth retardation: a prospective study. *Am J Obstet Gynecol* 1988; **158**: 1149–1153.
45. Gaziano E, Knox E, Wager GP, Bendel RP, Boyce DJ, Olsson J. The predictability of the small-for-gestational-age infant by real-time ultrasound-derived measurements combined with pulsed Doppler umbilical artery velocimetry. *Am J Obstet Gynecol* 1988; **158**: 1431–1439.
46. Dixon MY, Guidetti DA, Braverman JJ, Oberlander E, Langer O, Merkatz IR. Intrauterine growth retardation — a prospective study of the diagnostic value of real-time sonography combined with umbilical artery flow velocimetry. *Obstet Gynecol* 1988; **72**: 611–614.
47. Trudinger BJ, Cook CM, Giles WB, Connelly A, Thompson RS. Umbilical artery flow velocity waveforms in high-risk pregnancy. *Lancet* 1987; **i**: 188–190.

Discussion

Chairman: Dr N. Patel

HALL: I am not happy about using operative delivery for fetal distress as an outcome measure, because if you look at the literature on Caesarean section rates you could not really conclude that Caesarean sections were done because they were needed. There are babies with fetal distress who are not delivered by Caesarean section. I think that is a rather soft outcome to use.

MARŠÁL: We are aware of this weakness. We would have liked to have a better measurement of the outcome. But in our unit the rate of Caesarean sections is relatively low at about 8% which perhaps justifies the use of it.

CAMPBELL: I am disappointed that you do not find uterine waveforms successful. Do you just go on the placental side, or do you go on each side? Do you take the worst value, the mean or the best value?

MARŠÁL: We go on both sides and wc take the worst value. It is quite difficult when we get a normal signal because we do not see the vessel in most cases. If we get a normal signal we are quite sure that the signal comes from the intraplacental vessel. If we get a pathological pattern it is more difficult to be sure because it might be an error. We have been studying what might be the reason for the low predictive value of our results and we have considered two things. In methodology, we have been testing reproducibility for the umbilical artery because of the variation between ourselves which was 8%. However, for the uteroplacental artery it was 24% which is unacceptably high. The other possibility with regard to the methodological process might be that the uteroplacental artery is not always representative of the whole placenta. We just record velocities which belong to a small part of the placenta which is different from the umbilical artery where probably half of the placenta is represented.

CAMPBELL: I think that is the reason why, like Szulman, we are going lower now and getting the main branch of the uterine artery. So we are really going down into the groin which represents the sum of all the small arteries and vessels.

MARŠÁL: We are collecting normal data for our own normal population from the main branch of the uterine artery.

CAMPBELL: We have been criticised for failing to define small-for-dates or IUGR or hypertrophy. There are also great problems in definition of the indices we use in Doppler. As I understand it Dr Maršäl, it is not the mean of the maximum velocity nor the integral, but the time averaged maximum velocity. It is the mean of the maximum.

PATEL: It is the Gosling index.

CLAPP: It appears that in a percentage of cases in which there is evidence of retarded growth, presumably asymmetrical growth, there is a change in velocity waveform profiles and a change in total flow. There is a large fraction, about 30%

of the cases of small-for-dates babies, where you cannot tell morphometrically whether they are asymmetrically growth retarded or not, and in whom the method does not detect the fact that this growth retardation is present. The sensitivity and specificity of the methodology relative to the pathology involved in the individual cases requires consideration. Where in the process does the change occur? I would submit to you that all the physics data that I know of and all the data that I know of from a variety of labs, in the pregnant ewe where you can control exactly what downstream resistance is, the data strongly suggest that the ratios at least are not a linear function. They are at least a power function. A change in these ratios occurs long after there have been large changes in calculated placental vascular resistance from direct haemodynamic measurements. This is probably a late change in the process. I think that the burden of proof lies on the person who says that it is an early change, to prove it beyond a reasonable doubt in a prospective way in which serial measurements are taken. There were several things that were not mentioned that are of interest to me from a physiological point of view. I did not hear anyone say anything about the winking and blinking phenomenon in the arcuate arteries so beautifully described by Elizabeth Ramsay in the primate,(1) and I believe confirmed in the human by some people in Europe many years ago. The arcuate artery is not a flaccid open tube. The spiral artery is not a flaccid open tube. Intermittent perfusion of the intervillous space is characteristic of its flow. This should clearly have some effect on uterine artery waveforms in terms of downstream resistance. Likewise I heard nobody mention the effect of myometrial contractility on similar waveforms which I would think from a point of view of physics would have a distinct effect on the reflectance of waves in the uterine circulation. Doppler appears to be a technique that may well have great significant clinical promise, but you need to do some fairly in-depth longitudinal studies if you want to use it for a screening test in an unselected population. Certainly in the pathological pregnancies one must try to develop some better means of assessing the outcome parameters as determined ultrasonically, compared with some functional parameters of outcome. I would be very interested in terms of when change occurs in the course of pregnancy, to know how it correlates with things like biophysical profiles or breathing movements which may reflect something other than end stage deterioration in brain stem function. This is what many of the conventionally used tests for intervention now do.

PATEL: I think that most of the comments that you make are correct. What has been presented is the use of tests that are diagnostic tests in clinical situations rather than evaluation of these techniques in terms of studying pathophysiological conditions. I would add that it would be nice to hear what modulates or modifies the flow as you measure it even though you are using a diagnostic test.

CAMPBELL: Doppler examination would be an extremely bad test if it correlated very well with small-for-gestational-age fetuses. I am not interested in diagnosing small-for-gestational-age fetuses; I am interested in diagnosing hypoxic fetuses. All hypoxic fetuses in our experience have had some Doppler parameter in the fetus that is abnormal. We are not just studying velocity in the aorta, but also the common carotid, the middle cerebral and the renal arteries. Current Doppler allows you to do a complete survey of resistance to flow in the fetal organs. For instance, there is a very high correlation between resistance in the renal artery with hypoxia. So when you add up this profile of the fetal circulation in fetal hypoxaemia, where there is a low pO_2 you would always find an alteration in the fetal flow. That is why I am confident that it is an extremely viable test.

CLAPP: I would love to see this proved to be a very useful test. But you showed for cordocentesis that pO_2 outside the normal range occurred in less than 40% of the cases. If in the 40% that were outside the normal range you have a group of fetuses in whom growth retardation by morphometric parameters had already been established by you, it means several things to me. It means that there are growth retarded fetuses who are not hypoxic. Your other statement was that by the time you see a change in flow distribution they are hypoxic. To me that is a late change. If you can pick that up without having to do a cordocentesis I am sure that is of value because there must be some morbidity associated with the procedure.

CAMPBELL: We find flow changes some time before, but there is a false positive element. We find abnormal fetal flow changes where the pO_2 is normal, so it is either false positive or they may predate measurable changes in pO_2. Studying the fetus is the best way of assessing hypoxia. The umbilical artery is one degree less because abnormal resistance in the umbilical artery can be compensated by normal uterine flow which you sometimes get. I have seen a case of very severe loss of end-diastolic flow in the umbilical artery, but absolutely normal fetal flow because the uterine flow was normal. In other words the good flow in the intervillous space compensated for the resistance in the umbilical circulation. You have got to look at all the vessels to build up a complete Doppler picture of the situation

LEVENE: You are not using Doppler as a screening test as I understand it, but you are being triggered by those fetuses which you detect as being SGA. Can you tell us on a geographical basis in Malmö or wherever, what proportion of babies who are SGA are being detected ultrasonically?

MARŠÁL: Depending on the timing and the gestation when we do the screening — we perform it at 32 weeks' gestation — the cut-off level is about 50–55% on this basis.

LEVENE: So half of the small-for-gestational-age babies are going to be missed in your study. Why do you not expand the study and do what Professor Campbell is suggesting? Do it in the controlled way that you are proposing to do it in Sweden. Is that something that can be feasibly done in Sweden?

MARSAL: Not feasibly because you need the equipment to apply it to the whole population.

CHARD: I would like to pursue a point made by Professor Campbell, and it is a question to all the Doppler people. You said that you would not be at all happy if there were a relationship between fetal weight and Doppler measurements. In real life there is never such a thing as a perfect correlation because there is always going to be a variation. However, it is my impression that there is a very good correlation by which I mean about 0.8 between fetal weight and any of the Doppler indices which you care to choose. That applies to plumb normal populations. You just take any random 500 women. Can you guarantee that the bottom end of that is not simultaneously and dependently picking up the very small fetuses and the hypoxia which happens in those comparatively rare cases to be associated with whatever is the primary pathology? What I am saying to you is that the dependence which you do not want to exist does exist. Can you prove that it does not make it a test which is actually measuring something else?

CAMPBELL: Of babies diagnosed as small-for-gestational-age prenatally, about 45% have normal Doppler parameters. These babies deliver around term and complications in these cases are extremely rare. Conversely, where you have abnormal uterine and abnormal fetal flow patterns that is the group most at risk. They quickly go into hypoxic crisis with abnormal heart tracings and all the parameters we know, and need to be rescued by emergency Caesarean section. There is the divide. You have a group of SGA fetuses sent in for evaluation. If Doppler is normal they tend to deliver at term, often small babies, but they deliver at term. If Doppler is abnormal, the combination of abnormal uterine flow and abnormal fetal flow is the most severe combination of all.

CHARD: Is this an abnormal parameter for that preselected group, or an abnormal parameter relative to the unselected population? Otherwise, you are going to have a circular self-fulfilling prophecy.

CAMPBELL: The only routine screening we have done is this early prediction, because it seemed logical to me that somewhere non adaption of the spiral arteries may be a long term predictor of problems. It is not as perfect as we would want it to be as yet. But we are very early on. There are many other aspects of the uterine artery that we can study especially in response to stress. We have to add up the sensitivity for all the complications which are related to abnormal uterine flow, but there is something in it. But that is the only screening test we have done.

EIK-NES: I also think that we should use more of the information which is present in our Doppler signal. In the velocity tracing from the umbilical artery, for instance, we have the maximum velocity and the mean velocity. We have the complete frequency spectrum; we know that these curves look different in different fetuses. But we are using very little of that information. Actually the A/B ratio which is used mostly uses just two simple points on the curve of all that information. It is very easy to think that those two simple points will solve problems in obstetrics. I think that we should do some research in finding out what are the reasons for the changes or the variations in the signals, and also try to use more of the present information. That is what Dr Maršál has done with his visual evaluation of the Doppler signal. I am sure that by looking at the frequency spectrum which can be computerised, one can probably extract more information. There is also a comment on the biophysical profile. I discussed this with Frank Manning who developed the biophysical profile. In Trondheim I have a nonselected population of 3000 women to whom I can apply measurements, and he has something like that in Winnipeg also. We have discussed doing a combined study. We would do a biophysical profile and he promised to teach us the way he thinks it should be done.

There is a lot of variation there.

CLAPP: I view the fetus as very smart. If I were a fetus and I was getting in trouble with my supply line, I would stop moving, and I would do that fairly early on. I think that "kick count" data and all that early screening data suggests that if you took a more global view of fetal behaviour and could find a way to measure it; it might occur earlier than some of the things that you use now.

PATEL: A Swede, Leonard Nordstrom, who came to work with us from Dr Maršál's unit compared 57 high risk patients with both biophysical profiles and Doppler. The Doppler was better at identifying the fetuses that were at risk than was the biophysical profile.

EIK-NES: What about combined use adding Doppler later?

RUSH: If intrauterine growth retardation is a biological phenomenon for which there is no therapy, and very little in the way of any preventive strategy, it is just an interesting phenomenon about which we have spent a great deal of time talking. This is a biophysical technique to detect what appears to be a direct pathological situation in the fetus. Under what conditions would you find abnormality, Professor Campbell, and not intervene? Is this a red flag from which some clinical action must be taken? If that is so we are all again talking about different phenomena. Intrauterine growth retardation has been one of the most boring subjects of the last 20 years, it seems, as an observer. Because in "Chard's curve" it is something which has no therapeutic implications as far as I understand it (see Figure I).

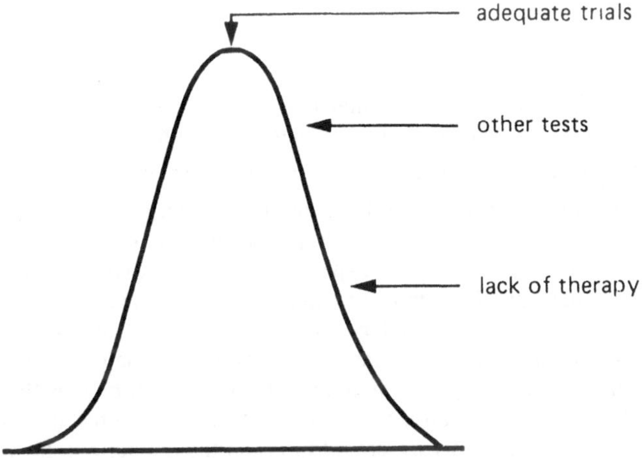

Figure I

Chard's curve. This is a graphical presentation of the life-history of a test of fetal wellbeing. After initial introduction there is increasing enthusiasm and a phase of rapid growth. This growth slows and stops when properly conducted trials shows that the test is less effective than was originally believed. The introduction of other tests then starts a decline. The process is completed when even larger trials show that performing the test makes no difference to fetal outcome, largely because of the lack of any specific therapy for the "at-risk" fetus.

CAMPBELL: If you have an abnormal uterine waveform it means that you watch that woman very carefully and monitor the fetus very carefully. If you have abnormal umbilical artery or fetal waveforms then you almost certainly have fetal hypoxia. Then you have to decide how severe the hypoxia is. Doppler of the fetus will give you an idea whether it is severe or not. But you cannot say if it is acidotic. The only way to find that out is by cordocentesis. If then by cordocentesis that fetus is acidotic you will deliver it straight away.

PATEL: Most people's experience has not been that a Doppler abnormal fetus when it is identified shows asphyxia at birth. Dr Maršál's data show that in fact sometimes Doppler is abnormal for as long as 33 days.

CAMPBELL: I am not saying that all hypoxic fetuses can go through labour and not survive. But the correlation between abnormal fetus by Doppler and hypoxia (not acidosis) is very high. If you do a cordocentesis and the fetus is acidotic you will deliver it. If you do it at 24 weeks and the fetus is hypoxic you can administer therapy which Dr Nicolaides will talk about later. You can give oxygen to the mother to breathe, and we believe that it works, but we have to do a randomised study to prove it. What you effectively do is push more oxygen across this very bad placenta into the fetus and keep it going for a few weeks until it is mature enough to deliver.

RUSH: This sounds to me like an issue of such deep importance that it should be amenable to trial. If this study group has a useful ending it might be to say that some sort of collaborative trial on this as a clinical tool should be pursued if it is not being done already.

PATEL: It is not being done. Are you recommending that whenever the Doppler is abnormal we do cordocentesis?

CAMPBELL: If you have abnormal Doppler you want to know the karyotype because Doppler abnormalities are associated also with genetic abnormality.

PATEL: You have not actually shown how much association there is.

CAMPBELL: I have not shown it yet, but there is an association between abnormal Doppler and abnormal fetal karyotype. We want to know the blood gases and we need to know it in a research capacity as well in a management capacity. For example, we have problems in that although we have a regional neonatal intensive care unit they very often cannot take our sick neonates because they are full up. So we have to send the mother out, and this is a problem which is not just confined to my hospital. We had a case not long ago of a very small baby with very severely abnormal Doppler. Normally, we would just have delivered that baby, but the neonatal unit was full and we were told to send the mother out. So we did cordocentesis and that fetus had a pH of 6.9. I refused to send the mother out and decided to deliver the baby straight away. The baby was resuscitated and we sent the baby straight from our delivery room to neonatal intensive care elsewhere. The baby has done very well. If we had sent that mother out without knowing that her baby's pH was 6.9 it would have been dead before delivery.

PATEL: I wonder what the long term outcome will be for that baby with a pH of 6.9.

STEWART: I should like to comment on the outcome measure and about trial of the uterine Doppler. The group at Port Royal in Paris, have actually been doing this and they have a group of survivors who had an abnormal measurement. Those were subjected to neurological examination after delivery and then followed up for one year. They found that only a very few of these children were abnormal at one year. It was a very small proportion. They did question how compromised these fetuses had been.

MARŠÁL: I cannot give you any results as yet, but we are doing a progress study of the 159 children born in the first study. The oldest of them are seven years old. We have quite a large protocol including neurological and psychological examination and we are anxiously waiting to see what we will find.

STEWART: This is what the Port Royal group found. They thought that this would pick out a group of really compromised fetuses, but it did not.

NICOLAIDES: The numbers of babies who would be so severely compromised would be extremely few. It would take several years before you could find any association. Also you would have a large number who would have a perfectly normal delivery. There is no association, for example, between long term outcome and cord pH, this strong end point that we have used in obstetrics for many years. Studies in Oxford and Sweden show that antenatal CTG abnormalities correlate with the long term prognosis, but not intrapatrum CTG abnormalities. I think that what fetal Doppler is primarily looking at is fetal response. We have known for years from animal studies the fetal responses to hypoxia. There is a good association between the various abnormalities and those Doppler parameters in the fetal circulation and the degree of hypoxia and acidosis in the extreme case, in a highly selected group on which we are doing fetal blood sampling. I also accept the criticism that if we look at the entire population as a method of screening we end up doing a large number of fetal blood samples that carry not just morbidity but actual mortality. I do not believe that should be part of routine practice in any way. I think that it should be confined to highly specialised centres. It should remain as an experimental technique that will allow us to find the various associations of the direct measurement of blood gases. In pO_2 we have a final end point. Unfortunately, at the moment the CTGs are proving not to be so sensitive in detecting hypoxia in these babies. Also the biophysical profile is not in our preliminary observations as useful as Doppler in predicting, in this highly preselected group, the degree of fetal compromise as measured by hypoxia.

CAMPBELL: We have a tremendous degree of elitism going on around this table! We have Dr Maršál saying "we do Doppler and it is quite useful. But nobody else should do Doppler." We have Dr Nicolaides saying "I do cordocentesis very successfully with very useful results. But nobody else should do cordocentesis." I went to the Third World recently to give some lectures and I suddenly realised that cordocentesis is a technique which is ideal for the Third World because it is very inexpensive. They all have their simple ultrasound machines and all they need is a spinal needle and they are in business. Most of the neonatal units have a blood gas analyser. If you train a very small cohort of people to do it, it has a low risk and a high amount of information.

HAN: The problem is that they do not have the end point to deal with it. Suppose that they have a hypoxic or an acidotic baby at 27 or 28 weeks, what are they going to do with it? They do not have the neonatal intensive care units to look after them.

CAMPBELL: As for Doppler, I can train a houseman to do umbilical artery Doppler in five minutes and that is a useful clinical tool. So I think that this is now a technique which is available to any hospital.

PATEL: In all fairness, what Dr Maršál said as I understood it was that it appears to be a valuable tool, but that it is not fully and properly evaluated to be used as a clinical tool for everybody. Are you saying that that is not the case?

CAMPBELL: I think that the information from the umbilical artery, a simple measurement of resistance, loss of end-diastolic flow—anybody can do that in five minutes. That information is invaluable, especially to the houseman in the middle of the night when he sees a strange heart tracing that he cannot interpret. When he puts on the Doppler transducer if there are end-diastolic frequencies he can go to sleep and sleep soundly, and so will I. If there are no end-diastolic frequencies then that baby should be delivered.

HALL: Have you tested that out? Because we have got to ask the question if that baby is really under threat of being compromised?

CHARD: Are there no false positives? If there are you going to be in an enormous amount of trouble.

CAMPBELL: Do you maintain that CTGs do not have any false positives?

CHARD: I am not denying that; they do.

CAMPBELL: We have techniques of diagnosing fetal hypoxia which are imperfect. I think that loss of end-diastolic flow in the umbilical artery is less imperfect than the other techniques .

CHARD: But you must know a false positive rate before you advocate something which will lead to a large number of extra Caesarean sections.

CAMPBELL: What is the false positive rate for an abnormal CTG? Nobody can tell you that.

CHARD: What is the false positive rate for the loss of end-diastolic flow? Can you define false positive? Is it a positive result in a case which would otherwise be normal? How do you define normality? You need to do a randomised controlled study.

CAMPBELL: The fetus is deoxygenated, compromised.

CHARD: How do you know that it was hypoxic *in utero*? You need a randomised prospective trial.

MARŠÁL: It was not my intention to say people should not use Doppler. I was trying to make the point that this is a sensitive method of assessing fetal condition and I agree that is probably a very late sign in the pathological process of developing hypoxia and asphyxia. However, in a clinical context I consider it to be an early sign when compared to other methods available to us as clinicians. But I would like to recommend a certain caution in application because we really do not know enough yet, for example, about the time relation between the CTG and blood velocity changes. I do not think that we really know what kind of management we should apply in various types of blood flow changes. That is what I think we should stress in our prospective trials before recommending everyone to use it. I do not think that five minutes is enough to understand the method. You can get signals, but for eliminating as many false positive findings as possible it is important that the operator knows what he is doing. It is also possible to get methodologically caused false positive findings.

HOWIE: One of the things that we have not defined is what we mean by "fetal compromise". There may be different types of abnormality measurements during pregnancy with different relationships to outcome. It may be that in the hypoxic fetus the problem may be that the baby may become acutely hypoxic in labour with the risk of intrapartum death. That is one type of compromise. There is a different type of compromise which may be the baby who finishes up with neurodevelopmental disability and who may never actually show evidence of hypoxia in labour. It is compromised because it simply has too few brain cells. So it finishes up with a poor outcome of a completely different type. What I think is essential is that whenever you are doing a test, whether it is Doppler flow in the umbilicus or the uterus or whatever, you define the bad feature clinically that is going to be related to it. If you talk about hypoxia it may be a bad immediate feature which does not relate later on. Before you start making any clinical recommendations about how the test should be used you have got to define how the abnormality that you are seeing is related to a developmental procedure which neonatalogists and the mothers themselves can understand. I do not think that we have even defined what we mean by a "compromised fetus". We are using the term as though it is one thing, while it may be a whole series of different things. You have got to relate what your test tells to subsequent outcome in real terms.

REFERENCE

1. Martin CB, McGaughey HS, Kaiser IH, Donner MW, Ramsay EM. Intermittent functioning of the uteroplacental arteries. *Am J Obstet Gynecol* 1964; **90:** 819–823.

Clinical dating and assessment

Dr M.H. Hall

Assessment of fetal growth requires the most accurate possible estimate of gestational age, for the midwife or obstetrician deciding upon investigation or intervention, for the neonatologist calculating survival and handicap rates, and for the epidemiologist studying the prevalence and aetiology. Unfortunately, the pursuit of precision often leads to the exclusion from published studies of women with uncertain gestation. In a study of 11 602 women in a total population in Aberdeen such uncertainty was associated with irregular menstruation (present in 10.2% of all women), with oral contraceptive use (reported by 11.0% of all women), and with an uncertain last menstrual period (LMP) (in 8.9% of all women),(1) and with various other factors such as lactational amenorrhoea. Women with uncertain gestation are not a homogenous group, but tend to have poorer outcomes, so that their exclusion would mean omitting 37% of perinatal deaths, 34% of those with low birthweight babies, and 37% of preterm labours.(2) This is clearly inappropriate and it is therefore necessary to continue to take a careful clinical history, to examine women carefully, and make full use of available biophysical and biochemical tests when clinically indicated.

GOLD STANDARDS FOR DATING

Time elapsed since LMP, as recommended by WHO(3) is inappropriate as it tends to overestimate gestation length.(1) Because of the well-established unreliability of menstrual data in some cases, only women with "immaculate" data have been used in most studies validating other methods of gestation assessment, such as scan measurements of crown rump length (CRL), biparietal diameter (BPD) or femoral length (FL). These methods have proved to correlate closely with certain menstrual data, but cannot logically be better.

Actual date of delivery has also been used as a gold standard. Because induction rates are quite high in some settings, and because the date of induction is obviously selected by the obstetrician, only cases of spontaneous onset of labour are used when actual date of delivery is used as an end point. However, this does not solve the problem, as gestation at delivery is earlier in spontaneous than induced cases in British Births 1970 data,(4) and in 16 959 women studied recently in Aberdeen (Figure I). There is no way of knowing what would have happened had no induction been done, except that average gestation length would be increased. Furthermore, boys deliver earlier than girls.(4,5) In any event gestation length is not normally distributed around 280 days; delivery is much more likely to occur very early than very late.

Paediatric maturity scoring(6,7) is also sometimes proposed for neonatal, clinical and epidemiological use.(8) It is certainly of value (though not to the obstetrician

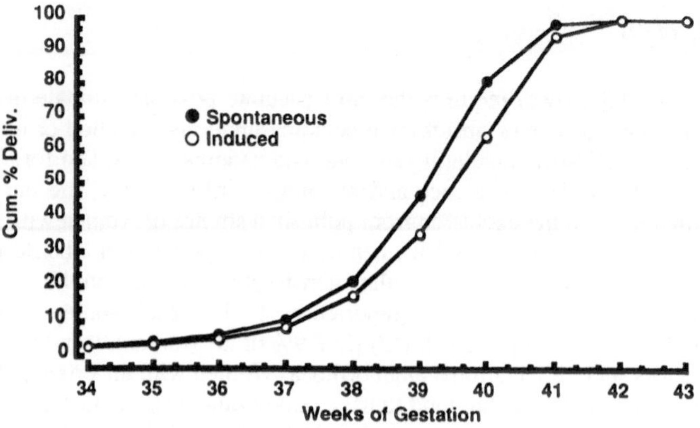

Figure I
Cumulative percentage of deliveries by weeks of gestation and whether spontaneous or induced.

antenatally) where gestation is uncertain, but should not be taken as more accurate than certain dates.

Given the absence of universal gold standards it would seem most sensible for the obstetrician and the epidemiologist to use a best clinical estimate, using all available information and which will usually be in close agreement with early scan measurements. However, the later the "dating" scan is done, the more likely it is that a divergence from average growth may already have occurred. If this happens, interpretation of the subsequent growth patterns will be inaccurate.

DEFINITIONS OF GESTATIONAL AGE

Naegele's rule assumes a gestation length of 266 days from conception or 280 days from the notional LMP. This calculation was of course contrived before it was possible to make any biophysical or biochemical measurements to sort out problems with uncertain gestation. Two hundred and eighty days divides neatly into 40 weeks, but 40 weeks of gestation are variously defined as 274–280 days (rounding up), from 280–286 days (rounding down) or 277–283 days (rounding to the nearest week). Hawkins[9] advocates the last of these, but though this is clearly more logical, it would preclude the use of birthweight for gestation tables based on completed weeks. In a study using 16 960 women with singleton live births in Aberdeen City and Suburbs 1976–85 (using certain gestations only so that days of gestation could be calculated) Campbell, Lemon and I analysed the cumulative percentage of women delivering by "completed" and "Hawkins" weeks of gestation. Clearly the distribution of gestation at delivery would be considerably changed by using "Hawkins" weeks (Figure II) and this should not be done unless birthweight for gestation tables, neonatal survival curves, etc. are similarly calculated.

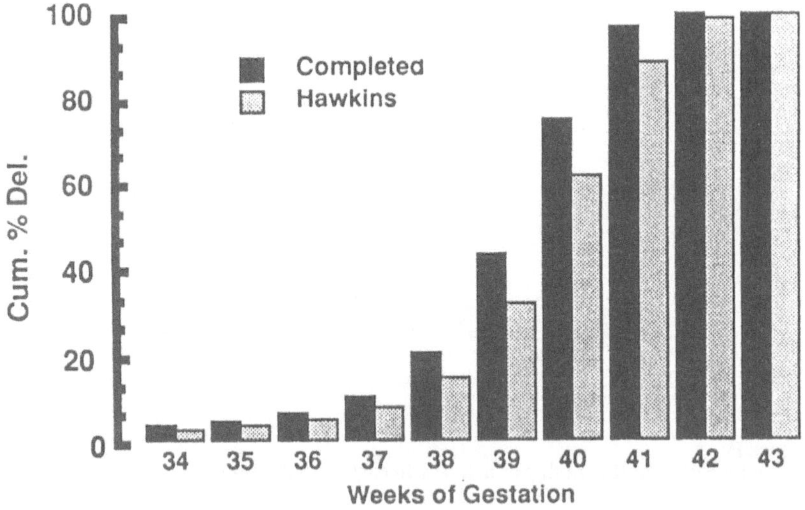

Figure II
Cumulative percentage of deliveries by weeks gestation using different definitions

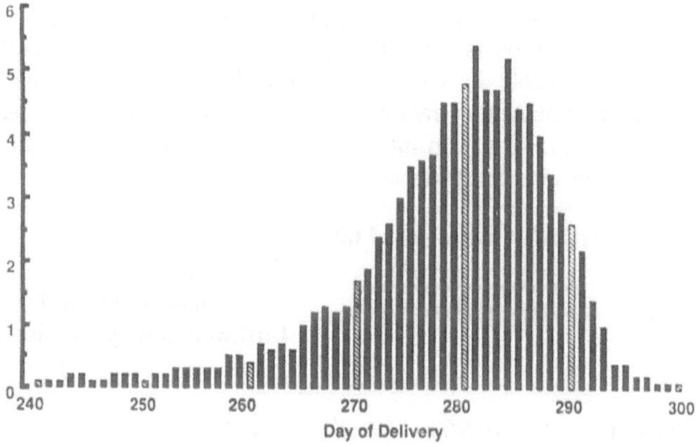

Figure III
Percentage distribution of day of delivery in cases of spontaneous onset of labour

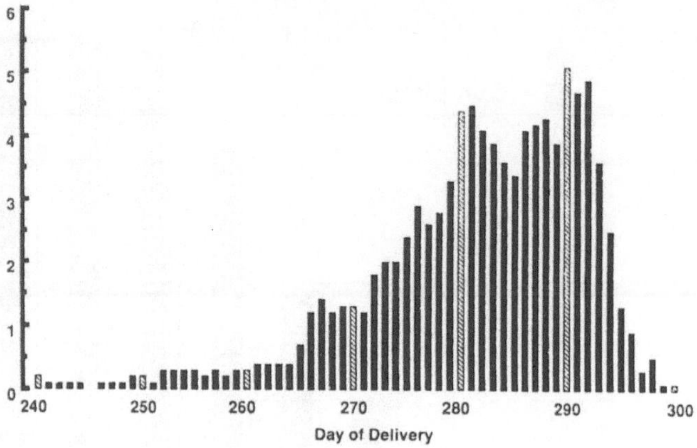

Figure IV
Percentage distribution of day of delivery in cases of induction

Looking at gestation length in days allowed us to look at the actual distribution of gestation length in detail, both in spontaneous onset of labour (Figure III) and in induced cases (Figure IV). Where labour starts spontaneously, the mode for gestation length is 281 days, but as expected it is considerably later in induced cases, suggesting that the "normal" length of gestation is actually more than 280 days. Another interesting point is that induced cases tend to cluster around the beginnings of completed weeks before 40 weeks and around the end of the 42nd week. This means that birthweight for weeks of gestation is bound to be slightly less in induced cases for that reason alone. However, we confirmed the previous finding[4] that birthweight for gestation is actually greater in spontaneous onset of labour than in induced cases (Table 1). Clearly induction because of suspected growth retardation may be a contributory factor, but not the whole story, as most inductions are done after term. This is in interesting contrast to the report that preterm infants are smaller than scan estimates of intrauterine weights.[10]

Table 1. Percentage of SGA by onset of labour

	Total	Less than 10th Centile Birthweight for Gestation	
		n	%
Spontaneous labour	10,968	868	8.1
Induced	6,261	688	11.0
Total	16,959	1,556	9.2

CLINICAL ASSESSMENT OF GROWTH

It is possible in early pregnancy to identify a number of risk factors for growth retardation or fetal macrosomy. Previous obstetric history of either event increases the likelihood of a recurrence,[11] but although a history of growth retardation is often used as a clinical indication for extra surveillance, it may be that the outcome is worse when growth retardation occurs in women with a previous average weight baby.[12] Maternal size (both height and weight) is associated with fetal birthweight for gestation, but again, it may be that this association describes normal physiology rather than pathology — at least some small women with small babies have not experienced growth retardation, and some large women with unusually large babies do not in fact show any pathology. The question of whether to adjust for maternal size when classifying birthweight for gestation is therefore not straightforward.[13]

It has been known for many years[14] that there is an association between poor maternal weight gain and low birthweight. High weight gain is also associated with fetal macrosomy.[15] However, the suspicion that "excessive" weight gain led to pre-eclampsia resulted in widespread dietary restriction in pregnancy and some American studies[16,17] of this practice are therefore of limited value, especially when total pregnancy weight gains are used (since this must be determined largely by gestation length, which itself relates to birthweight). A recent study[18] of very small numbers of highly selected, supposedly normal women (who nevertheless had 19% of babies less than the 10th centile) suggested study of weight gain between 28 and 32 weeks. However it has been estimated[19] that much larger data sets are required to establish reliable relationships between maternal weight gain and birthweight. This is partly because mean weekly weight gain varied considerably during pregnancy, and it is not known what is the best interval to use. Long intervals are probably more reliable than short intervals, and early intervals allow more time for intervention following a suspicion or diagnosis of growth retardation. Also maternal weight gain in early pregnancy is less influenced by the actual weight of the fetus.

Clinical assessment of the size of the uterus is rendered more precise by measuring the fundal height using a tape measure. Both unusually small and unusually large fetuses are often missed, however, and false positives are common.[20,21] In spite of this, it has been argued that the positive predictive value of clinical[22] measurements and risk factors is as good as that of more sophisticated techniques and that the latter should be used only selectively.

REFERENCES

1. Hall MH, Carr-Hill RA, Fraser C, Campbell D, Samphier ML. The extent and antecedents of uncertain gestation. *Br J Obstet Gynaecol* 1985; **92**: 445–451.
2. Hall MH, Carr-Hill RA. The significance of uncertain gestation for obstetric outcome. *Br J Obstet Gynaecol* 1985; **92**: 452–460.
3. World Health Organization Expert Committee on Maternal and Child Health. *Public Health Aspects of Low Birthweight. Third Report of the Expert*

Committee on Maternal and Child Health. Technical Report Series 1961. **217**: Geneva: WHO, 1961.

4. Chamberlain R. Birthweight and length of gestation. In: *British Births 1970, Vol. 1. The First Week of Life*. Eds. R Chamberlain, IG Chamber, B Howlett, A Claireux. London: Heinemann Medical, 1970.
5. Hall MH, Carr-Hill RA. Impact of sex ratio on onset and management of labour. *Br Med J* 1982; **285**: 401-403.
6. Farr V, Mitchell RG, Neligan GA, Parkin JM. The definition of some external characteristics used in the assessment of gestational age in the newborn infant. *Dev Med Child Neurol* 1966; **8**: 507–511.
7. Dubowitz LM, Dubowitz V, Golding C. Clinical assessment of gestational age in the newborn infants. *J Paediatr* 1970; **77**: 1–10.
8. Report of the FIGO Sub-Committee on Perinatal Epidemiology and Health Statistics following a Workship in Cairo November 11–18 1984. *Methodology of Measurement and Recording of Infant Growth in the Perinatal Period*. FIGO, 1986.
9. Hawkins DF. "Gestation" and "completed" weeks. *J Obstet Gynecol* 1988; **4**: 1.
10. Secher NJ, Kern Hansen P, Thomsen BL, Keiding N. Growth retardation in preterm infants. *Br J Obstet Gynaecol* 1987; **94**: 115–120.
11. Bakketeig LS, Hoffman HJ, Harley EE. The tendency to repeat gestational age and birthweight in successive births. *Am J Obstet Gynecol* 1979; **135**: 1086–1103.
12. Ounsted M. Small-for-dates babies: a developmental update. *Paediatric and Perinatal Epidemiology* 1988; **2**: 203–207.
13. Carr-Hill RA, Pritchard C. *The Development and Exploitation of Empirical Birthweight Standards*. Basingstoke: Macmillan Press Ltd, 1985.
14. Thomson AM, Billewicz WZ. Clinical significance of weight trends during pregnancy *Lancet* 1953; **i**: 243–247.
15. Boyd ME, Usher RH, McLean FH. Fetal macrosomia: prediction risks, proposed management. *Obstet Gynecol* 1983; **61**: 715–722.
16. Eastman NJ, Jackson E. Weight relationships in pregnancy. *Obstet Gynecol Surv* 1968; **23**: 1003–1025.
17. Niswander K, Jackson EC. Physical characteristics of the gravida and their association with birthweight and perinatal death. *Am J Obstet Gynecol* 1974; **119**: 306–313.
18. Lawton FG, Mason CG, Kelly KA, Ramsay IN, Morewood GA. Poor maternal weight gain between 28 and 32 weeks gestation may predict small-for-gestational-age infants. *Br J Obstet Gynaecol* 1988; **95**: 884–887.
19. Campbell DM, Carr-Hill RA, Knox A, Lemon J. Hypertension, maternal weight gain and birthweight. *Clin Exp Hyperten* 1987; **2**: 299–310.
20. Svigos JM. The macrosomic infants: a high risk complication. *Med J Aust* 1981; **1**: 245–246.
21. Hepburn M, Rosenberg K. An audit of the detection and management of small-for-gestational-age babies. *Br J Obstet Gynaecol* 1986; **93**: 212–216.
22. Villar J, Belizan JM. The evaluation of the methods used in the diagnosis of intrauterine growth retardation. *Obstet Gynecol Surv* 1986; **41**: 187–199.

Discussion

Chairman: Dr N. Patel

PERSSON: This discussion took place some 10 years ago in Sweden, but it is still going on in the UK and is starting in the United States. With ultrasound you will predict the date of delivery with an error of plus or minus seven days standard deviation. Using only the last menstrual period you predict with an error of 13 days. Now 13 days is about two and a half times worse than seven days if you compare variance. We studied this in depth and the result was that the best prediction was ultrasound. After that came the woman's own statement of when she became pregnant. After that it was the last menstrual period. Even later in the chain came the last menstrual period if you correct for anything other than 14 days of preovulatory interval. The clinical estimation of gestational age was well out. The maximum error that you have by clinical estimation was up to 13 weeks. It was not unusual for it to be 8 weeks. This means that any other clinical evidence, using all available information, makes the situation worse than if you just rely on last menstrual period. No other correction is valid.

HALL: What is your gold standard?

PERSSON: The date of delivery if you do not induce labour.

HALL: So there is no such thing as pre term labour in Sweden?

PERSSON: Yes, of course there is. If you assume that a pregnancy is 34 weeks of age and you have dating by ultrasound then you can be assured that it is at least 32 weeks. But if you use clinical estimates of gestational age and you believe that it is 34 weeks then there is a 10% chance that it is 28 weeks or earlier. If you are going to use modern obstetrics you have to date the pregnancy very carefully. Otherwise you should go back to the old obstetrics where the best thing an obstetrician could do was just sit down and wait for the future to come. I must also oppose very strongly the thinking that a fetus that is 3500 g is mature and it is ready to be born. The most important things in all these discussions we have had is actually maturity and gestational age. It is not the case that the fetus will come when it has an adequate weight. If you were to deliver every fetus weighing 3.5 kg then you will end up in very serious trouble. There is another problem — why screen? Two-thirds of the conditions that a fetus could suffer from are not clincially detectable. To detect these you will have to make a tremendous number of ultrasound examinations. Consider Denmark. If you take the examinations in excess of five done on clinical grounds, then there would be one examination for each Danish woman. So if you allow every clinical complication in pregnancy to have at least five ultrasound examinations there will still be one for all the other Danish women and you will be able to detect somewhat more of the complicated pregnancies than what you do by clinical means. That is one reason to organise the examination, as a means of saving examinations. In my mind this is the only reason for doing screening.

PATEL: I think that Dr Hall was talking about Professor Campbell's remarks regarding not routinely doing a second stage screen, not one scan.

CAMPBELL: Could I just stress that I am not saying that a second routine examination would not be valuable; I think that it would be. It would probably detect a small additional number of small-for-gestational-age fetuses. Also it would pick up some anomalies that you had missed at the 18/20 week scan. It is just that we have only got so many resources, and I would much rather that they spend 15 more minutes on the 18/20 week scan than cut it short and do a second scan, because the first scan is the most important.

RUSH: Professor Persson, if you have the tighter standard deviation of 7 days versus 13 days, is the major value therefore keeping the obstetrician from inducing labour and doing Caesarean section inappropriately? Is that the utility of having the precise dating?

PERSSON: That is one of the reasons but it is not the main one. The main reason is that if you practice active obstetrics then you must know. In some places it is accepted practice to deliver twins at 36 weeks, and if you do not date it properly some of these twins, approximately 10%, would be younger than 30 weeks. It is our responsibility to do the least harm possible. If you look at Swedish conditions, without ultrasound assessment and without routinely inducing post term pregnancies, we killed approximately four infants every year in Sweden for every two saved.

CLAPP: I just wanted to make a point about clinical screening in relation to the discussion of weight gain. It concerns the way one decides what normal is in terms of trying to assess the value of any parameter and a deviation of the parameter from normal. In all of the studies used the standard deviation for the population is so broad that you lose its ability to detect abnormality, because you would include a lot of the abnormality in your normality. My approach has been different, and that has been to pick out a group of women who are clinically very low risk people prior to pregnancy, who have a normal pregnancy that lasts the appropriate period of time and whose baby's birthweight is between the 25th and 75th centile. Then I go back and look at weight gain and various other morphometric parameters in those women serially before, during and after pregnancy. Then I think that you get an idea of a normal standard to which you can compare. You would find that if you did that then you might be able to be able to get much more mileage in terms of clinical screening out of specific weight gain in pregnancy. Until you take that approach you are never going to know whether it is valid. That is true of a lot of parameters in pregnancy, such as blood glucose.

HALL: The problem with that is that you cannot assume that what you have described and observed in a group of highly selected women actually does apply to the rest of the population. This is the problem with using the actual date of delivery. You really did not respond to that at all, Professor Persson. What length of gestation did you use? What did you assume was the normal length of gestation when you were making your predictions? You observed the actual date of delivery, but then your scan measurement is based on some notional appropriate length of gestation. People who have looked at actual length of gestation know the actual date of onset of labour and then frequently they say that the point at the bottom end of the gestation distribution looks pretty untidy and so they miss them out. But you cannot miss them out because you then are going to be using those standards for a population in which people do deliver pre term. You are not going to tell me that you do not have any 28-week gestation babies in Sweden. When they come out at 28 weeks they are not 40 weeks.

PERSSON: A baby at 30 weeks will not weigh 5 kg. What we are assuming is that gestational length is about 280–281 days.

HALL: So 281 days was your assumption? I think that is probably wrong; I think that it is probably longer than that.

PERSSON: It does not matter really because if a woman says she had her last menstrual period at that time, then there is a certain numbers of days left until she will deliver. It is the same thing for morphometry. If you do an examination and find a certain value then there is a certain number of days left until she will deliver. The actual date of gestation is somewhat academic in that sense.

CAMPBELL: You are using exactly the same parameters for predicting from the first day of the last menstrual period as from the morphometry. You do exactly the same in predicting the specific date. Because we had plus or minus 2 weeks the pre term ones do not come into that. You are determining how many will deliver within that time frame.

HALL: You excluded the pre term ones.

CAMPBELL: We had plus or minus 2 weeks; we had plus or minus 3 weeks; we had plus or minus 4 weeks, we had all these. There was a difference at all the cut-off points.

LIND: You have to have a gold standard. Sonar can never be better than your primary thing because the assumption that I guess you are making is that the interval from conception to delivery is fixed. I know of no data whatsoever which would support the concept that while from menstruation to ovulation is variable, the interval from ovulation to spontaneous onset of labour is fixed to within plus or minus 7 days. Guerrero and Florez published a letter in the Lancet(1) based on data from 1408 women (they actually started with something like 13 000 women) whom they asked to record the date of their basal body temperature rise. From the day of menstruation on to the rise of basal body temperature the standard deviations are actually quite tight at from 4 days to about 16 days. From the time of basal body temperature rise to delivery actually has a standard deviation of nearly 12 days. So biologically I would put to you that it is of no relevance how much the standard deviation is from the first day of period to when you ovulate. There is a biological variation from conception to the time of delivery.

HALL: Even then, women who will actually record this data using the temperature charts are not necessarily going to be the same as the population. I agree that it is an interesting and useful piece of data.

LIND: That is *reductio ad absurdum!* Of course you will get to the stage where no data is worth having because whoever offered it to you used a selected population.

PERSSON: You are certainly familiar with a German study from the First World War when the men had one day leave now and then. They related this one day leave to the last menstrual period and dated the pregnancy and there was absolutely no peak in relation to the last menstrual period when the man had been at home. The spread was enormous meaning that women did not really know when they became pregnant. There are many biases also in basal temperature measurements.

LIND: You started off at a point; your assumption I would argue is based on no data whatsoever. Namely, that the time of conception to the time of spontaneous onset of labour has to be within plus or minus 7 days.

PERSSON: No I did not say that.

LIND: Well how do you derive it then? What Dr Hall asked was, "what do you use in your original equation that allows you to calculate EDD?" It has to be fixed on some basis.

PERSSON: It is a population study earlier in this series showing that when you have this value for some fetal parameter then it is in the average a number of days left until delivery. That is how we do it.

LIND: Yes, but it still has to be based on something.

CAMPBELL: The simple matter is that I have experienced obstetrics before there was ultrasound dating and it absolutely revolutionised obstetrics. The other thing is that we are talking about small-for-gestational-age now, not intrauterine growth retardation. You cannot diagnose small-for-gestational-age unless you know the gestational age. No matter what convolutions of discussion we go through there is only one accurate way of diagnosing small-for-gestational-age and that is ultrasound.

HALL: If your one and only ultrasound is done at 20 weeks, which seems to be what you are advocating, so that you can kill two birds with one stone and look for abnormality, then as you pointed out there is a risk that you will be flattening the curve by assuming that some small-for-dates babies are less far on than they really are; and assuming that some already large-for-dates babies are further on than they are. The further along you go from the last menstrual period with your scan the more that will be the case. In the women who appear late for booking it is always going to be a problem.

STEER: Most midwives that I am aware of, indeed most doctors, use Naegele's rule when they are calculating EDD from the LMP. Certainly that is true in our hospital and in the other hospitals in the North West Thames region. So when there is a box that says "EDD from LMP" it is actually plus or minus 3 days because it depends on the length of the months that you use. One of the things that is important is to determine whether people are using Naegele's rule, because if you were to take the EDD from the LMP from clinical data there is a built-in variance of plus or minus 3 days. It is not an accurate way of calculating gestational age.

RUSH: The question is what really leaves the patient best off. I understand that there are ways to avoid intervention and avoid inappropriate procedures. It is really not interesting in this context what normal biology is. You have a mechanism that allows you to use fewer procedures and have a less interfered with healthier population and that seems to be appropriate. This is what I hear from Professor Persson, that it allows the obstetrician to forego intervention when you otherwise would be too anxious not to forego intervention. So in some ways it appears overly academic to worry about what the normal biology of the situation is.

HALL: I hear that the Caesarean section rate in Sweden is quite high.

PERSSON: It is about 8% The incidence of instrumental deliveries is about half that.

REFERENCE

1. Guerrero R, Florez PE. The duration of pregnancy. *Lancet* 1969; **ii:** 268–269.

SECTION 6

CLINICAL IMPLICATIONS OF FETAL UNDERGROWTH (Continued)

Treatment of fetal growth retardation

Mr K.H. Nicolaides, Mr D.L. Economides and Mr G. Thorpe-Beeston

INTRODUCTION

In the management of pregnancies with small for gestational age (SGA) fetuses the main aim is to distinguish between normal small fetuses, not at increased risk of perinatal death or chronic handicap, and fetuses that are growth retarded due to uteroplacental or fetal insufficiency. For the growth retarded fetus, antenatal surveillance is mainly aimed at determining the optimum time, mode and place for delivery. In cases of severe early onset growth retardation with a high risk of perinatal death a number of experimental approaches at improving fetal health and growth have been undertaken, but their success has been limited. More recently cordocentesis has provided access to the fetal circulation and a better understanding of fetal physiology. This knowledge will hopefully lead to the development of more successful methods of treatment.

IMPROVEMENT OF MATERNAL HEALTH

Cigarette smoking

Although the effect of smoking on pregnancy is difficult to isolate from other adverse socio-economic factors, recent studies have shown that infants born to smoking mothers are 150–440 g lighter than infants born to non-smokers. Furthermore, there is a strong dose–response relationship between smoking, early fetal loss, late fetal death and early neonatal death.[1]

Women who stop smoking before or during pregnancy deliver infants whose mean birthweight is greater than infants of women who continue to smoke. This apparent beneficial effect is observed even in women who stop smoking in the third trimester of pregnancy.[2,3] However, there are no studies that have examined or demonstrated an improvement in fetal growth or wellbeing by cessation of maternal smoking in pregnancies where SGA had been diagnosed.

Drug addiction

Maternal ingestion of drugs may affect the fetus directly after transplacental transfer or indirectly by affecting the uteroplacental vessels. In mothers with opiate addiction approximately 25% of pregnancies are complicated by the birth of small-for-dates infants.[4] In contrast, heroin addicts treated with low dose methadone throughout pregnancy deliver infants of comparable weight to those of non-addicted women of similar socio-medical status.[5]

Alcoholism

The incidence of perinatal death in alcoholic women is much higher than in their non-drinking relatives.[6] Furthermore, heavy alcohol consumption is associated with the fetal alcohol syndrome (growth impairment, neurological abnormalities and abnormal facies). In this condition the failure of postnatal catch-up growth[7] and the symmetrical nature of growth retardation point to periconceptual damage in fetal growth potential and it is unlikely that cessation of drinking in the third trimester will restore fetal growth.

Maternal disease

Anaemia

In maternal anaemia the oxygen carrying capacity of blood and the supply of oxygen to the feto-placental unit is reduced. However, there is controversy as to whether the incidence of intrauterine growth retardation is increased. In sickle cell disease, sickling in maternal venous sinuses of the placenta and severe maternal anaemia have been suggested as the underlying causes of the associated increase in the incidence of intrauterine growth retardation.[8] The extent to which growth retardation can be prevented by prophylactic exchange transfusions remains controversial.

Hypertension

Although maternal hypertension is commonly associated with intrauterine growth retardation there is no convincing evidence that treatment of hypertension will either prevent the development of proteinuria or improve fetal growth.[9]

Renal disease

In mothers with renal disease, perinatal mortality and the incidence of pre-term deliveries and small-for-dates infants are higher than in healthy pregnancies.[10] Antenatal management is aimed at early detection and treatment of superimposed pre-eclampsia and fetal surveillance for timely delivery rather than improvement of fetal growth and wellbeing.

Diabetes mellitus

Diabetic nephropathy is associated with fetal growth retardation. Although good diabetic control before and during pregnancy is essential in order to reduce the incidence of congenital abnormalities, fetal macrosomia and perhaps late intrauterine death, it has not been shown to improve the maternal nephropathy and vasculopathy which are responsible for growth retardation.[11]

Heart and lung disease

In severe cases of chronic lung disease and cyanotic heart disease the spontaneous abortion rate and incidence of intrauterine growth retardation is increased, presumably due to the maternal systemic hypoxaemia, and in coarctation of the aorta due to inadequate placental perfusion.[12] Pre-pregnancy cardiac surgery improves maternal health and is associated with a good pregnancy outcome.[13]

IMPROVEMENT OF UTEROPLACENTAL BLOOD FLOW

Bed rest

Bed rest is widely advocated in a variety of complications in pregnancy, including intrauterine growth retardation. It has been suggested that bed rest improves uterine blood flow by reducing sympathetic tone and endogenous catecholamine release.[14] Indeed, studies using radioisotope scanning have demonstrated that bed rest improves uterine blood flow both in normal pregnancies and those complicated by chronic hypertension.[15] Bed rest has also been claimed to improve placental function as demonstrated by an increase in maternal urinary oestriol excretion.[16] However the extent to which bed rest improves fetal growth and wellbeing in pregnancies with documented intrauterine growth retardation remains to be determined.

Betamimetics

It has been speculated that long term oral administration of these agents may promote fetal growth. Indeed ritodrine has been shown to increase significantly uterine blood flow in third trimester pregnancies complicated by hypertension. However, although animal studies have shown an increase in fetal birthweight after treatment with ritodrine or terbutaline, the effect on birthweight in human pregnancies is disputed.[17]

Anticoagulants

Prophylactic administration of dipyridamole (300 mg daily) and aspirin (150 mg daily) from 12 weeks' gestation, to a group of women at high risk of pre-eclampsia and fetal growth retardation has been shown to protect against the recurrence of these complications.[18] Similarly, prophylactic administration of aspirin (60 mg daily) from 28 weeks' gestation to angiotensin-sensitive primigravidae may prevent the development of pre-eclampsia.[19] More recently, Trudinger *et al.*[20] reported on a placebo-controlled, double blind trial of aspirin (150 mg daily) in women with a high (> 95th centile) umbilical arterial flow velocity wave form systolic/diastolic ratio. Although in the majority of patients the indication for the Doppler studies was the clinical suspicion of growth retardation, no data is provided on the estimated fetal size at the time of entry to the study. The mean birthweight of infants of mothers who received aspirin was 516 g heavier than the placebo group. The suggested mechanism of action of low dose aspirin is the differential inhibition of thromboxane A_2 production and restoration of the normal prostacyclin–thromboxane balance.

Solcoseryl

Solcoseryl is a protein-free and antigen-free haemodialysate derived from calf blood. It is thought to: (i) activate the cellular respiratory chain leading to better oxygen utilisation by the tissues, (ii) increase the energy reserves of the cells, (iii) decrease the total peripheral resistance of the arteries and (iv) stimulate the contractile heart force. Kaplinski and Kurjak[21] have investigated the effects of solcoseryl therapy in a comparative study of pregnancies with growth retardation diagnosed by ultrasound measurement of hPL in maternal serum and amniotic fluid, measurement of oestriol in maternal serum and urine, and cardiotocography. Twenty-seven patients were treated with daily intravenous infusion of solcoseryl in addition to bedrest; 92% of the patients delivered infants with birthweights above the 10th centile. Twenty-five women were treated with bedrest alone; 30% delivered infants above the 10th centile.

Allylestrenol

Allylestrenol is a synthetic progestogen thought to have pregnancy-maintaining and weight-promoting properties. It has been used in the treatment of threatened abortion and an increase in the urinary secretion of hCG, hPL, pregnanediol and oestriol have been reported after allylestrenol therapy in the first half of pregnancy.[22] In a prospective, placebo-controlled trial of 30 patients in whom the fetal weight estimated by ultrasonography was below the 10th centile, the administration of allylestrenol (30 mg daily) was associated with a significantly greater fetal weight gain. Indeed, it was reported that 53% of the infants' birthweights were above the 10th centile.[23] More recently, Pearce *et al.*[24] reported the findings of a prospective placebo-controlled study of allylestrenol in 11 patients with ultrasonically diagnosed growth retardation. The impedence to flow in the uterine artery (RI), measured by Doppler, in the control group increased significantly with time, but in the treated group it did not change. It was suggested that allylestrenol may improve or at least prevent deterioration of the maternal uteroplacental circulation either by alpha-receptor blockade or by an anti-platelet function.

FETAL NUTRIENT SUPPLEMENTATION

Maternal

Beischer *et al.* [16] investigated the value of bed rest and intravenous administration of hypertonic dextrose and/or amino acid solution to 635 women with persistently low oestriol excretion as an alternative to preterm delivery. In 65% of the patients oestriol excretion improved and entered the normal range. This regime of bed rest and hyperalimentation was associated with a reduction in the incidence of perinatal death. In those women whose oestriol excretion entered the normal range the perinatal mortality was 1.1% compared to 10.5% in those who failed to respond.

Intrapartum infusions of 10% intralipid to mothers with normal pregnancies is associated with an increase in umbilical cord blood free fatty acid, glycerol and beta-hydroxybutyrate levels.[25] It was suggested that maternal infusion of intralipid should be considered as a possible approach to the treatment of growth retarded fetuses.

Fetal

Animals

In chronic sheep preparations nutrients such as amino acids or glucose can be administered to the fetus by intra-amniotic, fefal gastrointestinal, or fetal intravenous administration without obvious adverse effect. Furthermore, fetal nutritional supplementation improves growth and development in experimentally induced growth retardation in fetal lambs.[26]

Humans

In human studies intermittent intra-amniotic administration of amino acids is associated with a rapid uptake by the placenta and an increase in maternal and fetal blood concentrations.[27-29] Amino acid uptake by the fetus may be by swallowing amniotic fluid or by absorption through the umbilical cord. In three pregnancies complicated by growth retardation, diagnosed by low 24-hour maternal oestriol excretion and fetal biparietal diameter, Renaud *et al.* administered up to 14 intra-amniotic injections of amino acids between 30 and 38 weeks.[27] There was normalisation of maternal urinary oestriol levels and in one case the rate of increase in the biparietal diameter, which had previously shown a plateau, was also normalised.

MATERNAL HYPEROXYGENATION

Animal studies have demonstrated that maternal hyperoxygenation has little effect on normally oxygenated fetuses. However, in hypoxaemic fetuses maternal hyperoxygenation restores the frequency of fetal breathing movements to normal.[30,31] Similarly, in humans Ritchie and Lakhani[32] reported that in normal pregnancies maternal inhalation of 50% oxygen had no significant effect on the incidence of fetal breathing movements. Conversely, in pregnancies complicated by severe pre-eclampsia or growth retardation, within 20 min of maternal hyperoxygenation there was an increase in fetal breathing movements to normal. Arduini *et al.*[33] in 10 growth retarded fetuses with abnormal Doppler findings of the fetal circulation (high pulsatility index in the aorta and low in the internal carotid artery) showed that maternal hyperoxygenation was associated with a tendency for normalisation of these Doppler parameters.

In a study of severely SGA second trimester fetuses with abnormal Doppler measurements of the fetal circulation and where fetal hypoxia was documented by blood gas analysis of samples obtained by cordocentesis, maternal hyperoxygenation for 10 min resulted in: (i) an increase in fetal pO_2 above normal indicating that placental transfer was unimpaired, suggesting that in these cases chronic maternal hyperoxygenation was contra-indicated in view of the potential adverse effects of oxygen on the premature fetus; (ii) an increase in the fetal pO_2 to within the normal range; (iii) no increase in fetal pO_2, presumably because the disease was too severe, suggesting that such babies require delivery.[34] Furthermore, in a study of 19 severely growth retarded fetuses with abnormal Doppler measurements and documented fetal hypoxaemia, humidified oxygen (55%) was administered to the mothers through an MC face mask for 24 hours a day. Fetal oxygenation was monitored by measurement of the mean blood velocity in the fetal thoracic aorta. In four cases there was a rise in the aortic velocity which was sustained for several days or weeks and all infants survived. In six cases there was no improvement in aortic velocity and in this group there were one intrauterine and four neonatal deaths. In a third group of nine cases there was a temporary improvement and subsequent deterioration in the aortic velocity: six infants survived, one baby died *in utero* and four died in the neonatal period.

These preliminary observations suggest that in some growth retarded fetuses maternal hyperoxygenation can improve fetal oxygenation and that this improvement may allow delivery to be delayed until the fetus has reached the stage of viability. However, the benefit of maternal oxygen therapy has not been proven.

BLOOD SAMPLING IN SMALL FETUSES

Cordocentesis

Cordocentesis has provided access to the fetal circulation and made possible the investigation of fetal cytogenetic, acid-base and metabolic status. There follows a summary of data derived from cordocentesis performed at King's College Hospital, London in 263 SGA fetuses. The results are compared to reference ranges of blood gases and metabolites for gestation that were constructed from the study of fetuses that were appropriate for gestational age (AGA) at the time of cordocentesis. These latter fetuses had cordocentesis for prenatal diagnosis and were subsequently found to be cytogenetically normal and not to be affected by the genetic disease for which they were investigated. Better understanding of the pathophysiology of the disease hopefully will lead to the development of better corrective strategies.

All SGA fetuses were referred from other centres and therefore preselected. This is reflected in: (i) the severity of growth retardation (fetal abdominal circumference 2–8 SDs below the normal mean for gestation); (ii) reduced amniotic fluid, or oligohydramnios in 162 or 62% of the cases; (iii) abnormal Doppler findings in the uterine artery (62%), umbilical artery (59%), or fetal vessels (68%); and (iv) the high incidence of chromosomal abnormalities (16%).

Technique of cordocentesis

Cordocentesis is performed as a single operator, out-patient procedure.[35] The site and direction of the umbilical cord at its insertion into the placenta are identified by ultrasound scanning with a curvilinear transducer. With the transducer in one hand, held parallel to the intended course of the needle, the chosen site of entry on the maternal abdomen is cleaned with antiseptic solution and local anaesthetic infiltrated down to the myometrium. A 20G needle is then introduced either transplacentally or transamniotically into the umbilical cord. The umbilical cord vessel sampled is identified as artery or vein by the turbulence seen ultrasonically when sterile saline (200–400 µl) is injected intravascularly through the sampling needle.

Risks of cordocentesis

The risk of fetal death after cordocentesis depends on the indication for sampling and the experience of the operator. In a series of 553 cases sampled in our centre for prenatal diagnosis of genetic disease (e.g. thalassaemia), or for karotyping in cases of minor fetal malformations (eg. hydronephrosis) the procedure-related fetal loss rate was less than 1% (4 of 469 pregnancies which did not undergo subsequent elective abortion). These four losses occurred as a result of chorioamnionitis or fetal haemorrhage. Similarly, Daffos *et al.*[36] in a series of 562 cases, sampled primarily for diagnosis of toxoplasmosis, reported seven fetal losses.

Blood gases, pH and lactate

AGA fetuses

The umbilical venous and arterial pO_2 and pH decrease with gestational age while pCO_2 increases and blood lactate concentration does not change.[37,38] The changes with gestation are compatible with the pO_2, PCO_2 and pH measurements at hysterotomy in early gestation[39] and at elective Caesarean section at term.[40] Other studies of samples obtained at cordocentesis have demonstrated similar values and trends, although the umbilical venous and arterial pH and the arterial pO_2 did not decrease with gestation.[41] Weiner examined 31 umbilical venous and 10 umbilical arterial samples and did not find any significant changes with gestation.[42]

The oxygen tension in fetal blood is much lower than in maternal blood, and it has been suggested that this is due either to incomplete venous equilibration of uterine and umbilical circulations, or to high placental oxygen consumption. However, the high affinity of fetal haemoglobin for oxygen, together with the high fetal cardiac output in relation to oxygen demand compensates for the low fetal pO_2.[43] The decrease in fetal blood pO_2 with gestation is steeper in the umbilical vein than artery. Since the uteroplacental blood flow per kilogram does not change with gestation, this decrease must reflect increased placental oxygen consumption with advancing gestation. Indeed, the umbilical arteriovenous oxygen difference decreases with gestation, and since umbilical blood flow per kilogram does not increase,[44] then umbilical oxygen uptake, and therefore fetal oxygen consumption, is reduced with advancing gestation.

Despite the decrease in fetal pO_2 with gestational age, the umbilical venous blood oxygen content remains the same because the fetal haemoglobin concentration rises with gestational age.[45] This is probably mediated by erythropoietin since its concentration is higher in the cord blood of normal term than premature infants.[46]

Fetal blood lactate concentration does not change with gestation and the values are similar to those in samples obtained at elective Caesarean section at term.[40] The umbilical venous concentration (mean 0.99, SD 0.32 mmol/l) is higher than the umbilical arterial (mean 0.92, SD 0.21 mmol/l) suggesting that the normoxaemic human fetus is, like the sheep fetus,[47] a net consumer of lactate. Furthermore, the concentration of lactate in umbilical cord blood is higher than in maternal blood and the two are correlated significantly. This suggests a common source of lactate, which is likely to be the placenta. Indeed, the human placenta has been shown to produce lactate which is secreted into both fetal and maternal circulations.[48]

SGA fetuses

Some SGA fetuses are hypoxaemic, hypercapnic, hyperlacticaemic and acidotic (Figures I–III).[38,49] These findings demonstrate that asphyxia manifested at birth may not be due to the process of birth itself, but rather it may exist antenatally. The degree of acidosis correlates significantly with both hypercapnia and hyperlacticaemia. Furthermore, both respiratory and metabolic acidosis increase with hypoxaemia. The carbon dioxide accumulation is presumably the result of reduced exchange between the uteroplacental and fetal circulations, due to reduced blood flow. Decreased blood velocity in the descending fetal aorta(50) and increased resistance in the umbilical(51) and uterine arteries(52) in SGA pregnancies correlate significantly with fetal hypoxaemia, hypercapnia and acidosis.

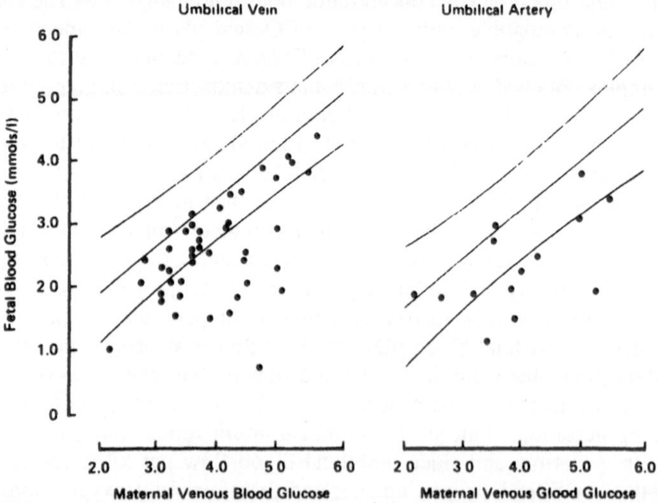

Figure I
Reference ranges (mean and individual 95% confidence intervals) for umbilical venous and arterial blood oxygen tension (mmHg) with gestation in appropriate-for-gestational age fetuses, and the individual values (●) of small-for-gestational-age fetuses.

In umbilical venous blood mild hypoxaemia may be present in the absence of hypercapnia or acidosis, while in umbilical arterial hypoxaemia there is a linear increase in the degrees of hypercapnia and acidosis (Figures II, III). Indeed, in the umbilical artery the pCO_2 exceeds the 97.5th centile of the reference range before the development of significant hypoxaemia. Thus, in mild uteroplacental insufficiency the carbon dioxide that accumulates in umbilical–arterial blood is cleared by a single passage through the placenta, and this is probably the result of the greater speed of diffusion of carbon dioxide compared to oxygen. In contrast, hyperlacticaemia is present in borderline hypoxaemia and is an early biochemical sign of oxygen deficit. In severe uteroplacental insufficiency the rate of clearance of carbon dioxide is exceeded by the rate of production and umbilical venous hypercapnia and acidosis increase exponentially. Thus the best determinants of uteroplacental insufficiency are umbilical venous hypoxaemia or hyperlacticaemia and umbilical arterial hypercapnia or acidosis.

Some SGA fetuses are hyperlacticaemic (Figure IV). This has also been demonstrated in fetal sheep subjected to acute hypoxia(53) or which were growth retarded.(54) When there is inadequate oxygen supply the Krebs cycle is inhibited, and pyruvic acid is converted to lactic acid by the action of lactate dehydrogenase. The

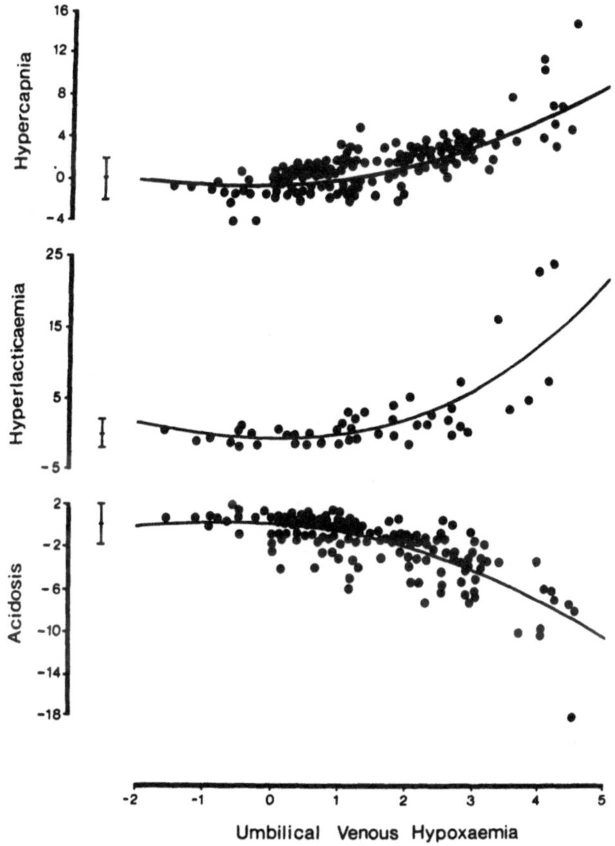

Figure II
The correlations between umbilical venous hypoxaemia and hypercapnia, hyperlacticaemia or acidosis in small-for-gestational-age fetuses.

correlation between hypoxaemia and hyperlacticaemia supports the concept of reduced oxidative metabolism of lactate. Alternatively, hyperlacticaemia could be the result of impaired fetal gluconeogenesis, resulting in decreased utilisation of lactate. Indeed, gluconeogenic substrates are increased in SGA infants[55] which also have decreased gluconeogenic ability.[56] A third possible mechanism producing hyperlacticaemia is increased placental production of lactate. Hypoglycaemia in SGA fetuses is probably caused by a reduction in the supply of glucose to the fetoplacental unit.[57] It is possible that there is a compensatory increase in the pla-

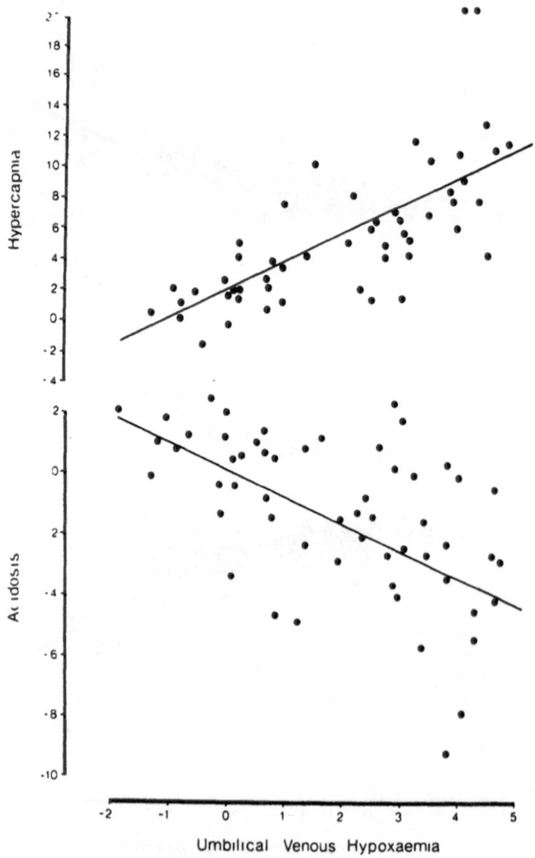

Figure III
The correlations between umbilical arterial hypoxaemia and hypercapnia or acidosis in small-for-gestational-age fetuses.

cental production of lactate, for the fetus to utilise as an alternative energy substrate to glucose. This is supported by studies in the sheep, where experimentally induced growth retarded fetuses show increased consumption and the placenta increased production of lactate.[58] However, since maternal blood lactate is not higher in the SGA than AGA groups, and since there is no correlation between fetal and maternal blood lactate it is unlikely that the high fetal blood lactate is of placental origin.

Blood glucose and plasma insulin

Until recently, knowledge of fetal glucose metabolism was mainly derived from

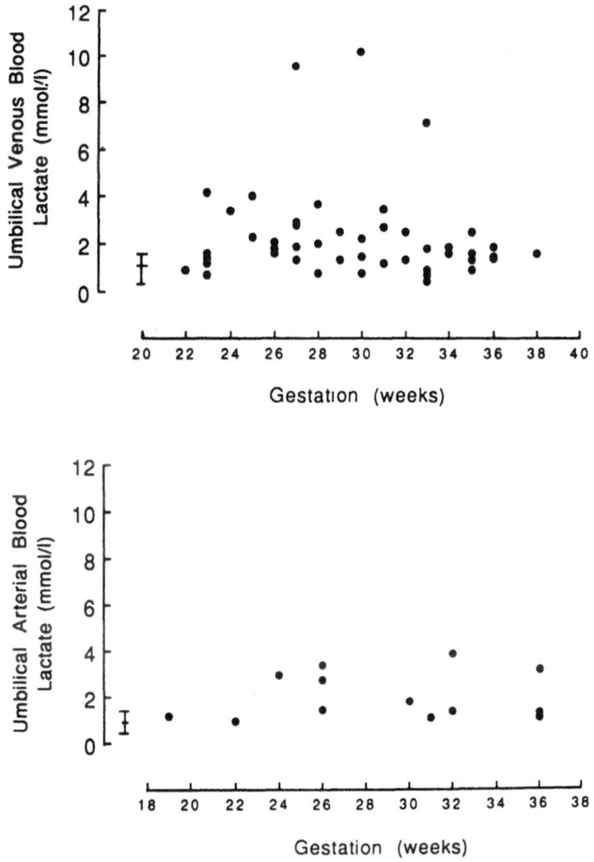

Figure IV
Umbilical venous and arterial blood lactate concentration (mmol/l) in small-for-gestational-age fetuses. The vertical lines represent the mean + 2SDs in appropriate-for-gestational-age fetuses.

animal experiments and human studies in labour or at delivery.[59–61] These studies have established that the transport of glucose across the placenta is by carrier-mediated facilitated diffusion[62] and that the glucose uptake into the umbilical vein from the placenta is directly related to the maternal concentration and to the transplacental glucose gradient.[60] More recently examination of fetal blood samples obtained by cordocentesis has allowed the study of fetal blood glucose and insulin, both in AGA and SGA fetuses.

AGA fetuses

The mean umbilical venous blood glucose concentration (Figure V) is higher than in the umbilical artery indicating that there is fetal glucose uptake from the placenta.(57) Similarly, the maternal glucose concentration is higher than the fetal and the levels in the two compartments are significantly correlated, confirming that the major source of fetal glucose is the mother. In experimental animals glucose uptake into the umbilical vein from the placenta is directly related to the maternal arterial blood glucose concentration and to the transplacental gradient.(60)

The umbilical venous plasma insulin concentration and the fetal insulin to glucose ratio increase exponentially with gestation.(63) These findings presumably reflect the progressive maturation of the endocrine activity in the human fetal pancreas. Although insulin has been demonstrated in the fetal pancreas and circulation as early as ten weeks' gestation, it was previously suggested that insulin release by the pancreas is glucose insensitive before 28 weeks.(64) Thus, although maternal administration of glucose at term results in increase of both glucose and insulin in fetal scalp blood in labour(65) or cord blood at delivery,(66) Adam *et al.*(67) were unable to demonstrate insulin release by infusing glucose into 15 to 20 weeks' gestation human fetuses exposed at hysterotomy before elective abortion.

Although the fetal plasma insulin concentration correlates with the maternal hormone level, this is not due to placental transfer but simply reflects the good correlation between fetal and maternal glucose.(63) Indeed, fetal glucose is better correlated with maternal glucose than with fetal insulin, suggesting that the main determinant of fetal blood glucose level is the maternal blood glucose concentration.

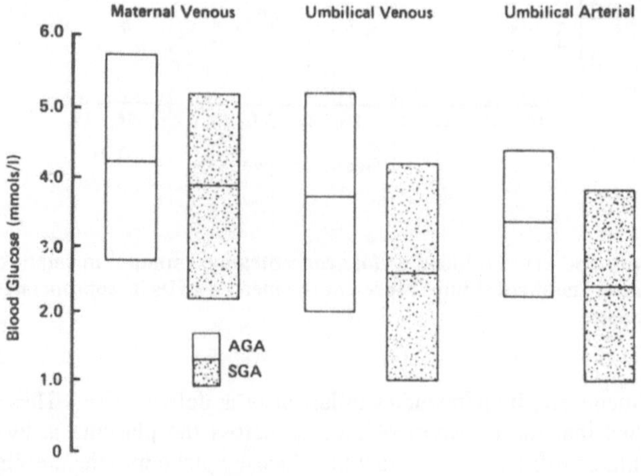

Figure V

The maternal, umbilical venous and umbilical arterial blood glucose concentration (mmol/l) in appropriate- and small-for-gestational-age pregnancies.

SGA fetuses

Some small for gestational age neonates are at increased risk of hypoglycaemia and it has been suggested that the causes are depletion of liver glycogen stores[68] and impaired hepatic gluconeogenesis[55]. However, hypoglycaemia has also been demonstrated in intrauterine life both in experimental animals and in SGA human fetuses (Figure VI).[49,54]

Possible causes of fetal hypoglycaemia are inadequate maternal supply of glucose to the feto-placental unit, either because of decreased maternal glucose concentration or impaired placental perfusion; decreased fetal gluconeogenesis or increased fetal glucose consumption. The maternal blood glucose in our SGA group was significantly lower than the controls (Figure V) and this is thought to be the result of relative hyperinsulinaemia due to decreased placental production of diabetogenic hormones.[69] However, the observed decrease in maternal glucose is too small to account for the severity of fetal hypoglycaemia.

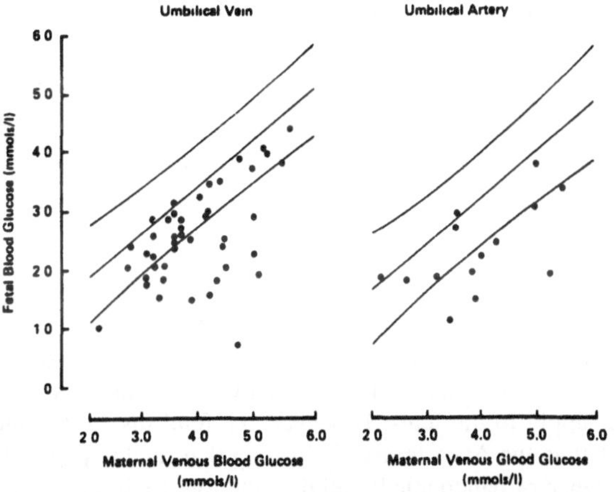

Figure VI
Reference ranges (mean and individual 95% confidence intervals) of fetal with maternal blood glucose concentration (mmol/l) in pregnancies with appropriate-for-gestational age fetuses, and the individual values (●) in those with small-for-gestational-age fetuses.

In the SGA fetuses, the degree of hypoxaemia correlates with the maternal-fetal glucose gradient in both the umbilical vein and umbilical artery. The two lines describing these correlations are parallel. Therefore, the major cause of fetal hypoglycaemia is unlikely to be decreased endogenous production or increased consumption of glucose. In sheep, restriction of placental growth by removal of endometrial caruncles produces growth retarded fetuses that are also hypoxaemic and hypoglycaemic.[58] However, hypoglycaemia is not due to increased glucose consumption as a result of hypoxaemia because in experimental fetal growth retardation produced by prolonged maternal hypobaric hypoxia the fetuses are hypoxaemic but not hypoglycaemic.[70] Placental transfer of glucose does not require oxygen. Furthermore, placental glucose consumption in experimental growth retardation is not increased.[58] Therefore, it is likely that the major cause of hypoglycaemia in SGA fetuses is reduced glucose supply from the mother and that the maternal to fetal glucose gradient is a measure of impaired placental perfusion.

Intrauterine growth is determined by the influence of nutritional and endocrine factors on the genetic potential of the fetus.[71] Although maternal nutrition *per se* has a marginal effect on human fetal size, uteroplacental blood flow and therefore nutrient supply to the fetoplacental unit plays a major role. With regard to anabolic hormones, the fetoplacental unit is essentially self-contained because the placenta is largely impermeable to maternal peptides. Hormones important in postnatal growth, such as growth hormone and thyroxine, are present in the human fetus from early gestation but their influence on fetal growth is minor. However, insulin is thought to have a major fetal growth-promoting action. There is controversy as to whether this is the result of its well recognised anabolic activities or a consequence of an independent growth-promoting activity, such as stimulation of the release of somatomedins.[64]

Fetal blood sampling by cordocentesis has demonstrated that some SGA fetuses are hypoinsulinaemic.[63] This finding supports the results of previous studies. Thus, congenital absence[72] or experimental chemical ablation of the pancreas[73] is associated with intrauterine growth retardation. Similarly, restriction of placental growth in sheep, by removal of endometrial caruncles, produces growth retarded fetuses that are also hypoinsulinaemic.[54] Low plasma insulin has also been demonstrated in SGA neonates.[74]

In samples obtained by cordocentesis from SGA fetuses, the degree of hypoinsulinaemia correlates significantly with the degree of fetal hypoglycaemia.[63] Since the major cause of hypoglycaemia in SGA fetuses is reduced uteroplacental blood flow, this suggests that hypoinsulinaemia is the result of reduced glucose supply to the fetus. However, the fetal insulin to glucose ratio is lower in the SGA than the AGA fetuses indicating that fetal hypoinsulinaemia may also be a consequence of pancreatic β-cell dysfunction. Reduced endocrine pancreatic tissue was found at autopsy in growth retarded infants.[75]

Fetal insulin does not correlate with the degree of fetal smallness suggesting that insulin is not the primary determinant of fetal size.[63] Instead, insulin may influence fetal growth through its action on nutrient uptake and utilisation. Hypoinsulinaemia in the fetus will direct nutrients away from the insulin sensitive tissues, such as skeletal muscle, liver and adipose tissue. The result will be decreased glycogen and fat stores and impaired fetal growth.

Plasma cortisol and ACTH

AGA fetuses

Plasma cortisol is present in the fetal circulation and the concentration (Figure VII) does not change between 18 and 36 weeks' gestation.[76] This is in agreement with the findings of Nahoul *et al.* [77] who also measured plasma cortisol in samples obtained by cordocentesis between 21 and 30 weeks. In contrast, Murphy[78] examined samples obtained at hysterotomy and Caesarean delivery and reported a midtrimester fall and a subsequent late gestational rise in fetal plasma cortisol. It was suggested that the rise in plasma cortisol concentration may contribute to the maturation of fetal tissues. Indeed, in animals, a wide variety of maturational processes can be accelerated by stimulation of the fetal adrenals or by administration of corticosteroids.[79] However, in human fetuses there is no fetal cortisol surge before 36 weeks' gestation, by which time most fetal organs are mature. Furthermore, maturation of human fetuses can take place in the absence of adrenal glands.[80] This evidence suggests that a late cortisol surge may not be necessary for organ maturation in human fetuses.

In animals, the prepartum corticosteroid surge is a dramatic event in which the plasma levels of cortisol increase exponentially within a few days of term, and which is thought to be involved in the initiation of labour. In humans, the fetal corticosteroid surge is less marked. Although cord blood levels of cortisol at term are higher in infants delivered after labour than after elective Caesarean section, studies comparing cord cortisol levels in induced and spontaneous labour have come to opposite conclusions regarding the role of cortisol in the initiation of labour.[81,82] Umbilical cord plasma cortisol concentration obtained at Caesarean section at 38 weeks was higher than in cordocentesis samples, but the highest fetal plasma cortisol concentration was in samples obtained at vaginal delivery at term. Furthermore, there was a significant correlation between maternal and fetal cortisol at term suggesting that the high fetal cortisol concentration in cord blood at vaginal delivery is simply a result of the high maternal cortisol rather than instrumental in initiating labour.

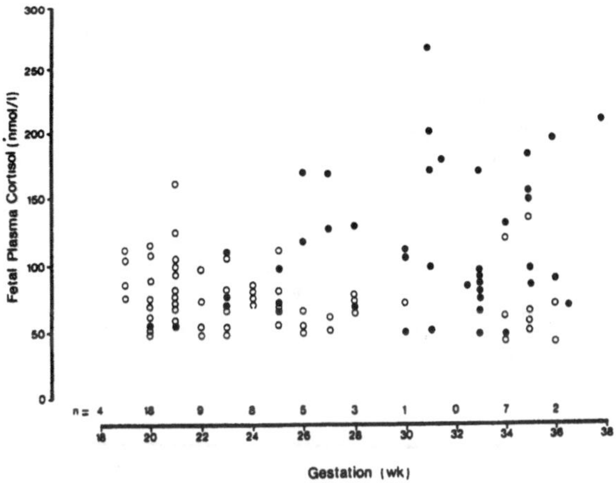

Figure VII
Plasma cortisol concentration (nmol/l) in appropriate- (○) and small-for-gestational-age (●) fetuses.

ACTH is present in the plasma of the midtrimester human fetus and the concentration increases with gestation.(76) Maternal ACTH does not cross the placenta to the fetus(83) but the placenta is capable of producing ACTH.(84) However, it is not known whether fetal plasma ACTH originates from the fetal pituitary, the placenta, or both.

There is no significant correlation between ACTH and cortisol levels in fetal blood,(76) suggesting that the fetal pituitary-adrenal axis may be relatively immature. The lack of correlation between cortisol and ACTH has also been shown in the sheep(85) where the adrenal becomes sensitive to ACTH stimulation only in very late gestation.(79) Alternatively, the findings could be explained if a major source of ACTH is the placenta;(84) placental secretion of ACTH is insensitive to negative feedback by steroids.(86)

SGA fetuses

In SGA fetuses plasma cortisol concentration is increased, presumably in an effort to combat the accompanying hypoglycaemia (Figure VIII).(76) This was also found in experimentally induced growth retarded sheep fetuses, which responded to acute hypoxaemia by increasing both plasma cortisol and ACTH levels.(85) However, in human SGA fetuses, the plasma ACTH concentration is decreased.(76) Therefore, the most likely explanation for the raised plasma cortisol is increased adrenal blood flow, the consequence of redistribution in fetal circulation in response to hypoxaemia.(87) The reduced plasma ACTH levels in SGA fetuses may be the result of negative feedback of cortisol on pituitary ACTH secretion, or a direct consequence of the reduced placental size and therefore decreased placental production of ACTH, corticotrophin-releasing hormone, or both.

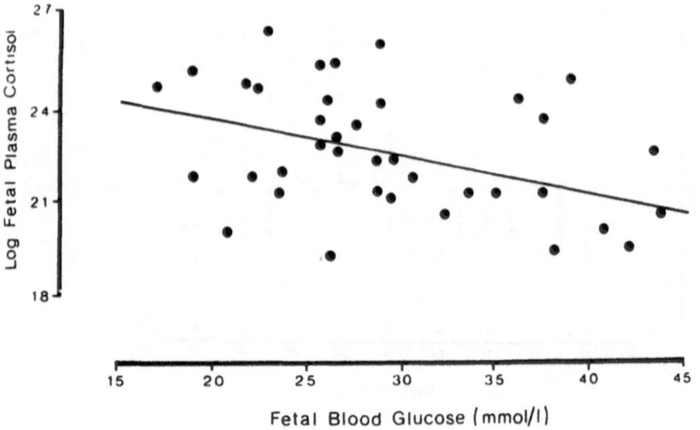

Figure VIII
The correlation between fetal cortisol and glucose in small-for-gestational-age fetuses.

Plasma lipids

AGA fetuses

Lipid metabolism is of major importance for fetal cell and organ growth and in later fetal life there are increasing requirements of lipids for special functions in the brain, lung and adipose tissue.[88] Fetal plasma triglyceride concentration decreases exponentially with gestation (Figure IX). [89] This observation is compatible with reported levels in cord blood at the time of delivery. Thus, premature infants of 25–26 weeks had higher cord triglyceride concentration than did those delivered after 27 weeks.[90] There is no correlation between fetal and maternal trilyceride levels suggesting that there is no significant transplacental transport of these lipids, and that the fetal levels reflect fetal metabolism. Fetal tissues are capable of synthesising triglyceride from at least 12 weeks' gestation.[91,92] However, deposition of adipose tissue begins after 24 weeks and increases exponentially so that at 32 weeks the fetal fat content is 3.5%, and at 40 weeks 16% of the body weight.[94] Therefore, the observed decrease in plasma triglyceride concentration with gestation may be the result of increased utilisation by the fetus for deposition into adipose tissue.

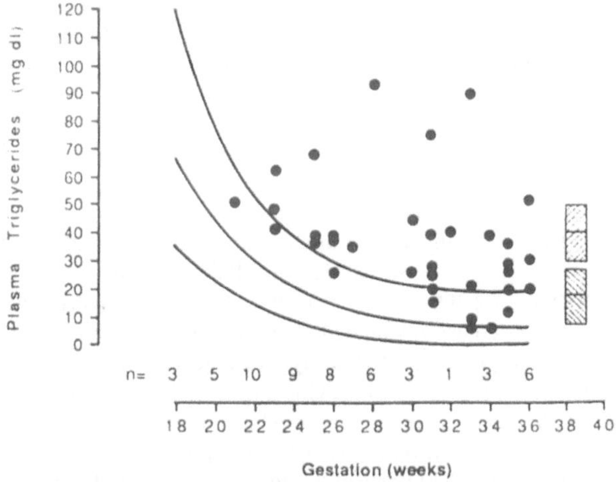

Figure IX
Reference ranges (mean and individual 95% confidence intervals) of fetal plasma triglyceride concentration (mg/dl) with gestation, and the individual values of small-for-gestational-age (●) fetuses. The mean (SD) of umbilical cord plasma triglyceride concentration from vaginal (▨) and elective Caesarean (▧) deliveries are also shown.

The cord plasma triglyceride concentrations at elective Caesarean section are similar to the levels in samples obtained by cordocentesis in late gestation. However the cord triglyceride and NEFA levels at vaginal delivey are significantly higher than those at Caesarean section (Figure IX). [89] Therefore, the stress of labour is associated with an increase in plasma non-esterified fatty acid (NEFA) and triglyceride concentrations and this is likely to be the result of stress-mediated lipolysis.[94]

The plasma NEFA levels, although present in low concentrations in the fetus, correlate significantly with the maternal levels suggesting that there is placental transfer of fatty acids. In contrast, the maternal and fetal glycerol concentrations are not significantly correlated. On the basis of umbilical arterio-venous differences in humans at the time of elective Caesarean section, it has also been inferred that NEFA may cross the placenta in significant amounts.[95] However, studies of the perfused human placenta[96] have shown that the rate of NEFA transfer from mother to the fetus was approximately 20% of that required for adipose tissue deposition, and therefore the major source of fetal NEFA is endogenous synthesis. The low fetal NEFA compared to the maternal and the decrease in umbilical venous plasma concentration with gestation may be the result of utilisation of NEFA for fat deposition.

SGA fetuses

In hypoxaemic SGA fetuses the plasma triglyceride concentration is increased (Figure X) and the blood glucose and plasma insulin decreased; plasma NEFA and glycerol levels are not disturbed.[89] The possible mechanisms of the hypertriglyceridaemia are mobilisation of fat stores or reduced utilisation of triglycerides.

In intrauterine life the energy requirements of the fetus are met largely by the oxidation of glucose.[59] At birth the glucose supply from the mother suddenly ceases and within a few hours there is a dramatic rise in plasma triglycerides and NEFA.[97] This biochemical change is thought to result from lipolysis of fetal adipose tissue and is mediated by the release of catecholamines.[98] The resultant high levels of circulating NEFA may exert a glucose-sparing action via the glucose–fatty acid cycle, resulting in diminished peripheral utilisation of glucose, thereby making more glucose available for metabolism in the brain.[99] Lipolysis may also be responsible for the high NEFA, glycerol and triglyceride levels found in cord blood samples from asphyxiated neonates at birth.[100,101] Thus, it is thought that in the presence of perinatal asphyxia glycogen stores are rapidly depleted and lipids are mobilised from fat stores to provide substrate for oxidation.[98] However, in hypoxaemic SGA fetuses the plasma levels of NEFA and glycerol are not increased, suggesting that in chronic intrauterine hypoxia and hypoglycaemia the major cause of the observed hypertriglyceridaemia is unlikely to be increased lipolysis.

An alternative mechanism for hypertriglyceridaemia in hypoxaemic SGA fetuses is decreased utilisation of triglycerides, due either to impaired oxidation of lipids or to reduced uptake into adipose tissue. In AGA fetuses the plasma triglyceride concentration decreases exponentially with gestation and this decrease coincides with increased deposition of fat.[93] Therefore, failure of the normal process of fat deposition will be accompanied by failure of triglyceride levels to decline.This may be analogous to the situation in low birthweight infants and in children with marasmus where the ability to clear intralipid from the circulation is reduced.[102–104]

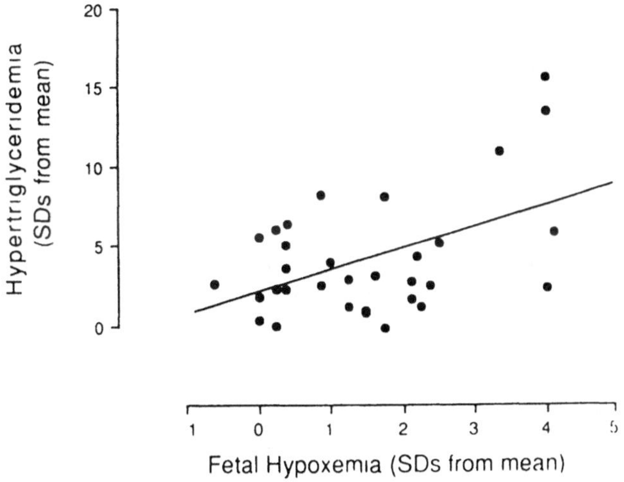

Figure X
The correlation between fetal hypoxaemia and hypertriglyceridaemia in small-for-gestational-age fetuses.

Plasma amino acids

AGA fetuses

The fetal plasma aminogram has been extensively studied in the past in cord blood samples obtained at hysterotomy, Caesarean section or vaginal delivery.[105–108] These studies have shown that the fetal levels are higher than the maternal, providing supporting evidence for active transport across the placenta.[111] In conditions where placental function is impaired fetal amino acid metabolism is disturbed[105] and SGA infants have abnormal amino acid profiles[110, 111]

Recently, studies in samples obtained by cordocentesis have demonstrated that there is a significant correlation between fetal and maternal levels for individual amino acids and that the concentration in the fetus is higher than in the mother.[112] Furthermore, the feto-maternal amino acid ratio decreases with advancing gestation implying increased consumption by the fetoplacental unit.[112] This increase in metabolic activity is compatible with the increased oxygen consumption by the fetoplacental unit and the decrease in fetal blood pO_2 with advancing gestation.[37, 38]

SGA fetuses.

In pregnancies complicated by fetal hypoxaemia and growth retardation there is a disturbance in both maternal and fetal plasma amino acid profiles. Furthermore, there are significant correlations between the change in maternal or fetal plasma amino acid concentrations and the degree of fetal hypoxaemia.[112,113]

The maternal plasma concentration of both essential and non-essential amino acids is increased in fetal hypoxaemia (Figure XI), and this is compatible with the concept that in uteroplacental insufficiency there is a reduction in both the supply and therefore the consumption of amino acids by the fetoplacental unit.

The fetal plasma concentration and feto-maternal ratio of essential amino acids is decreased (Figure XII). These findings could be the result of either increased fetoplacental consumption of these amino acids or reduced perfusion and transport across the placenta. In uteroplacental insufficiency the supply of both oxygen and glucose to the fetoplacental unit is reduced.[(57)] In sheep, removal of endometrial caruncles results in fetal hypoxaemia, hypoglycaemia and growth retardation.[(58)] In this situation the production of lactate by the placenta is increased, presumably to provide the hypoglycaemic fetus with an alternative substrate for oxidation. It has been suggested that the excess lactate is the result of increased placental consumption of amino acids.[(58)]

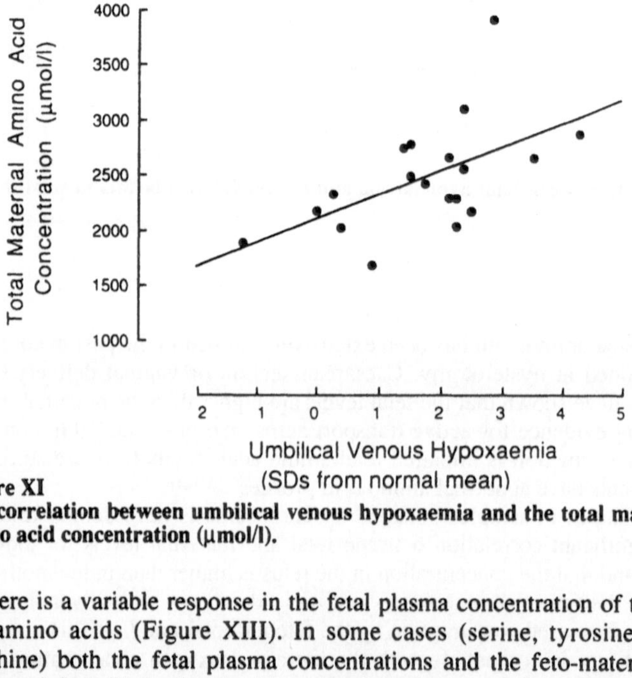

Figure XI
The correlation between umbilical venous hypoxaemia and the total maternal plasma amino acid concentration (μmol/l).

There is a variable response in the fetal plasma concentration of the non-essential amino acids (Figure XIII). In some cases (serine, tyrosine, taurine and ornithine) both the fetal plasma concentrations and the feto-maternal ratios are decreased. It is likely that the biosynthetic pathways of these amino acids are not fully established in intrauterine life and therefore they may be considered to be essential for the fetus. Some non-essential amino acids increase in SGA fetuses and this may be the result of: (i) tissue breakdown; during maternal fasting in the sheep, there is a net flow of amino acids away from the fetal hind limb, suggesting that the fetus is capable of diverting amino acids away from areas of tissue growth;[(114)] (ii) decreased utilisation for protein synthesis, because of the reduced supply of the essential amino acids. Indeed, this may be the explanation for a similar increase in some non-essential amino acids observed in children with protein malnutrition.[(115)] (iii) decreased utilization for oxidation; when fetal sheep are subjected to prolonged hypobaric hypoxia,[(70)] and when human neonates are asphyxi-

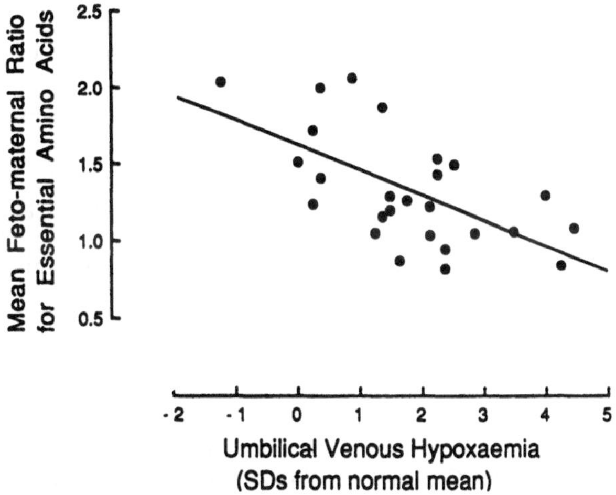

Figure XII
The correlation between umbilical venous hypoxaemia and the mean feto-maternal ratio of essential amino acids in small-for-gestational-age fetuses.

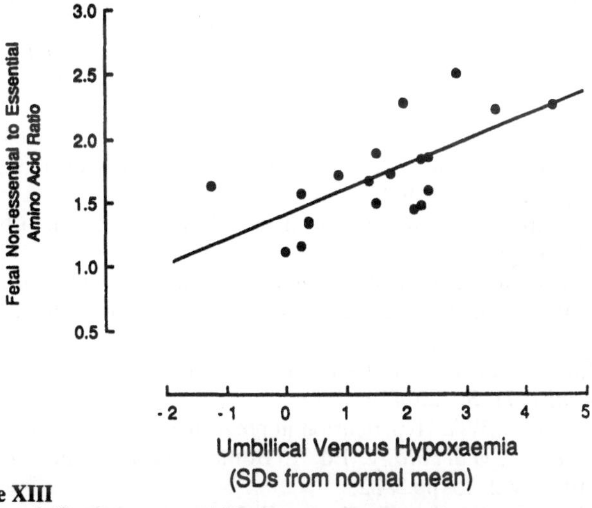

Figure XIII
The correlation between umbilical venous hypoxaemia and the plasma non essential to essential amino acid ratio in small-for-gestational-age fetuses.

ated at birth,(116) the plasma levels of alanine are increased, (iv) decreased utilization for gluconeogenesis; the gluconeogenic amino acids, such as alanine and glycine are increased in growth retarded neonates(55) and infusion of alanine in these infants fails to raise the glucose level suggesting impaired gluconeogenesis.(56)

CONCLUSION

Fetal blood sampling by cordocentesis has provided evidence that severe early onset fetal growth retardation is commonly associated with chromosomal abnormalities. Furthermore, some small fetuses are hypoxaemic, hypercapnic, hyperlacticaemic and acidaemic, and they have disturbed carbohydrate, lipid and protein metabolism. Attempts at improving the growth and wellbeing of SGA fetuses include the treatment of maternal disease, maternal-fetal nutrient and oxygen supplementation and uteroplacental vascular dilatation. Although there is a rational basis for most of these attempts, to date there is no conclusive prospective controlled study to demonstrate beneficial effects in the growth retarded fetus.

REFERENCES

1. Murphy JF. The effects of maternal smoking on the unborn child. In: *Progress in Obstetrics and Gynaecology*. Edinburgh: Churchill Livingstone, 1984; Vol. 4: pp.36–51.
2. Rantakallio P. The effect of maternal smoking on birth weight and the subsequent health of the child. *Early Hum Dev* 1978; **24:** 371–382.
3. Macarthur C, Knox EG. Smoking in pregnancy: effects of stopping at different stages. *Br J Obstet Gynaecol* 1988; **95:** 551–555.
4. Ellwood DA. Maternal narcotic addiction. In: *Progress in Obstetrics and Gynaecology*. Ed. J Studd. Edinburgh: Churchill Livingstone, 1989; Vol. 7: pp.91–103.
5. Strauss ME, Andresko M, Stryker JC, Wardell JN, Dunkel LD. Methadone maintenance during pregnancy: Pregnancy, birth, and neonate characteristics. *Am J Obstet Gynecol* 1974; **120:** 895–900.
6. Sullivan WL. A note on the influence of maternal inebriety on the offspring. *J Ment Sci* 1899; **45:** 489–503.
7. Wright JT, Barrison IG. Alcohol and the fetus. In: *Progress in Obstetrics and Gynaecology*. Ed. J Studd. Edinburgh: Churchill Livingstone, 1984, Vol 4: pp.25–36.
8. Perkins RP. Inherited disorders of haemoglobin synthesis and pregnancy. *A m J Obstet Gynecol* 1971; **3:** 120–159.
9. Moore MP, Redman CWG. Hypertension in pregnancy. In: *Recent Advances in Obstetrics and Gynaecology*. Ed. J. Bonnar. Edinburgh: Churchill Livingstone, 1987; Vol. 15: pp.3–32.
10. Katz AI, Davison JM, Hayslett JP, Singson E, Lindheimer MD. Pregnancy in women with kidney disease. *Kidney International* 1980; **18:** 192–206.
11. Watkins PJ. Diagnosis and treatment of diabetic nephropathy. *Med Intern* 1985; **13:** 554–556.
12. Benny PS, Prasao J, MacVicar J. Pregnancy and coarctation of the aorta. *B r J Obstet Gynaecol* 1980; **87:** 1159–1161.
13. Singh H, Bolton PJ, Oakley CM. Pregnancy after surgical correction of tetralogy of Fallot. *Br Med J* 1982; **285:** 168–170.

14. Zuspan FP. Chronic hypertension in pregnancy. *Clin Obstet Gynecol* 1984; **27:** 854–873.
15. Lunell NO, Nylund LE, Lewander R, Sarby B, Thornstom S. Utero-placental blood flow in pre-eclampsia measurements with indium-113m and a computer-linked gamma camera. *Clinical and Experimental Hypertension* 1981; **B1:** 105–117.
16. Beischer NA, Abell DA, Drew JH. Intra-uterine growth retardation. In: *Progress in Obstetrics and Gynaecology* Ed. J Studd. Edinburgh: Churchill Livingstone, 1984: Vol 4: pp.82–92.
17. Brettes JP, Renaud R, Gandar R. A double blind investigation into the effects of ritodrine on uterine blood flow during the third trimester of pregnancy. *A m J Obstet Gynecol* 1975; **124:** 164–168.
18. Beaufils M, Uzan S, Donsimoni R, Colau JC. Prevention of pre-eclampsia by early antiplatelet therapy. *Lancet* 1985; **i:** 840–842.
19. Wallenburg HCS, Dekker GA, Makowitz JW, Rotmans P. Low-dose aspirin prevents pregnancy-induced hypertension and pre-eclampsia in angiotensin-sensitive primigravidae. *Lancet* 1986; **i:** 1–3.
20. Trudinger BJ, Cook CM, Thompson RS, Giles WB, Connelly A. Low-dose aspirin therapy improves fetal weight in umbilical placental insufficiency. *A m J Obstet Gynecol* 1988; **159:** 681–685.
21. Kaplinski AK, Kurjak A. The treatment of growth retarded fetuses with haemodiaslysate (Solcoseryl): ultrasonic control. In: *Recent Advances in Ultrasound Diagnosis*. Eds. A Kurjak, G Kossoff. Edinburgh: Churchill Livingstone, 1984; Vol. 4: p.174.
22. Kurjak A, Kaplinski AK. In-utero treatment of the fetus with growth retardation. In: *The Fetus as a Patient*. Ed. A Kurjak. Amsterdam: Elsevier, 1985: pp.86–101.
23. Kaneoka T, Taguchi S, Shimizu H, Shirakawa K. Prenatal diagnosis and treatment of intrauterine growth retardation. *J Perinat Med* 1983; **11:** 204.
24. Pearce JM. Effects of Allylestrenol on deteriorating utero-placental circulation. *Lancet* 1988; **ii:** 1252.
25. Rubaltelli FF, Enzi G, De Biasi F, Bondio M, Rondinelli M. Effect of lipid loading on fetal uptake of free fatty acids, glycerol and beta-hydroxybutyrate. *Biol Neonate* 1978; **33:** 320–326.
26. Charlton V. Fetal nutritional supplementation. *Sem Perinatal* 1984; **8:** 25–30.
27. Renaud R, Kirschtetter L, Koehl C. Amino acid intra-amniotic injections. In: *Recent Progress in Obstetrics and Gynecology*. Eds. L Persianov, T Chervakova, J Presl. Proceedings of the VII World Congress of Obstetrics and Gynecology, Prague, Excerpta Medica: pp.234–256.
28. Heller L. Intrauterine amino acid feeding of the fetus. In: *Parental Nutrition in Infancy and Childhood*. New York: Plenum Press, 1974: pp.206–213.
29. Saling E, Dudenhausen JW, Kynast G. Basic investigation about intra-amniotic compensatory nutrition of the malnourished fetus. In: *Recent Progress in Obstetrics and Gynecology*. Eds. L Persianov, T Chervakova, J Presl. Proceedings of the VII World Congress of Obstetrics and Gynecology,

Prague, Excerpta Medica: pp.227–233.
30. Boddy K, Dawes GS, Fisher R, Pinter S, Robinson JS. Fetal respiratory movements. Electrocortical and cardiovascular responses to hypoxaemia and hypercapnia in sheep. *J Physiol* 1974; **234:** 599–618.
31. Dawes GS. Breathing and rapid eye movements before birth. In: *Fetal and Neonatal Physiology*. Eds. RS Comline, DW Gross, GS Dawes, PS Nathanielsz. Cambridge: Cambridge University Press, 1973: p.360.
32. Ritchie JWK, Lakhani K. Fetal breathing movements and maternal hyperoxia. *Br J Obstet Gynaecol* 1980; **87:** 1084–1086.
33. Arduini D, Rizzo G, Mancuso S, Romanini C. Short-term effects of maternal oxygen administration on blood flow velocity waveforms in healthy and growth-retarded fetuses. *Am J Obstet Gynecol* 1988; **159:** 1077–1180.
34. Nicolaides KH, Campbell S, Bradley RJ, Bilardo CM, Soothill PW, Gibb D. Maternal oxygen therapy for intrauterine growth retardation. *Lancet* 1987; **i:** 942–945.
35. Nicolaides KH, Soothill PW, Rodeck CH, Campbell S. Ultrasound-guided sampling of umbilical cord and placental blood to assess fetal wellbeing. *Lancet* 1986; **i:** 1065–1067.
36. Daffos F, Capela-Pavlovsky M, Forestier F. Fetal blood sampling during pregnancy with use of a needle guided by ultrasound: A study of 606 consecutive cases. *Am J Obstet Gynecol* 1985; **153:** 655–660.
37. Soothill PW, Nicolaides KH, Rodeck CH, Campbell S. Effect of gestational age on fetal and intervillous blood gas and acid-base values in human pregnancy. *Fetal Therapy* 1986; **1:** 168–175.
38. Nicolaides KH, Economides DL, Soothill PW. Blood gases and pH in appropriate and small for gestational age fetuses. *Am J Obstet Gynecol* 1989; In press.
39. Rudolph AM, Heyman MA, Teramo KAW, Barrett CT, Raiha NCR. Studies on the circulation of the previable human fetus. *Pediatr Res* 1971; **5:** 452–465.
40. Pardi G, Buscaglia M, Ferrazzi E, Bozzetti P, Marconi AM, Cetin I, Battaglia FC, Makowski EL. Cord sampling for the evaluation of oxygenation and acid-base balance in growth-retarded human fetuses. *Am J Obstet Gynecol* 1987; **157:** 1221–1228.
41. Cox WL, Daffos F, Forestier F, Descombey D, Aufrant C, Auger MC, Gaschard JC. Physiology and management of intrauterine growth retardation: a biologic approach with fetal blood sampling. *Am J Obstet Gynecol* 1988; **159:** 36–41.
42. Weiner CP. Cordocentesis for diagnostic indications: two years' experience. *Obstet Gynecol* 1987; **70:** 664–667.
43. Battaglia FC, Meschia G. *An Introduction to Fetal Physiology*. London: Academic Press, 1986: pp.154–167.
44. Gerson AG, Wallace DA, Stiller RJ, Paul D, Weiner S, Bolognese RJ. Doppler evaluation of umbilical venous and arterial blood flow in the second and third trimesters of normal pregnancy. *Obstet Gynecol* 1987: **70**:622–662.
45. Nicolaides KH, Soothill PW, Clewell WH, Rodeck CH, Mibashan RS.

Campbell S. Fetal haemoglobin measurement in the assessment of red cell isoimmunisation. *Lancet* 1988; **i**:1073–1075.
46. Finne PH. Erythropoetin levels in cord blood as an indicator of intrauterine hypoxia. *Acta Pediatr Scand* 1986; **55**:478–489.
47. Burd LI, Jones MD, Simmons MA. Placental production and fetal utilisation of lactate and pyruvate. Nature 1975; **254**:210–211.
48. Holzman IR, Philips AF, Battaglia FC. Glucose metabolism, lactate and ammonia production by the human placenta in vivo. *Pediatr Res* 1979; **13**:117–120.
49. Soothill PW, Nicolaides KH, Campbell S. Prenatal asphyxia, hyperlacticaemia, hypoglycaemia and erythroblastosis in growth retarded fetuses. *B r Med J* 1987; **294**:1051–1053.
50. Soothill PW, Nicolaides KH, Bilardo CM, Campbell S. Relation of fetal hypoxia in growth retardation to mean blood velocity in the fetal aorta. *Lancet* 1986; **ii**: 1118–1119.
51. Nicolaides KH, Bilardo CM, Soothill PW, Campbell S. Absence of end diastolic frequencies in the umbilical artery: a sign of fetal hypoxia and acidosis. *Br Med J* 1988; **297**:1026–1027.
52. Soothill PW, Nicolaides KH, Bilardo C, Hackett G, Campbell S. Utero-placental blood velocity resistance index and umbilical venous pO_2 . pCO_2 pH, lactate and erythroblast count in growth retarded fetuses. *Fetal Therapy* 1986; **1**: 176–179.
53. Jones CT. The development of some metabolic responses to hypoxia in the fetal sheep. *J Physiol* 1977; **265**: 743–762.
54. Robinson JS, Kingston EJ, Jones CT, Thornburg GD. Studies on experimental growth retardation in sheep. The effect of removal of endometrial caruncles on fetal size and metabolism. *J Dev Physiol* 1979; **1**: 379–398.
55. Haymond MW, Karl IE, Pagliara AS. Increased gluconeogenic substrates in the smal!-for-gestational age infant. *New Engl J Med* 1974; **291**: 322–328.
56. Mestyan J, Schultz K, Horvath M. Comparative glycemic responses to alanine in normal term and small-for-gestational-age infants. *J Pediatr* 1974; **85**: 276–278.
57. Economides DL, Nicolaides KH. Blood glucose and oxygen tension in small for gestational age fetuses. *Am J Obstet Gynecol* 1989; **160**: 385–389.
58. Owens JA, Falconer J, Robinson JS. Effect of restriction of placental growth on fetal and uteroplacental metabolism. *J Dev Physiol* 1987; **9**: 225–238.
59. James EJ, Raye JR, Gresham EL, Makowski EL, Meschia G, Battaglia FC. Fetal oxygen consumption, carbon dioxide production and glucose uptake in a chronic sheep preparation. *Pediatrics* 1972; **50**: 361–371.
60. Hay WW, Sparks JW, Randall BW, Battaglia FC, Meschia G. Fetal glucose uptake and utilisation as functions of maternal glucose concentration. *Am J Physiol* 1981; **246**: E237–E242.
61. Spellacy WN, Goetz FC, Greenberg BZ, Ellis J. The human placental gradient for plasma insulin and blood glucose. *Am J Obstet Gynecol* 1964; **90**:753-757.
62. Widdas WF. Inability of diffusion to account for placental glucose transfer in

the sheep and consideration of the kinetics of a possible carrier transfer. *J Physiol* 1952; **118**:23-29.

63. Economides DL, Proudler A, Nicolaides KH. Plasma insulin in appropriate and small for gestational age fetuses. *Am J Obstet Gynecol* 1989; In press.
64. Hill DJ, Milner RDG. The role of peptide growth factors and hormones in the control of fetal growth. In: *Recent Advances in Perinatal Medicine*. Ed. MI Chiswick. Edinburgh: Churchill Livingstone, 1987: pp. 79-102.
65. Coltart RM, Beard RW, Turner RC, Oakley NW. Blood glucose and insulin relationships in the human mother and fetus before onset of labour. *Br Med J* 1969; **4**:17-19.
66. Milner RD, Hales CN. Effect of intravenous glucose on concentration of insulin in maternal and umbilical-cord plasma. *Brit Med J* 1965; **5430:** 284–286.
67. Adam PAJ, Teramo K, Raiha N, Gitlin D, Schartz R. Human fetal insulin metabolism early in gestation. *Diabetes* 1969; **18**:409-416.
68. Shelley HJ, Neligan GA. Neonatal hypoglycaemia. *Br Med Bull* 1966; **22:** 34–39.
69. Khouzami VA, Ginsburg DS, Daikoku NH, Johnson JW. The glucose tolerance test as a means of identifying intrauterine growth retardation. *Am J Obstet Gynecol* 1981;**139**:423-426.
70. Jacobs R, Owens JA, Falconer J, Webster MED, Robinson JS. Changes to metabolite concentration in fetal sheep subjected to prolonged hypobaric hypoxia. *J Dev Physiol* 1988; **10**:113-121.
71. Gluckman PD, Liggins GC. Regulations of fetal growth. In: *Fetal Physiology and Medicine*. Ed. RW Beard, PW Nathanielz. 2nd edition. New York: Dekker, 1984: pp. 511-557.
72. Lemons JA, Ridenour R, Orsini EN. Congenital absence of the pancreas and intrauterine growth retardation. *Pediatrics*, 1979; 64: 255–257.
73. Hill DE, Holt AB, Reba R, Cheek DB. Alteration in the growth pattern of fetal rhesus monkey following in utero injection of streptozotocin. *Pediatr Res* 1972; **6**:336-340.
74. Lin C, Moawad AH, River PH, Blix P, Abraham M, Rubenstein AH. Amniotic fluid C-peptide as an index for intrauterine fetal growth. *Am J Obstet Gynecol* 1981; **139**:390-396.
75. Van Assche JA, De Prins F, Aerts L, Verjans M. The endocrine pancreas in small for dates infants. *Br J Obstet Gynaecol* 1977; **84**:751-753
76. Economides DL, Nicolaides KH, Linton EA, Perry LA, Chard T. Plasma cortisol and ACTH in appropriate and small for gestational age fetuses. *Fetal Therapy* 1989; In press.
77. Nahoul K, Daffos F, Forestier F, Scholler R. Corisol, cortisone and dehydroepiandrosterone sulphate levels in umbilical cord and maternal plasma between 21 and 30 weeks of pregnancy. *J Steroid Biochem* 1985; **23:**445-450.
78. Murphy BEP. Human fetal serum cortisol levels related to gestational age: Evidence of a midgestational fall and a steep late gestational rise, independent of sex or mode of delivery. *Am J Obstet Gynecol* 1982; **144**:276-282.

79. Liggins GC. Adrenocortical-related maturational events in the fetus. *Am J Obstet Gynecol* 1976; **126**:931-941.
80. Liggins GC. The influence of the fetal hypothalamus and pituitary on growth. In: *Size At Birth.* Eds. K Elliot, J Knight. Ciba Foundation Symposium 27. Amsterdam: Elsevier, 1974: pp. 165-183.
81. Murphy BE. Does the human adrenal play a role in parturition? *Am J Obstet Gynecol* 1973; **115**:521-525.
82. Sybulski S, Maughan GB. Cortisol levels in umbilical cord plasma in relation to labor and delivery. *Am J Obstet Gynecol* 1976; **125**:236-238.
83. Allen JP, Cook DM, Kendall JW, McGilvray R. Maternal-fetal ACTH relationship in man. *J Clin Endocrinol Metab* 1973; **37**:230-234.
84. Liotta AS, Osathanondh R, Ryan KJ. Presence of corticotropin in human placenta: demonstration of in vivo synthesis. *Endocrinology* 1977; **101**:1152-1158.
85. Robinson JS, Jones CT, Kingston EJ. Studies on experimental growth retardation in sheep. The effects of maternal hypoxaemia. *J Dev Physiol* 1983; **5**:89-100.
86. Petraglia F, Sawchenko PE, Rivier J, Vale W. Evidence for local stimulation of ACHT secretion by corticotropin-releasing factor in human placenta. *Nature* 1987; **328**:717-719.
87. Peeters LLH, Sheldon RF, Jones MD, Makowski EL, Meschia G. Blood flow to fetal organs as a function of arterial oxygen content. *Am J Obstet Gynecol* 1979; **135**:639-646.
88. Warshaw JB. Fatty acid metabolism during development. *Sem Perinatol* 1979; **3**:131-139.
89. Economides DL, Crook D, Nicolaides KH. Hypertriglyceridaemia and hypoxaemia in small for gestational age fetuses. *Am J Gynecol* 1989; In press.
90. Dhanireddy R, Hamosh M, Siva KN, Chowdry P, Scanlon JW, Hamosh P. Postheparin lipolytic activity and intralipid clearance in very low-birth-weight infants. *J Pediatr* 1981; **98**:617-622.
91. Yoshioka T, Roux JF. In vitro metabolism of palmitic acid in human fetal tissues. *Pediatr Res* 1972; **6**:675-681.
92. Vilee CA, Loring JM. Alternative pathways of carbohydrate metabolism in fetal and adult tissues. *Biochem J* 1961; **81**:488-494.
93. Widdowson EM. Growth and composition of the fetus and newborn. In: *Biology of Gestation..* Ed. NS Assali. New York: Academic Press, 1968: p.23.
94. Dawkins MJR. Changes in blood glucose and non-esterified fatty acids in the foetal and newborn lamb after injection of adrenaline. *Biol Neonate* 1964; **7**:160-166.
95. Elphick MC, Hull D, Sanders RR. Concentration of free fatty acids in maternal and umbilical cord blood during elective Caesarean section. *Br J Obstet Gynaecol* 1976; **83**:539-544.
96. Dancis J, Jansen V, Kayden HJ, Schneider H, Levitz M. Transfer across perfused human placenta II. Free fatty acids. *Pediatr Res* 1973; **7**:192-197.
97. Van Duyne CM, Havel RJ. Plasma unesterified fatty acid concentration in

fetal and neonatal life. *Proc Soc Exp Biol Med* 1959; **102**:559-602.
98. Tsang R, Glueck J, Evans G, Steiner PM. (1974) Cord blood hypertriglyceridemia. *Am J Dis Child;* **127**: 78-82.
99. Randle PJ, Garland PB, Hales CN, Newsholme EA. The glucose-fatty acid cycle. Its role in insulin sensivity and the metabolic disturbances of diabetes mellitus. *Lancet* 1963; **i**:785.
100. Sabata V, Stembera ZK, Novak M. Levels of unesterified and esterified fatty acids in umbilical blood of hypoxic fetuses. *Biol Neonate* 1968; **12**:194-200.
101. Sabata V, Wolf H, Lausmann S. Glycerol levels in the maternal and umbilical cord blood under various conditions. *Biol Neonate* 1970; **15**:123-127.
102. Gustafson A, Kjellmer I, Olegard R, Victorin L. Nutrition in low birth weight infants. *Acta Pediatr Scand* 1972; **61**:149-158.
103. Gurson C, Saner G. Lipoprotein lipase activity in marasmic type of protein calorie malnutrition. *Arch Dis Child* 1969; **44**:765-768.
104. Shennan AT, Bryan MH, Angel A. The effect of gestational age on intralipid tolerance in newborn infants. *J Pediatr* 1977; **91**:134-137.
105. Young M, Prenton MA. Maternal and fetal plasma amino acid concentrations during gestation and in retarded fetal growth. *J Obstet Gynaecol Br Commonw* 1969; **76**:333-334.
106. Cockburn F, Robins SP, Forfar JO. Free amino acid concentrations in fetal fluids. *Br Med J* 1970; **3**:747-750.
107. Lindblad BS, Baldesden A. The normal plasma free amino acid levels of non-pregnant women and of mother and child during delivery. *Acta Pediatr Scand* 1967, **56**:37-38.
108. Cockburn F, Blagden A, Michie EA, Forfar JO. The influence on preeclampsia and diabetes mellitus on plasma free amino acids in maternal umbilical vein and infant blood. *J Obstet Gynaecol Br Commonw* 1971; **78**:215-231.
109. Enders RH, Judd RM, Donohue TM, Smith CH. Placental amino acid uptake. III. Transport systems for neutral amino acids. *Am J Physiol* 1976; **230**:706-710.
110. Lindblad BS, Zetterström R. The venous plasma free amino acid levels of mother and child during delivery. II After short gestation and gestation complicated by hypertension with special reference to the "small for dates" syndrome. *Acta Pediatr Scand* 1968; **57**:195-204.
111. Cetin I, Marconi AM, Bozzetti P, Sereni LP, Corbetta C, Pardi G, Battaglia FC. Umbilical amino acid concentrations in appropriate and small for gestational age infants: a biochemical difference present in utero. *Am J Obstet Gynecol* 1988; **158**:120-126.
112. Economides DL, Nicolaides KH, Gahl W, Bernardini I, Evans M. Plasma amino acids in appropriate and small for gestational age fetuses. *Am J Obstet Gynecol* 1989; In press.
113. Economides DL, Nicolaides KH, Gahl W, Bernardini I, Bottoms SF, Evans M. Cordocentesis in the diagnosis of fetal starvation. *Am J Obstet Gynecol* 1989; In press.
114. Liechty EA, Lemons JA. Changes in ovine fetal hindlimb amino acid

metabolism during maternal fąsting. *Am J Physiol* 1984; **246**: E459-E466.
115. Holt LE, Snyderman SE, Norton PM, Roitman E, Finch J. Plasma aminogram in Kwashiorkor. *Lancet* 1963; **ii**: 1345-1348.
116. Schultz K, Mestyan J, Solesz G. The effect of birth asphyxia on plasma free amino acids in preterm newborn infants. *Acta Paediatr Acad Sci Hung* 1977; **18**:123-130.

Fetal activity and biophysical evaluation in IUGR

Dr M. J. Whittle

The maternal appreciation of fetal life has been, since ancient times, a traditional indication that the baby is in good condition. Attempts to use the observation in a scientific way to identify a group of babies at risk of intrauterine death has met with mixed success. The principle has been extended to use modern technology in the form of ultrasound and certainly the ability to observe directly fetal activity has broadened the scope. Nevertheless there are conflicting data and the use of fetal movements as reliable indicators of impending fetal demise remains to be substantiated.

This chapter examines the use of monitoring fetal activity as a method of assessing the condition of the growth retarded fetus but although the method has been offered as appropriate there are no prospective large studies to support that view.

ANIMAL EVIDENCE

Evidence that intrauterine fetal breathing actually occurred was disputed at first although chest wall movements had been seen in fetal lambs delivered into waterbaths. In the more mature fetal lamb these chest wall movements were only seen when the fetal cord was clamped and the fetus asphyxiated,. The questionable validity of these early observations meant that breathing came to be regarded as abnormal and it was some years later before new technology was available to show that in fact fetal breathing was not only normally present but could be observed throughout pregnancy.(1) Various factors influenced the frequency of chest wall movements including gestational age, diurnal rhythm, maternal nutritional state and, importantly, the blood gases. Thus it was observed that chest wall movements increased when the fetus was hypercapnic but decreased or disappeared completely when there was hypoxia; in fact in the very hypoxic fetus gasping movements were observed.

Other types of fetal activity include forelimb movements which have been observed in the exteriorised fetal lamb.(2) This group also noted that the movements were influenced by a number of factors, including hypoxia, although they were unable to define a diurnal rhythm. These changes could be correlated with the pattern of eye movements and thus with the natural rest/activity cycles which become a feature of a normally functioning central nervous system and are increasingly prominent as the fetus ages.

BEHAVIOURAL STATE

Since the various forms of fetal activity appear to be influenced by the particular behavioural state in which the fetus exists it is important to realise how these are devised. Four states have been described(3) and relate to those seen in the neonate (Table 1). Only 1F and 2F exist for sufficient time to be identified for certain in the

Table 1. Fetal behavioural activity

	1F	2F	3F	4F
Body movements	Incidental	Periodic	Absent	Continuous
Eye movements	Absent	Present	Present	Present
Heart rate patterns	Stable; few accelerations	Frequent accelerations	Stable; no accelerations	Large accelerations

fetus and these are characterised by the following: State 1F, quiescence which can be regularly interrupted by body movements, absent eye movements, and a stable heart pattern with a small oscillation band-width; State 2F, frequent and periodic gross body movements, continuous eye movements and a heart rate with a broad band-width and frequent accelerations. States 3F and 4F occur infrequently in the fetus, do not show a developmental course and so are not considered further. As gestational age advances the various components gel so that they appear simultaneously with increasing frequency, so called coincidence. Thus, while at 32 weeks a recognisable State 1F exists only 29% of the time, this rises to 67% by 38 weeks.[3] These changes presumably relate to increasing maturation in the central nervous system.

The use of alterations in behavioural state as a method of fetal monitoring does not seem to have been considered practicable. Long periods of observation appear to be necessary. In any case significant periods of coincidence do not develop until later in pregnancy, probably after 34 weeks. The problem of data handling is certainly surmountable with the use of suitable computer programs[4] but even so the relevance of the data remains unclear.

Abnormalities in behavioural state have been noted in the growth retarded fetus[5] and it would appear that the increasing frequency of coincidence which is usually seen as gestation advances does not occur. Fetal behavioural change as such does not necessarily reflect hypoxia although this might be anticipated to have some significant effects.

FETAL ACTIVITY

The clinical use of fetal movements as a method of fetal evaluation was described by Sadovsky and Yaffe[6] who used a series of case reports to demonstrate that fetal movements, as perceived by the mother, appeared to become markedly reduced or even cease days or occasionally only hours before fetal death. Pearson and Weaver[7] described the use of a fetal movement count chart, often called the Kick Chart, which allowed the mother to record the time at which she had felt 10 kicks over a 12-hour span. The results suggested that movements seemed to cease about 12 to 48 hours before death. Of some relevance is the fact that 5/12 of the babies born following reduction in their movements had birthweights below the 5th centile. Conversely Mathews[8] found no difference in birthweight between those babies thought to be moving vigorously and those with reduced movements although the outcome in those babies not moving was much worse, in terms of fetal distress in labour and low Apgar scores in both appropriately grown and small-for-dates babies.

These observations led to the view that fetal activity indicated fetal health and, further, that a reduction in this activity preceded fetal death by a reasonable margin. Thus fetal movement should theoretically provide a warning system that indicates impending fetal demise in sufficient time for some effective action to be taken. Some support for this comes from a prospective randomised study involving 2250 patients[9] in which all the eight intrauterine deaths occurred in the non-counting group. In the counting group there were nine cases with reduced fetal movement, six of which were delivered by Caesarean section; there were no deaths in this group but two babies developed respiratory distress syndrome. The implication from this study is that these nine cases would have died if they had not been delivered at the appropriate time.

Whilst the maternal appreciation of fetal movement provides a simple method of assessing fetal condition on a day-to-day basis, it is relatively crude and gives no indication of the individual fetal activities. With the development of real time ultrasound technology it became possible to observe these movements and Manning *et al.*[10] described a biophysical assessment or *Planning Score*. The components of this score (Table 2) were fetal heart reactivity, fetal breathing movements, gross body movements, fetal tone and amniotic fluid pool depth. They assigned an arbitrary value to each component which, like the Apgar score, comprised a 0 or 2, so that the minimum score was 0 and the maximum 10. Changes have been noted also in discrete forms of fetal activity.

Table 2. Fetal biophysical score (Manning *et al*).[10]

Variable	Score 2	Score 0
Cardiotocography	At least 2 accelerations of 15 bpm, lasting 15 s in 20 min sessions.	No accelerations
Fetal breathing	At least 30 s of sustained breathing in 30 min	< 30 s breathing
Fetal movements	3 or more gross body movements in 30 min	< 3 movements
Fetal tone	At least one motion of limb from flexion to extension and back.	No movements
Amniotic fluid volume	A pocket of fluid at least 1 cm^2	< 1 cm^2 fluid

INDICATIONS FOR BIOPHYSICAL ASSESSMENT

In Manning's original description common indications for study were the post dates pregnancy and maternal diabetes. Since that time larger series have included suspected small-for-dates fetuses and pregnancies complicated by hypertension.

Other indications include those circumstances in which the cardiotocograph (CTG) is equivocal, altered by drug treatment, i.e. beta-blockers, complicated by the presence of variable decelerations or uninterpretable because of early gestational age. Alternatively the profile may be indicated because the mother reports reduced fetal movements or as a means of monitoring the fetal condition during treatment, as in rhesus disease.

METHOD OF BIOPHYSICAL ASSESSMENT

Using real time ultrasound the fetus may have to be observed for up to half an hour before the criteria are met for a normal result (Table 2). Although it has been proposed that the test interval of a week is adequate, this has been disputed,(11) the suggestion being that the interval may have to be less than this and should depend upon the underlying clinical problem.

The order in which the tests are performed is not really important, although Manning *et al.*(12) took the view that if all four ultrasound components of the profile were normal, fetal heart rate testing was not necessary and, indeed, in their study the CTG was always reactive in these circumstances. They found that when any one component was abnormal 64% of CTGs were normal, while if more than two were abnormal the CTGs were non-reactive. The one single component most likely to be associated with an abnormal CTG was reduced amniotic fluid volume. The single component most likely to be absent was fetal breathing (72%) with a non-reactive CTG being found in 24% of cases. Very rarely was absent fetal tone or reduced amniotic fluid volume the single missing component.

Conversely, Vintzileos *et al.*(13) considered the CTG to be an integral part of the profile which needed to be retained. Although the observation of fetal activity, i.e. breathing, body and limb movement, may take some time, it is important that short cuts are avoided. The assessment of fetal tone is not as difficult as it sounds and in fact the appearance of the hands and feet is the important feature. Thus fine movements of the fingers and dorsiflexion of the foot indicate normal tone.

The measurement of amniotic fluid volume is very subjective and many consider the original description of a significantly reduced volume of <1cm to be too rigorous. Indeed this description probably reflected the original use of this technique in the evaluation of the post dates pregnancy, and others(13) have considered <2cms to be significant (Table 3), but even this degree of oligohydramnios would be considered by many to be profound. One criticism of much that has been written concerning the biophysical profile relates to a lack of regard for the gestational age at the time of the assessment and this applies particularly to amniotic fluid volume which can change markedly with gestational age. Thus a 2 cm pool may be acceptable at term but almost certainly is not so at, say, 33 weeks.

Placental grading(14) is also assessed in the profile proposed by Vintzileos but

Table 3. Criteria for scoring biophysical variables (Vintzileos *et al*).[13]

Nonstress test (NST)	
Score 2 (NST 2):	> 5 FHR accelerations of at least 15 bpm in amplitude and at least 15 s duration associated with fetal movements in a 20- min period.
Score 1 (NST 1):	2 – 4 accelerations of at least 15 bpm in amplitude and at least 15 s duration associated with fetal movements in a 20-min period.
Score 0 (NST 0):	≤ 1 accelerations in a 20-min period.
Fetal movements (FM)	
Score 2(FM 2):	At least 3 gross (trunk and limbs) episodes of fetal movements within 30 min. Simultaneous limb and trunk movements were counted as a single movement.
Score 1 (FM 1):	1 or 2 fetal movements within 30 min.
Score 0 (FM 0):	Absence of fetal movements within 30 min.
Fetal breathing movements (FBM)	
Score 2 (FBM 2):	At least 1 episode of fetal breathing of at least 60 s duration within a 30-min observation period.
Score 1 (FBM 1):	At least 1 episode of fetal breathing lasting 30 – 60 s within a 30-min observation period.
Score 0 (FBM 0):	Absence of fetal breathing or breathing lasting less than 30 s within a 30-min observation period.
Fetal tone (FT)	
Score 2 (FT 2):	At least 1 episode of extension of extremities with return to position of flexion, and also 1 episode of extension of spine with return to position of flexion.
Score 1 (FT 1):	At least 1 episode of extension of extremities with return to position of flexion, or 1 episode of extension of spine with return to position flexion.
Score 0 (FT 0):	Extremities in extension. Fetal movements not followed by return. Open hand.
Amniotic fluid volume (AF)	
Score 2 (AF 2):	Fluid evident throughout the uterine cavity. A pocket that measures > 2cm in vertical diameter.
Score 1 (AF 1):	A pocket that measures < 2 cm but > 1 cm in vertical diameter.
Score 0 (AF 0):	Crowding of fetal small parts. Largest pocket < 1 cm in vertical diameter.
Placental grading (PL)	
Score 2 (PL 2):	Placental grading 0, 1 or 2.
Score 1 (PL 1):	Placenta posterior difficult to evaluate.
Score 0 (PL 0):	Placental grading 3.

whether this is a helpful addition or not is uncertain; Vintzileos *et al.*(13) suggest that a Grade 3 placental grading has a significant association with intrapartum distress and placental abruption.

RESULTS OF BIOPHYSICAL ASSESSMENT

The results of biophysical testing appear to be remarkably impressive. Table 4 indicates the expected outcome in a large number of high risk cases referred for evaluation by the profile.(15) It is seen that when the score is ten the outcome is excellent; this also applies with a score of eight provided the two points lost are not because the amniotic fluid volume is reduced. Under those circumstances the perinatal loss rate rises dramatically. Scores that are less than eight are associated with an increasingly high loss rate, four to six demanding a repeat evaluation and two or zero indicating the need to deliver. One important point is the need to establish fetal normality when the profile score is abnormal, and particularly if the amniotic fluid volume is reduced; renal agenesis features strongly in one series.(16)

Table 4. Expected outcome following biophysical scoring (Manning *et al.*)(15)

Score	PNM within a week
10/10 8/10	} < 1/1000
8/10 AFV = 0	89/1000
6/10, AFV = 2	Variable - re-test within 24 hours
6/10, AFV = 0	89/1000
4/10	91/1000
2/10	125/1000
0/10	600/1000

AFV = Amniotic fluid volume
PNM = Perinatal mortality

Looking specifically at the problem of the growth retarded fetus, Manning *et al.*(17) observed that five of nine babies in the group with a false negative result were either probably or definitely growth retarded. The implications of this are unclear and the reasons for the babies being small-for-dates are not stated, although fetal abnormality, as such, had been excluded. It may be of significance that all these losses followed the use of the modified profile i.e. without CTG, although no comment is made concerning this. Further, the test interval was 7 days in three of the cases and this may be inappropriately long when growth retardation is suspected. Manning *et al.*(15) using a group of neonatal proven growth retarded babies as the denominator estimated that the perinatal mortality rate was 27/1000 in babies suspected as small-for-dates and managed prospectively with the profile.

Whether the growth retarded fetus does have different patterns of activity is unclear, but other groups have suggested that this is possible. Thus the frequency of fetal breathing movements in response to maternal starvation(18) was noted to be significantly reduced in the growth retarded compared to the normal fetus. Further, fetal movement was diminished when growth retardation was associated with fetal heart decelerations.(19)

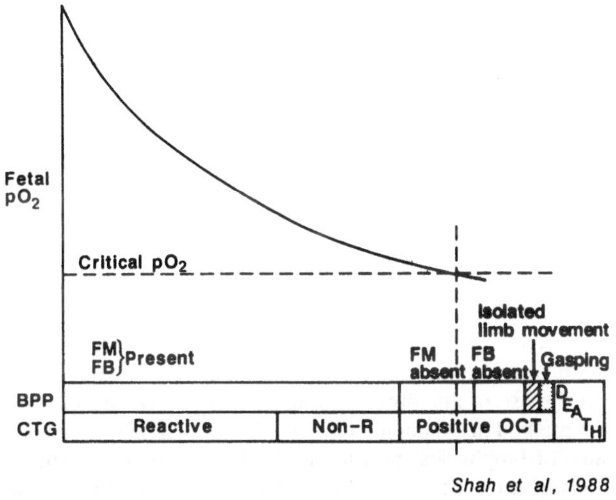

Figure I. The correlation of biophysical activity with fetal hypoxia
(Shah *et al.*)(23)
FM= fetal movement
FB = fetal breathing
CTG = cardiotocograph
BPP = biophysical profile
OCT = oxytocin challenge test

The other approach to the biophysical profile has been the evaluation of each component and it was found(13) that although loss of fetal breathing occurred in many babies with impaired outcome (high sensitivity), it had a low positive predictive value. Conversely, loss of fetal tone was a very good predictor of a very poor fetal outcome, and usually profound hypoxia. However, by the time the baby has reached this stage it may well be impossible to salvage.

The association of the various components of the profile with hypoxia demonstrated a high predictive value for the baby with marked acidosis.[20] In this study an abnormal profile score was predictive of a cord pH <7.20 in 82% of cases (Table 5). The fetal activity components of the score all provided a reasonable predictive value for acidosis, the weakest being absent fetal breathing and the strongest absent fetal tone.

Table 5. Components of the biophysical profile as predictors of fetal acidosis (pH < 7.2). (Vintzileos *et al.*)[20]

	Positive predictive value
Non reactive nonstress test	44%
Absent fetal breathing	35%
Absent body movements	71%
Absent fetal tone	100%
Amniotic volume < 2 cm	38%
Placental grade	14%
Biophysical score < 7/12	82%

DISCUSSION

The use of fetal activity to monitor fetal wellbeing in the potentially or actually growth retarded fetus does not appear to be well documented. Although there is a large database for the use of the biophysical profile in general, information on the specific use of the method in evaluating the growth retarded baby seems sparse.

Before the value of biophysical profile monitoring can be established the endpoints to be observed must be well defined. The correlates between the profile score and endpoint variables such as perinatal death, low cord blood pH or low Apgar scores are interesting but tell little about the use of the test in the specific problem of growth retardation. One study attempted to establish the ability of the biophysical profile to identify the small-for-dates fetus[21] and although the test seemed better than the CTG alone the small number of cases made meaningful interpretation impossible.

To some extent the use of the biophysical profile needs to be defined as well as the endpoints. Should the test be used primarily as a screening test or as a method of evaluating the at-risk pregnancy? Certainly its use as a screening test would seem impractical since it takes too long to perform and can only be done effectively by staff with a reasonable experience in ultrasound technique. Its advantage as a diagnostic test is that it does provide a semi-quantitative assessment of fetal condition which at least theoretically allows the progress of the pregnancy to be followed.[22]

What does the profile tell us of the fetal condition? It has been proposed[11] that the different components of the profile relate to the functioning of various parts of the fetal central nervous system. Thus brainstem function may be most sensitive to hypoxia, which would first produce changes in the CTG followed by loss of breathing movements. As hypoxia deepens the higher centres associated with movement and the maintenance of tone cease to function, and the baby stops moving; the next stage is death (Figure I).[23] Although this hypothesis is attractive it does not fully explain the observation in the hypoxic adult in whom movement may cease early on in hypoxia but whose brainstem function is maintained. It would seem likely that what is being observed is the effect of progressive hypoxia on the central nervous system as a whole and probably not in the selective way proposed.

If the observations of fetal activity give an indication of the relatively acute response of the fetus to hypoxia, the amniotic fluid volume reflects the effect of chronic hypoxia. Why amniotic fluid volume should decrease in growth retardation is not clear, but it has been proposed that it is the result of reduced fetal urine output in the face of a redistributed blood flow. Although this may be the case in some circumstances it cannot be the answer for all, since it is a common observation that perfectly adequate fetal activity is seen in oligohydramnios.

One serious criticism of the biophysical profile is that the various components are given the same weight. This dates back to the origins of the test as an assessment of the intrauterine Apgar score, but with the evidence now available from a very large experience in the use of the profile perhaps the scoring system should be modified.

The advantages of the biophysical profile are that it provides a non-invasive method of fetal evaluation which if necessary can be performed daily or more often. Further it provides a biological assessment of the fetal condition in that it seems reasonable to assume that if the fetus is moving and breathing it will usually be in good condition.[11] Although fetal blood sampling by cordocentesis may provide useful information in the growth retarded fetus[24,25] a disadvantage is that it gives information only at one point in time. Further, and perhaps more importantly, it assumes that the growth retarded baby with disordered gases is about to die and needs to be delivered. Whilst there is no doubt that these babies are in serious trouble, lack of knowledge about the aetiology and pathogenesis of fetal growth retardation makes interpretation of these data difficult. For example it may be that these babies can adjust their metabolism sufficiently to maintain an intrauterine existance even though the gases are deranged. A normal profile under these circumstances would indicate the need to prolong the pregnancy since functionally the baby's condition would be satisfactory.

CONCLUSIONS

The biophysical profile has been used successfully in a variety of obstetric complications. Its value in the specific circumstance of growth retardation has been less clearly defined, but the indications are that it should be effective since it provides an insight into the biological condition of the fetal central nervous system. The major advantages of the test are that it can be repeated as often as required and that it should provide important information about the progress of deterioration in the fetal condition.

REFERENCES

1. Boddy K. Fetal circulation and breathing movements. In: *Fetal Physiology and Medicine*. Eds. RW Beard, PW Nathanielsz. London: WB Saunders, 1976; pp.302–328.
2. Natale R, Clelow F, Dawes GS. Measurement of fetal forelimb movements in the lamb in utero. *Am J Obstet Gynecol* 1981; **140**: 545–551.
3. Nijuis J , Prechtl HFR, Martin CB, Bots RSGM. Are there behavioural states in the human fetus? *Early Hum Dev* 1982; **6**: 177–195.
4. Rizzo G, Arduini D, Mancuso S, Romanini C. Computer-assisted analysis of fetal behavioural states. *Prenat Diagn* 1988; **8**: 479–484.
5. Rizzo G, Arduini D, Pennestri F, Romanini C, Mancuso S. Fetal behaviour in growth retardation; its relationship to fetal blood flow. *Prenat Diagn* 1987; **7**: 229–238.
6. Sadovsky E, Yaffe H. Daily fetal movement recording and fetal progress. *Obstet Gynecol* 1973; **41**: 845–850.
7. Pearson JF, Weaver JB. Fetal activity and fetal wellbeing: an evaluation. *B r Med J* 1976; **1**: 1305–1307.
8. Mathews DD. Maternal assessment of fetal activity in small-for-dates infants. *Obstet Gynecol* 1975; **45**: 488–493.
9. Neldum S. Fetal movements as an indicator of fetal wellbeing. *Lancet* 1980; **i**: 1222–1223.
10. Manning FA, Platt LD, Sipos L. Antepartum fetal evaluation: development of a fetal biophysical profile. *Am J Obstet Gynecol* 1980; **136**: 787–795.
11. Vintzileos AM, Campbell WA, Nochimson DJ, Weinbaum PJ. The use and misuse of the fetal biophysical profile. *Am J Obstet Gynecol* 1987; **156**: 527–533.
12. Manning FA, Morrison I, Lange IR, Harman CR, Chamberlain PF. Fetal biophysical profile scoring; selective use of the nonstress test. *Am J Obstet Gynecol* 1987; **156**: 709–712.
13. Vintzileos AM, Campbell WA, Ingardia CJ, Nochimson DJ. The fetal biophysical profile and its predictive value. *Obstet Gynecol* 1983; **62**: 271–278.
14. Grannum PAT, Berkowitz RL, Hobbins JC. The ultrasound changes in the maturing placenta and their relation to pulmonic maturity. *Am J Obstet Gynecol* 1979; **133**: 915–922.
15. Manning FA, Menticoglou S, Harman CR, Morrison I, Lange IR. Antepartum fetal risk assessment: the role of the biophysical profile score. In: *Fetal Monitoring*. Ed. M J Whittle. London: Baillière Tindall, 1987: pp.55–72.
16. Manning FA, Hill LM, Platt LD. Qualitative amniotic fluid volume determination by ultrasound: antepartum detection of intrauterine growth retardation. *Am J Obstet Gynecol* 1981; **139**: 254–258.
17. Manning FA, Morrison I, Harman CR, Lange IR, Menticoglou S. Fetal assessment based on fetal biophysical profile scoring: experience in 19,221 referred high-risk pregnancies. *Am J Obstet Gynecol* 1987; **157**: 880–884.
18. Dornan JC, Ritchie JWK, Ruff S. The rate and regularity of breathing movements in the normal and growth retarded fetus. II. An analysis of false-nega-

tive fetal deaths. *Br J Obstet Gynaecol* 1984; **91**: 31–36.
19. Bekedam DJ, Visser GHA, Mulder EJH, Poelmann-Weesjes G. Heart rate variation and movement incidence in growth retarded fetuses: The significance of antenatal late heart rate decelerations. *Am J Obstet Gynecol* 1987; **157**: 126–133.
20. Vintzileos AM, Gaffney SE, Salinger LM, Kontopoulos VG, Campbell WA, Nochimson DJ. The relationships among the fetal biophysical profile, umbilical cord pH and Apgar scores. *Am J Obstet Gynecol* 1987; **157**: 627–631.
21. Platt LD, Walla CA, Paul RH, Trujillo ME, Loesser CV, Jacobs ND, Broussard PM. A prospective trial of the biophysical profile versus the non stress test in the management of high-risk pregnancies. *Am J Obstet Gynecol* 1985; **153**: 624–632.
22. Druzin ML, Lockshin M, Edersheim TG, Hutson JM, Krauss AL, Kogut E. Second-trimester fetal monitoring and preterm delivery in pregnancies with systemic lupus erythematosus and/or circulating anticoagulant. *Am J Obstet Gynecol* 1987; **157**: 1503–1510.
23. Shah DM, Brown JE, Boehm FH. *A simplified biophysical profile.* Abstract presented to Society of Perinatal Obstetricians, Las Vegas, February 1988.
24. Pearce JM, Chamberlain GV. Ultrasonically guided percutaneous umbilical blood sampling in the management of intrauterine growth retardation. *Br J Obstet Gynaecol* 1987; **94**: 318–321.
25. Cox WL, Daffos F, Forestier F, Descombey D, Aufront C, Auger MC, Gasschard JC. Physiology and management of intrauterine growth retardation. A biologic approach with fetal blood sampling. *Am J Obstet Gynecol* 1988; **159**: 36–41.

Discussion

Chairman: Professor P.W. Howie

HOWIE: We should begin to try to identify certain areas which are of particular concern and that could point the way for our own discipline to move forward in the whole area of intrauterine growth retardation. I would like to put forward a starting point as to how we might bring together some of our thoughts and try to identify the tasks. We are talking about clinical implications of fetal undergrowth. What are the tasks that actually face the clinician? We have talked about the baby that is "compromised " and the baby that is "getting into trouble" and we have used those terms very loosely without being at all specific about what we mean. What do we mean by "trouble"? It seems to me that clinicians are trying to do a number of things. We want to try to diagnose the condition because it may be very difficult to identify the baby who may have a problem. That may require a strategy, different tests and different trial models. We must decide how best to diagnose a condition, and that may involve screening. The second task is to try to deliver the baby before it dies because we know that some fetuses with intrauterine growth retardation die before they are delivered. The third task is to avoid anoxic damage. The baby *in utero* that is growth retarded is at risk of anoxia and if it becomes anoxic it may get specific anoxic damage which may be acute. There is a fourth thing which is to avoid starvation effects. The fetus that is already very small has had maybe weeks of starvation and may never make up the insult in starvation terms. Whether it is anoxic or not that fetus may go on being sick because it has been deprived. These are all different things but they are all linked in together. To reiterate we have four tasks: to diagnose the condition, because if you cannot diagnose you cannot do anything; to deliver the baby before it dies; to avoid the baby getting an acute anoxic insult, possibly during delivery; and to avoid the starvation effects suffered by the baby who may end up with cerebral or developmental disability because it has been starved.

COCKBURN: I think that Mr Nicolaides' data have very elegantly pointed out that the key perhaps to the whole thing is that the fetus is a completely anabolic creature; it is geared to anabolism and tissue growth. What he has shown is that the failure of growth is in a very high proportion of cases associated with a catabolic state. The fetus is just not geared to a catabolic state. He showed that the cortisol and the adrenalin were up and the insulin was down. In that situation it cannot grow. He showed that the fetus was releasing fatty acids probably from its own tissues and amino acids from its own tissues, and that there was a preponderance of certain amino acids in the fetus. That would mean that the fetus was living off its own reserves. If this is happening very early in pregnancy there is no way that a fetus has got the reserves to last more than hour or two. If it happens later in fetal life there is some degree of ability to survive on certain reserves of fat, glycogen and other material. You have evidence of a catabolic state *in utero* and as soon as you find that evidence you have an abnormal, dangerous situation in that fetus. If you add to that an acute hypoxaemic state you switch the fetus into a state where, for example, it is wasting what reserves of glycogen it has in anaerobic metabolism. It is just producing lactic acid and making its perfusion problem that much worse. So the basic thing is fetal starvation, a catabolic state and hypoxia on top of that which is critical. Early in pregnancy if you find that there is a catabolic state there is not a lot you can do about it unless you do what we can do outside the uterus; that is to ventilate the baby or give it oxygen and infuse complete parenteral nutrition. That is the only way that you will keep that early embryo going. In later gestation you may be able to calculate how much reserve there is and how much time you have got, because we know pretty well what reserves of energy there are in fetuses at different stages.

HAY: I should like to comment on Mr Nicolaides' data and also focus on the previous comments. I want to make a plea on the side of the neonatologists simply to be cautious, and to ask for sustained data over time. Our nurseries around the world are full of babies delivered with all good intentions who are extremely sick, and who do not grow well because we do not have the means of taking good care of them in spite of the great strides in neonatal medicine. I really do not think that we should start looking for different tools and different concepts to try to deliver babies earlier and earlier because we think that they may be getting into trouble. The message is to try to identify the baby that really is in trouble for whom we cannot do anything more under the circumstances. I have some questions about the data presented by Mr Nicolaides; one is related to the continued demonstration of norms that were shown, and the babies outside those norms. I am concerned that these norms are not identified very well. Could you show me how they are produced, how comparable they are from centre to centre and on what numbers they are based? Secondly, when you show babies that have one condition, for example hypoglycaemia, do those same infants have other abnormalities? You have quite a mixture of data and I do not see that there is a comparable infant that fits into all groups. You may be mixing a lot of different conditions.

NICOLAIDES: The normal data is derived from patients who have had cordocentesis for a number of reasons. Some of them are truly normal because they are having a fetal blood sample for prenatal diagnosis of genetic disease such as thalassaemia or haemophilia and have been found not to have the conditions for which they were being investigated. That is the major group in the gestations of 17–24 weeks. Beyond that is a group of fetuses that have various malformations detected by ultrasound where there is a high risk of an associated chromosomal abnormality. In the absence of an associated chromosomal abnormality, and having excluded fetuses that have obvious conditions that may affect oxygenation and metabolism (hydrops and major cardiac abnormalities, for example) those are assumed to be normal. We have some evidence that that is the case because if we take specific malformations like renal malformations that are spread in our population throughout pregnancy, and we compare the results with fetuses with renal malformations at 20–24 weeks with those at risk of haemophilia, their values are the same.

Therefore we are making a major assumption that a lot of these babies are abnormal. That is why you are sampling them. Metabolically they are not abnormal. The small-for-gestational-age babies are very highly preselected and different centres have used different criteria for their preselection. We are a referral centre, and less than 2% of those data were derived from patients whom we identified from our own centre. What is interesting to me is how excellent whatever these mechanisms of preselection are in the various regional hospitals, because they are picking up 15–20% of the babies with chromosomal abnormalities. They are picking up 30–50% of the babies in the SGA group that have hypoxaemia, those with metabolic changes. So whatever their system, it seems to be working. We have a problem, and that is the volume of blood that we can take. You can do karyotyping usually on 0.5 μl; you need to spend another 200–300 μl on blood gases, another 200–300 μl on ensuring that the blood sample was fetal. You are left with not more than 1 or in late gestation 2 μl blood to do the various metabolic studies. Some of them are done on the same group of fetuses, but others are separate. In the glucose and insulin studies there was an overlap which allowed us to have the correlations between hypoglycaemia, hyperinsulinaemia and increased severity of hyperinsulinaemia related to hypoglycaemia.

STEWART: You have a veritable welter of data. I accept the liability to death of all these deviations from accepted standards. But having said that, I am concerned because I would like to know what the consequence is for a survivor of having any of the parameters that you were talking about outside what you believe to be the normal standards. For example, the pH of less than 7.2. The mean pH in the average low birthweight baby is actually 7. So I am wondering what is the consequence of having hypoxaemia if he survives, the amino acids are at an acceptable standard, and so on? Do you have that data?

NICOLAIDES: That would take about 10 years.

STEWART: No; you get a very good idea within one year after the birth of the affected child.

NICOLAIDES: How many of the abnormalities that you are observing at the first year persist at the age of 10?

STEWART: You can get a very strong correlation between neurological impairment in the strict sense of the word, and I am not talking about cerebro-motor impairment, but rather neurological impairment and its later outcome in a number of different ways. If you had looked at your cohort very carefully over the first year you would know an enormous amount about them.

HOWIE: This is an extremely important point and we look forward to hearing more about it in your presentation later.

STEWART: There is a very central issue which I want to raise in broad terms. It is the question of whether these deviations are affecting mortality and morbidity in the same way. I think that we have to question that. I entirely accept that some of these fetuses will die, so they have to be delivered. But what sort of individuals are we delivering? Are we getting individuals who are so damaged that there is not a hope of doing anything for them, or are they delivered in such a way that the neonatologist can have some reasonable chance of treating them?

LEVENE: I think that this is a particularly important point because many obstetricians and neonatologists believe prematurity to be a continuum—death, handicap, normality. Eut in the condition we are talking about, severe growth retardation, it is not a continuity. Obstetricians are worried about the fetus dying before they can deliver it. Once the fetus is delivered the chance of death is extremely small in modern neonatal units. But we are very concerned about long term developmental problems and I think it is going to take years for us to know whether these children have an IQ deficit of, say, 10 points which is the sort of area we are probably looking at with the majority of them. We are not talking about cerebral palsy. I do not believe that there is a direct relationship between intrauterine growth retardation and cerebral palsy, although there are clearly some children with IUGR who do develop it. The strategy that we need to develop in this particular case, in terms of our end point for any studies that we are setting up, has to be very carefully thought out in terms of the short term outcome, i.e. death; and the long term outcome, i.e. developmental or intellectual problems.

HOWIE: Can you expand on that please? This is absolutely critical; if we are doing anything we have really got to have a morbidity end point. I see this in virtually every paper I read. We have got to have this kind of follow-up, and virtually nobody does it. Have you any suggestions on the way that we should go forward?

LEVENE: I was going to ask both the speakers, because I think that they have both highlighted the fact that there is no controlled data here at all. To my mind the only way that we can start to answer these questions is to set up carefully controlled studies with defined end points. Those end points must be neurodevelopmental; there is no point in obstetricians saying that this baby was born with a good Apgar score, and therefore we did a good job. We need to be thinking quite a long way down the line. Perhaps we need to decide what those end points are; I would say that a year is far too early in intrauterine growth retardation. Could I ask both the speakers if they could identify perhaps one area that they think a controlled study should be addressing, and then we can think about what the specific end points are.

MILNER: While the points that Professor Levene is making are very important, I think that the consequences of being a graduate from neonatal intensive care are much broader than neurological. If we are looking at the quality of life for the long term survivor we need to concentrate on the quality of respiratory life and the quality of gastrointestinal life, for example. There are significant percentages of survivors now with bronchopulmonary dysplasia, subglottic tracheal stenosis and major bowel resection. They have to be added into the equation because it focusses back on the central theme of this discussion of how one assesses the quality of fetal life and what action you should take upon it. The second point is that if you take a community such as Sheffield with a relatively stable population and take the 5-year olds who are neurodevelopmentally handicapped, only 10% have got anything that is retrospectively associated with the kind of obstetric and perinatal information that we are talking about. Ninety percent of the otherwise undiagnosable neurodevelopmental handicap at age 5 is a "black box" in the kind of aetiological concepts that we are discussing. I was listening to what Mr Nicolaides was saying with particular interest because it seemed to be giving me for the first time the sort of information in the human species that hitherto has only been available to us from animal species.

RUSH: I do not think that it is IUGR. I think again that it is extremes of birthweight. The data from studies of sib pairs many years ago showed absolutely no difference in neurodevelopmental outcome, with up to 1000 g difference in birthweight between sib pairs, and showed only miniscule differences with 1500 g difference. We have seen data of developmental disability in IUGR. IUGR is strongly socioeconomically related. We are talking about extremes of very low birthweight and very short gestation; that is where neurodevelopmental disability occurs. Also the studies of surviving twin pairs suggest that it is almost exactly the same thing. Very small twins whose co-twin died in the perinantal period were developmentally identical to singletons, i.e. much of the deficit in twins is clearly due to the postnatal environment in the twin world rather than the intrauterine growth retardation of the twins.

LIND: With these tests we have got to be very careful that we do not get a high false positive rate, because the picture that Professor Cockburn described is dramatic and urgent and we need to do something about it. But what is going to happen if we get these tests wrong and start to give our paediatric colleagues babies that would have done perfectly well *in utero*? Any sort of needling technique will give you transient information when all the metabolic parameters may seem horrendous, and 5 minutes later may give you an entirely different story. Coming back to the biophysical profile, perhaps we need a less sensitive index. What we want is a test that is so crude that by the time it does go positive you can be absolutely certain that the baby is in deep trouble, rather than a highly sensitive index with a high false positive rate.

FRASER: Regarding the value of the screening diagnostic tests, perhaps we should think again about Chard's curve. I think that the progress in new diagnostic tests must be very carefully evaluated by those who innovate the test, and the evaluation should include its applicability outside the specialist centre. Obviously, one has a major concern about amateurs doing cordocentesis, for example. When you have got a test like the Manning test which is a score with multiple observations involved you multiply the potential for observer error. What is the observer error and how reproducible is it outside their own hands? The next stage is to validate that test in a properly designed prospective and randomised trial against the existing gold standard of diagnostic tests for the condition we are talking about.

WHITTLE: There are very few data about reproducibility with the Manning and Vintzileos work and in fact only two main centres reporting about the usefulness or applicability of the test in clinical practice. A few other groups have reported but nothing like their numbers. I would agree with you entirely. I think that it is always one of the big failings in practice that people dream up tests which are good in their hands, but then on general release give unsatisfactory results. Coming back to the point that you were making, Professor Howie, I think that if there is anything to come out of this Study Group for our colleagues who are not in specialist centres, I do think that we need to provide some sort of indication of the sort of test that might be helpful. If those tests cannot be done in a busy District General Hospital or even a busy Central Hospital, then perhaps there should be some indication about the wisdom of referring patients to a place where the test can be performed. I think that the problem is that we really do not know whether a given test will help us at all in the evaluation of this particular problem.

HOWIE: Mr Nicolaides, you said that there were no controlled trials. You made no mention of the randomised studies in hypertensive women who were given low dose aspirins. This did improve both placental weight and birthweight. These are in fact controlled trials which have now given rise to the Clasp study which is ongoing in the UK at the moment. One may criticise it, but it is looking both at the hypertensive, and suspected fetal growth retardation. The question is whether that trial has got its end points right. I do not think that it is going to follow through in the way that Professor Levene and Dr Stewart were suggesting. Very recently Trudinger reported that women with umbilical artery Doppler flow abnormalities at 28 weeks were randomised either to aspirin or placebo and the aspirin treated group produced both bigger babies and larger placentae. So there are some controlled trials, but whether they are appropriate or what clinical credence you give to them is debatable.

Intrapartum monitoring in IUGR

Mr P.J.Steer

INTRODUCTION

The definition of intrauterine growth retardation (IUGR) remains a matter of controversy. The most common definition classifies a baby as "growth retarded" if it has a birthweight less than the tenth centile, corrected for sex and gestational age.[1] In fact, many babies with such a birthweight behave and develop normally and are probably simply genetically small.[2] In addition, there are many causes of true intrauterine growth retardation, such as genetic abnormality, intrauterine infection, maternal nutritional deprivation, placental blood flow impairment due to vascular disorders (as in pre-eclampsia) or restriction of maternal cardiac output (as in maternal cardiac disease), etc. Thus it is preferable to use the term "small-for-gestational-age" (SGA) rather than IUGR when discussing babies defined as abnormal using centile birthweight classification and reserve the latter term for babies in which a specific diagnosis of growth retardation is reached based on more specific criteria, such as a fall-off in intrauterine growth, oligohydramnios, neonatal hypoglycaemia, low neonatal ponderal index, absence of subcutaneous fat stores, etc.

Most studies of intrapartum monitoring have compared SGA babies with those of more average weight (AGA), rather than looking at babies who are specifically IUGR. This reflects the difficulty of making the more specific diagnosis on a large enough scale to make statistical comparisons possible. It follows that their findings are general in nature and may not apply to every category of growth retarded baby. However, provided this limitation is borne in mind, the findings have clinical value in that a precise pathological classification of IUGR is often not possible until after delivery, and sometimes not until some years after birth. Thus, clinical management has in any case to depend on the crude classification by weight for gestational age alone. In the study reported here this convention is therefore followed using throughout the expression "SGA" rather than "IUGR".

At St Mary's Hospital in Paddington we have developed a computerised obstetric data collection system[3] which is now in use throughout the North West Thames Regional Health Authority. Systematic data collection began in 1976 and went "on-line" in 1982. In addition, in 1984, for six months from 1st June to 30th November, we attempted to obtain complete cord blood pH and blood gas analysis on all babies delivered; in the event this was achieved in 748 of 1206 (61%). The sampled cases included a high proportion of the abnormal deliveries as most of those missed were normal deliveries at night.

For the purposes of this study group, therefore, all deliveries at St Mary's during 1984 have been analysed and classified by centile birthweight, with particular reference to those where cord blood pH and gas values are available. Initial analysis showed that significant differences in intrapartum variables and cord blood parameters could only be demonstrated when birthweight was less than the 5th centile. For example, for babies between the 5th and 10th centile, mean arterial cord blood pH was 7.26, identical to that for babies above the 10th percentile. However, if birthweight was <5th centile, mean pH was significantly reduced to 7.24. Thus the groups selected were <5th centile (SGA) and equal to or more than the 5th centile (AGA).

PATIENTS AND METHODS

Selected data from all the deliveries entered on the St Mary's Hospital data collection system for 1984 (n=2126) were transferred to an IBM PC. Data from the cord blood study, which included a detailed analysis of the cardiotocograph tracing, were merged, cross-referencing by hospital number and the first two letters of first and family names.

Babies were defined as small-for-gestational-age (SGA) if they fell below the 5th centile, weight for gestational age, as determined using the Altman and Coles nomograms. (4)

Statistical analysis was performed using SPSS (PC version). Values for all variables were not available for every baby; the number available is given separately for each analysis.

RESULTS

Seventy-eight of 2,126 babies (3.7%) were identified as SGA on the above criteria; the remaining 2,048 were classified as AGA. Mean gestational age was similar in both groups (39.13 weeks, SD 2.02, compared with 39.19 weeks, SD 2.35) but birthweight in the SGA group was more than a kilogram less than in the AGA group (2.11 SD, 0.37 kg, compared with 3.26 SD, 0.55 kg).

SGA fetuses were more than twice as likely as AGA fetuses to develop abnormal cardiotocograms (CTGs) in labour; 30 of 70 (43%) SGA babies with inter-

Table 1. Interaction of CTG with SGA

Percent with Apgar score <7 at one minute

	Trace normal % (n)	Trace abnormal % (n)	Chi²	p
AGA	11 (166/1533)	28 (111/394)	77	<0.0005
SGA	15 (6/40)	45 (13/29)	7.5	<0.0125
Chi ²	0.7	3.6		
p	NS	0.057		

pretable CTGs had abnormal patterns compared with only 394 of 1,928 (20%) AGA babies (Chi squared 20, p<0.0001). Similarly 28 of 78 (36%) SGA babies produced meconium staining of the liquor compared with only 356 of 2,044 (17%) AGA babies (Chi squared 17.3, p <0.0001). These abnormalities were reflected in an almost doubled rate of emergency Caesarean section, 14 of 78 (18%) compared with 200 of 2,048 (9.8%) (Chi squared 5.6, p <0.025).

Overall, SGA babies were significantly more likely to have low Apgar scores at one minute (one minute score <7, SGA 20 of 75 or 27%), compared with AGA 297 of 2,041 (15%); Chi squared 8.3, p<0.005). However, this difference largely disappeared if allowance was made for CTG pattern (Table 1). A similar, although not so marked, effect was seen if allowance was made for meconium staining of the liquor (Table 2).

Table 2. Interaction of meconium with SGA

Percent with Apgar score <7 at one minute

	No meconium % (n)	Meconium present % (n)	Chi^2	p
AGA	12 (209/1684)	25 (88/354)	36	<0.0005
SGA	22 (11/49)	35 (9/26)	1.3	NS
Chi^2	4.3	1.2		
p	0.038	NS		

SGA fetuses were twice as likely to have fetal blood sampling performed, with a rate of 23% (18/78) compared with 12% (254/2,048) for AGA fetuses (Chi squared 7.7, p<0.005). The rates of sampling as a proportion of the fetuses with abnormal traces was similar in both groups, 18/30 (60%) in the SGA group and 254/394 (64%) in the AGA group. However the mean value of the lowest pH recorded for each labour was significantly less in the SGA group than the AGA group (7.25, SD 0.08, compared with 7.28, SD 0.08; t = 1.54, p = 0.01).

In the six-month subgroup, a detailed analysis was made of the characteristics of the CTG pattern in both first and second stages of labour (Table 3). The only distinguishing feature was an increased incidence of variable/late decelerations in the SGA group; other aspects such as the baseline rate and incidence of accelerations showed no difference. Cord artery measurement showed that SGA babies were significantly more likely to have a metabolic acidosis while the levels of pO_2 and pCO_2 were not different (Table 4).

Table 5 shows that the overall classification of the CTG interacted with centile birthweight such that a normal CTG predicted normal cord artery pH and Apgar

Table 3. CTG variables

First stage	AGA		SGA	
Number of cases	1009		58	
Baseline rate (bpm)	138	SD 15	138	SD 14
Reactive (%)	84		85	
Variability < 5 bpm (%)	11		5	
Early decelerations (%)	7		7	
Variable/late decel. (%)	10		17	
None (%)	83		76	
Second stage				
Number of cases	828		44	
Baseline rate (bpm)	138	SD 17	136	SD 15
Reactive (%)	74		86	
Variability < 5 bpm (%)	15		11	
Early decelerations (%)	18		9	Chi squared
Variable/late decel. (%)	31		52	8.8
None (%)	51		39	p = 0.012

All differences non-significant except as shown

scores in both SGA and AGA babies, but that if the CTG was abnormal, SGA babies were significantly more likely to have abnormal outcome measures.

DISCUSSION

The incidence of birthweight less than the 5th centile according to Altman and Coles' nomograms was significantly lower in our population than would have been expected, but this may have been due to chance (Chi squared 3.34, $p<0.1>0.05$, two tailed). Certainly the cut off defined a population at significant risk of intrapartum dysfunction, as assessed by CTG pattern and fetal blood sampling; the neonatal outcome measures supported the conclusion that these babies are about twice as likely to run into trouble as AGA babies. It is reassuring that a normal CTG pattern was as reliable at indicating normality in the SGA fetus as in the AGA fetus. However it is equally important to remember that if the CTG becomes abnormal, the SGA fetus is more likely to have an abnormal outcome than if a similar abnormality occurs in an AGA baby. Modanlou *et al.*[5] were among the first to point out an increased risk of low Apgar scores amongst the babies of high risk mothers, and to show that this was linked with intrapartum fetal acidosis. As in our study, there was a greater difference of pH and base deficit than of pO_2 and

Table 4. Umbilical arterial cord blood gas and pH values

	(n)	AGA		(n)	SGA		p
pO_2 mmHg	698	21	SD 8	39	21.5	SD 9	NS
pCO_2 mmHg	707	53	SD 13	40	53	SD 17	NS
pH	708	7.26	SD 0.09	40	7.23	SD 0.09	<0.05
Base deficit (mmol/L)	700	4.6	SD 3.5	36	6.5	SD 4.6	<0.05

Table 5. Relationship between cardiotocogram pattern cord artery pH, base deficit and Apgar scores in babies weighing less than the fifth centile, weight for gestational age

Cardiotocogram pattern	Normal		Abnormal S2		Abnormal S1	
Birthweight centile	AGA	SGA	AGA	SGA	AGA	SGA
Number of cases	393	16	138	11	129	11
Mean Arterial pH	7.28	7.31	7.24*	7.19	7.21	7.16
SD Arterial pH	0.07	0.05	0.08	0.07	0.11	0.09
Number with Apgar 1 <7 (%)	57 (15)	1 (6)	19 (14)	3 (27)	33 (26)*	6 (55)
Number with Apgar 5 <7 (%)	9 (2)	9 (0)	0 (0)	1 (9)	5 (4)*	2 (18)

* $p< 0.05$

pCO_2. Subsequently Low *et al.*[6] reported a relationship between decreasing weight–gestational centile of the fetus and increasing frequency of total and late decelerations of the fetal heart rate. As in our study they found no relation between centile birthweight and other fetal heart rate parameters such as baseline rate. They went on to demonstrate a significant relationship between low centile birthweight and acidosis, such that the probability of acidosis ranged from 15% in an AGA fetus to 50% in a very SGA fetus.[7]

Lin *et al.*[8] studied 37 babies <10th centile and compared them with 88 babies of average centile birthweight. As in our study, they found similar cord arterial pH values in the two groups if the CTG trace remained normal throughout labour, and a greater fall of pH in the SGA group than in the AGA group if the CTG trace was abnormal. They also measured cord arterial lactate concentrations and found similar values if the CTG was normal (SGA 23.4 and AGA 24.9 mg/100ml respectively), whereas if the CTG was abnormal the values rose to 49.3 mg/100ml in the SGA babies compared with only 31.2 mg/100ml in the AGA group. As in our study they found no significant differences in cord artery pO_2 and pCO_2. This dissociation between pO_2 levels and pH has recently been shown to be present even before the onset of labour in a study of growth retarded fetuses investigated by cordocentesis.[9] Thus it seems unlikely that the metabolic acidosis seen more often in SGA than AGA babies can be due simply to chronic hypoxia; rather it seems likely that there is some more complex underlying metabolic derangement.

In conclusion, we have shown that normal CTG patterns and absence of meconium staining of the liquor can be used safely to predict wellbeing in labour, even when the fetus is SGA. However, if the CTG become abnormal, or if there is meconium staining, the development of acidosis is more rapid and severe in the SGA than the AGA baby. This acidosis is not simply hypoxic in origin but also reflects a complex underlying metabolic dysfunction. Correspondingly, the characteristic abnormality of the CTG in SGA fetuses is the variable/late deceleration, rather than changes in baseline rate, variability or reactivity.

REFERENCES

1. Brar HS, Rutherford SE. Classification of intrauterine growth retardation. *Sem Perinatol* 1988; **12**: 2–10.
2. Teberg AJ, Walther FJ, Pena IC. Mortality, morbidity and outcome of the small for gestational age infant. *Sem Perinatol* 1988; **12**: 84–94.
3. Maresh M, Beard RW, Combe D, Dawson AM, Gillmer MDG, Smith G, Steer PJ. Selection of an obstetric database for a microcomputer and its use for on-line production of birth notification forms, discharge summaries and perinatal audit. *Br J Obstet Gynaecol* 1983; **90**: 227–231.
4. Altman DG, Coles EC. Nomograms for precise determination of birth weight for dates. *Br J Obstet Gynaecol* 1980; **87**: 81–86.
5. Modanlou H, Yeh SY, Hon EH. Fetal and neonatal acid-base balance in normal and high risk pregnancies. *Obstet Gynecol* 1974; **43**: 347–353.
6. Low JA, Pancham SR, Worthington D. Fetal heart deceleration patterns in relation to asphyxia and weight–gestational age percentile of the fetus. *Obstet Gynecol* 1976; **47**: 14–20.
7. Low JA, Karchmar J, Broekhoven L, Leonard T, McGrath MJ, Pancham SR, Piercy WN. The probability of fetal metabolic acidosis during labor in a population at risk as determined by clinical factors. *Am J Obstet Gynecol* 1981; **141**: 941–951.
8. Lin CC, Moawad AH, Rosenow PJ, River P. Acid–base characteristics of fetuses with intrauterine growth retardation during labor and delivery. *Am J Obstet Gynecol* 1980; **137**: 553–559.

9. Pardi G, Buscaglia M, Ferrazzi E, Bozzetti P, Marconi AM, Cetin I, Battaglia FC, Makowski EL. Cord sampling for the evaluation of oxygenation and acid–base balance in growth-retarded fetuses. *Am J Obstet Gynecol* 1987; **157**: 1221–1228.

Discussion

Chairman: Professor P.W. Howie

PATEL: I know that your talk was related to intrapartum care but I wonder if you have any assessment of parameters that you looked at in the neonatal period apart from the cord blood gases, such as ultrasonic measurements or neurological assessment?

STEER: The babies were twice as likely to end up in special care, but most of them did not, despite the fact that they had a mean birthweight of 2 kg. The policy of St Mary's would be to send them to transitional care, again because most of them were born in pretty good clinical condition.

PATEL: There was no structured assessment carried out?

STEER: No. Apart from the cord gases. This was not data that was collected as part of a prospective study, it was just part of our routine data collection system.

CHARD: Could I make a general point about diagnosis? All the speakers we have heard this morning have been presenting multi-parameter systems. Of course the problem with any multi-parameter system is that of reaching any overall conclusion when a series of observations are made, aspects of the biological profile, if you will, some of which are positive and others of which are negative. That is going to vary substantially between different individuals. Has anyone explored the use of Bayes' theorem in order to assemble an overall pattern of risk? May I enter a very strong plea that this be looked at, because Bayes' theorem, which is very widely used in other aspects of clinical medicine, is considered to be mathematically the most appropriate method of assembling a series of nondefinitive risks. If you have, taking as an example the biophysical profile, a series of parameters for each of which you can quote a sensitivity, a predictive value etc., but you want to assess the overall risk for a specific patient who has, say, three positive factors and three negative factors, that is the appropriate way to go.

STEER: I have not done that, but I think that it begs the question in one sense, in that it implies that I was describing what I would consider to be tests. I am not sure whether they were tests in the usual sense because we do not actually have an outcome. I would consider the Apgar score as much of a test relating to further development as the CTG, and similarly with the pH. What I was trying to describe was the interrelationship of various physiological variables insofar as we can measure them rather than describing "tests" which I would advocate people apply, other than simply to say that if a heart tracing is normal the chances of a poor outcome would seem to be very low whether the baby is SGA or not.

ALBERMAN: The way the literature on cerebral palsy is going leaves one with a very strong feeling that there is a reason for being SGA and that causes both the SGA and the asphyxia. Have you looked backwards at any of these babies or have there been ultrasound studies on them?

STEER: What you are suggesting is a hypothesis which is often true. When we see disturbances of acid base and CTGs in labour, with an SGA baby it is a manifestation of damage that has already occurred during pregnancy rather than damage actually occurring. Nonetheless I think that we have a duty to ensure that it does not become so severe that we add to the damage. Many of these babies who do perfectly well in labour turn up 3 or 4 years later quite seriously handicapped. One must appreciate that we are looking at disturbances of physiology which to some extent in the majority of cases may be quite peripheral to the long term outlook for the baby. To that extent I agree with you that longitudinal studies are badly needed, but it is generating the funds and the enthusiasm to do them that is the problem.

HOWIE: The point is a very important one from a medico-legal point of view because the assumption is that it is the hypoxia and the labour which does damage and not the insult which may have occurred many weeks before.

HAY: In relationship to your data on acid–base balance and lactate, and also this applies to the cordocentesis values, it is important to avoid overinterpreting one specific biochemical parameter. We interpret a change in lactate concentration in a child or an adult as implying hypoxia and oxygen insufficiency. This may not at all be the case in the fetus. Experimental studies in animals, for example, have demonstrated that you can infuse copious amounts of lactate into a fetus and the pH does not change at all. When infused as lactic acid the capacity for the fetal liver to extract lactate is excessive. You might suspect that a change in lactate represents either that the liver does not take up lactate as well or that blood flow has been shunted away for some other reason so that the capacity for the liver to clear is different. That redirects the question about individual value of lactate meaning something that a physician would act upon in the fetal condition differently from how they might in the postnatal condition.

PATEL: Except that in the animal situation you are infusing lactate in a well perfused placenta in a healthy fetus, while here we are talking about a fetus that presumably is unhealthy.

NICOLAIDES: A similar situation in the human is the Rhesus model. If you give a blood transfusion the blood is extremely acidotic with a pH of 6.9. My policy has been to transfuse big volumes quickly, expanding the fetal placental volume at a rate of 50% per minute. If you take a blood sample immediately at the end of that process the pH and the blood vessels are normal. As you said, in that case you have a normally functioning placenta. This may be an explanation for the high cortisol that we are finding in the absence of a low ACTH. It may not be a physiological endocrine response but it may reflect the redistribution in blood flow with an increased blood supply to the adrenal. Blood shunted away from the liver may explain the high lactate. From the antenatal data that I showed the lactate is above 2 standard deviations of the normal range before the pO_2 drops below 2 standard deviations of the normal range. That is much more marked in the umbilical artery than the umbilical vein.

CLAPP: There are a couple of things that have been said relative to redistribution of blood flow that I find disturbing in terms of the interpretation of the data, the last of which was the issue of the elevated cortisol. Cortisol is raised in a compartment. How much blood flow goes to the adrenal makes absolutely no difference. What you are looking at is a relationship between production and clearance; either clearance is down or production is up or you change the volume of distribution. So that when one sees an elevated cortisol you cannot explain that on the basis of flow redistribution. The same thing was mentioned relative to the partial pressure of oxygen in scalp blood. I think it has been well shown that the scalp responds and the skin responds in terms of a hypoxic stress in a similar fashion to the gut. It does not vasodilate, if anything it vasoconstricts, and this is where you are getting your blood sample from.

STEER: We took two samples from the cord artery.

CLAPP: So these are not in labour.

STEER: The fetal scalp blood samples were assessed simply for pH because these were recorded on our clinical data collections. All the blood gases that I showed you were from cord artery samples at delivery.

CLAPP: That makes the point even stronger. If you look at the pO_2, there is a standard relationship with the saturation of the blood. You can change content by changing the amount of haemoglobin in the system, but what that reflects in the artery is total extraction versus total delivery. You cannot explain that by a recirculation of blood; that has to represent a change in the total amount of oxygen that is being utilised by the system. When you show the same pO_2 that means that the system as a whole is using the same amount fractionally relative to what it gets. The third point has to do with the lactate. While what Dr Hay says is correct, I would draw your attention to some very old data generated by Huckabee and Barron[1] in the sheep model, where they found that the placenta is a lactate sink in that you can in the normal situation see lactate being taken up from the maternal circulation and disappearing into the fetal–placental unit. You can see lactate being cleared from the fetal compartment as well. I think that Huckabee did a series of experiments where he varied the oxygen tension in a calculated way, in those days in the equivalent of the intervillous space. He felt that at a pO_2 less than 40% in those experiments the data fit the concept that the placenta was clearing lactate from the fetal compartment and thereby paying off the "oxygen debt" of the fetus. He came up with the concept that fetal survival was not so much contingent in the short term on oxygen delivery to the fetus, but on oxygen delivery to the placenta. How applicable that information is to this situation and those values I do not know.

STEER: We have to be careful when we talk about hypoxia or hypoxaemia. We are talking about the partial pressure of oxygen which is not necessarily the same as oxygen saturation. It is not even necessarily very closely related to oxygen delivery to the tissues because that will depend on flow as well. So we must be specific when we are using these terms.

REFERENCE

1. Huckabee WE, Metcalfe J, Prystowsky H, Barron DH. Insufficiency of O_2 supply to the pregnant uterus. *Am J Physiol* 1960; **15:** 1139–1143.

Neonatal management of the SGA infant

Professor M.I. Levene

DEFINITIONS OF GROWTH RETARDATION AFTER BIRTH

The diagnosis of intrauterine growth retardation can be made in a variety of different ways, most of which are not available to the obstetrician. The simple definition of small-for-gestational-age (SGA) is one based on low weight for gestational age, and this is generally stated to occur when the infant's birthweight is below the tenth centile for gestational age. Severe intrauterine growth retardation (IUGR) may also be defined as weight below the third centile for gestational age. Provided that the gestational age is accurately known or can be clinically assessed these diagnostic categories are straightforward.

Other methods exist to define IUGR. The best known is the Ponderal Index (PI) and this refers to the infant's relative amount of soft-tissue mass. This is calculated by the formula:

$$\frac{\text{weight (g)}}{[\text{crown–heel length (cm)}]^3} \times 100$$

A low number represents a disproportionately long infant with little soft tissue mass. This suggests that the infant is wasted of fat but there has been sparing of length as would occur in cases of acute starvation. These are the infants with relatively normal head circumference whose growth retardation is asymmetrical. Charts showing the normative data for PI are available.(1)

A more direct method for assessing the amount of adipose tissue is to measure the amount of subcutaneous fat. This can be done in one of two ways. Mid-arm circumference will give a convenient and accurate measure to compare with normal data, but skin fold thickness is probably the method of choice. This measurement is made by a special spring-loaded caliper. A double layer of skin is gently pinched between the jaws of the instrument and a measurement read off in millimeters. The normative data for triceps skinfold thickness in full-term infants has been published by Oakley and colleagues.(2)

It is clear that two infants of identical weight and gestational age may be of different lengths, PIs and skin fold thicknesses but one may have suffered severe IUGR and have little soft tissue mass with low skinfold thickness, and the other may be shorter in length but well nourished. The neonatologist therefore has the advantage in being able to describe more carefully the dimensions of growth retardation and identify particular causes with different patterns of abnormal growth.

If IUGR is defined simply on the basis of birthweight below the 10th centile for gestational age, then the diagnostic accuracy antenatally appears to be relatively poor. Two relatively recent studies have reported the proportion of SGA infants detected antenatally. In one, only 37% of SGA infants were detected before birth(3) and the other diagnosed only 30% when the 5th centile was taken as the cut-off point.(4) The accuracy was improved somewhat to 44% when a lower cut-off point of below the 2.3rd centile was taken. The author is not aware of any published data reporting either the sensitivity or specificity of antenatal diagnosis of IUGR.

The complications that may develop in growth retarded infants are numerous and are described below. Many such complications are very obvious when they occur but others such as hypoglycaemia may be benign and of little clinical significance. It is therefore important to consider carefully the diagnostic criteria for the definition of IUGR when assessing the incidence of these complications.

BIRTH ASPHYXIA

The growth retarded fetus is born in a suboptimal condition and may withstand the rigours of labour in a less well adapted condition than the normally grown infant. There is no doubt that birth asphyxia occurs significantly more commonly in growth retarded fetuses. In a study of almost 20,000 full-term infants born in Leicester we found that 25% who had birth asphyxia (defined as post-asphyxial encephalopathy) were small for gestational age.(5)

Asphyxia is due to the simultaneous combination of hypoxia and hypoperfusion, and this is more likely to occur as an acute event in an already chronically asphyxiated infant. The incidence of birth asphyxia in growth retarded fetuses is not well known and will depend on both the definition of asphyxia as well as that for IUGR. In a study of over 38 000 consecutive deliveries, 1.2% of the babies developed birth asphyxia (defined as requiring positive pressure ventilation for more than one minute) compared with 4% of infants below the third weight centile for gestational age.(6) The same study reported that 34% of premature SGA infants were asphyxiated according to this definition. There is no published evidence that the severity of IUGR correlates with the severity of birth asphyxia.

The association between IUGR and asphyxia is a particularly important one because of the implications of early prenatal recognition of the compromised growth retarded fetus whose brain may be protected by careful delivery.

Once intrapartum asphyxia has occurred there are few specific therapeutic regimes that are known to reduce cerebral injury. It is important to maintain adequate oxygenation, fluids and temperature. Infection and hyperbilirubinaemia should be anticipated and avoided, or treated. Convulsions are treated with phenobarbitone as the first line drug; respiratory depression should be anticipated and the infant ventilated if necessary. The reader is referred elsewhere for a full description of the management of birth asphyxia.(7)

DISORDERS OF GLUCOSE METABOLISM

Hypoglycaemia

The association between hypoglycaemia and IUGR was first reported by Cornblath *et al.* in 1959(8) in eight small-for-gestational-age infants who developed symptomatic hypoglycaemia between 40 and 57 h after birth. The overall incidence of hypoglycaemia in SGA infants has been reported as up to 40% of premature SGA infants, compared to an incidence of only 3% in premature infants whose growth was appropriate for gestational age.

Those infants most at risk of hypoglycaemia appear to be the ones who have asymmetrical growth retardation and a low PI. In a prospective study, 23 out of 62 asymmetrically growth retarded infants had hypoglycaemia within 12 h of birth compared to only 8% of proportionately growth retarded infants. The loss of subcutaneous fat suggests rapid and possibly acute starvation with the depletion of glycogen stores. The lack of glycogen reserve is the cause of the predisposition to neonatal hypoglycaemia. In infants who have suffered IUGR the glycogen content per gram of tissue is the same as normally grown infants, but the total glycogen content has been reported to be substantially lower in SGA infants.(10)

There is some evidence that severe growth retardation may be associated with hyperinsulinaemia, (11,12) but this is likely to be clinically a considerably less important cause of the hypoglycaemia than low glycogen stores.

A distinction must be made between symptomatic hypoglycaemia (known to carry a bad prognosis) and asymptomatic hypoglycaemia which appears to be a benign condition. All growth retarded infants should be carefully monitored for hypoglycaemia and treated in an appropriate manner to avoid symptomatic hypoglycaemia. In a recent paper Jones and Roberton(4) reported that only 9% of growth retarded infants (<5th centile) developed hypoglycaemia and all but one were asymptomatic. The other was jittery and did not develop convulsions. Modern neonatal management should prevent hypoglycaemia as a cause of neurodevelopmental handicap.

Hyperglycaemia

Rarely the severely SGA infant may develop a transient form of diabetes mellitus. This is probably due to failure of the pancreas to produce adequate amounts of insulin. The infant presents with hyperglycaemia, glycosuria and polyuria. Ketonuria is not a feature, but the infant may rapidly develop severe dehydration.

The treatment is to use regular doses of subcutaneous soluble insulin together with appropriate rehydration. Insulin therapy is only necessary for 3–6 months as the islet cells recover normal function. Some infants have been successfully treated with chlorpropamide. There is often rapid catch up growth when insulin is started.

RESPIRATORY DISEASE

It has been recognised for many years that growth retarded infants have a lower risk of respiratory distress syndrome (RDS) than normally grown infants. This is probably related to the stress of placental insufficiency with release of corticosteroids from the maternal or fetal adrenal. In a retrospective study with matched controls the incidence of RDS in a group of premature SGA infants was 5% compared with an incidence of 74% for a matched group of appropriately grown infants. The reduced risk of RDS in SGA premature infants also makes many other neonatal complications less likely.

There are however a number of respiratory conditions which do occur more frequently in growth retarded infants.

Meconium aspiration

A common feature of full-term delivery is passage of meconium by the fetus. This is often associated with fetal distress but appears to be relatively non-specific. If intrapartum asphyxia is severe the fetus will start to gasp, and if thick meconium is present in the liquor then this may be aspirated deep into the bronchial tree. Some babies who have aspirated meconium then develop the meconium aspiration syndrome. This condition is characterised by severe shunting due to pulmonary hypertension. The babies are cyanosed and usually have severe respiratory distress. Pneumothorax is a common complication in this condition. The chest X-ray characteristically shows irregular opacities. Meconium aspiration has been reported in up to 18% of SGA infants.

The management is directed towards respiratory support which includes supplemental oxygen, mechanical ventilation at relatively high rates and tolazoline for pulmonary hypertension. The prognosis is usually good although these infants may develop very severe lung disease.

Recently it has been suggested that meconium aspiration syndrome has, in fact, little to do with meconium in the airways. Chronic fetal hypoxia leads to hypertrophy of the muscularis layer of the pulmonary arterioles with subsequent severe pulmonary hypertension.[(13)] It is this that is the important factor in the morbidity associated with this condition and not the meconium aspiration. This is probably the cause in a proportion of these children but it is also likely that meconium aspirated deep into the lungs causes an irritant pneumonitis with similar clinical features and a typical radiological appearance.

The prevention of meconium aspiration is by means of adequate suction of the oropharynx when the head is delivered. If there is thick meconium in the mouth, then intubation should be attempted and any meconium sucked out under direct vision. If meconium is found below the cords then the baby should be admitted to the neonatal unit for observation. There is no evidence that steroids are helpful in the management of this condition.

Pulmonary haemorrhage

This condition is well recognised in severely growth retarded infants. In the 1958 survey of British births, massive pulmonary haemorrhage accounted for 46 of the 852 first-week deaths (6%) and was the third commonest cause of death in SGA infants.[(14)] In Australia the incidence of this condition is reported to be 8 per 1000 SGA infants and was thought to be the second commonest cause of death in growth retarded infants.[(15)] They reported a 93% mortality for massive pulmonary haemorrhage.

The condition usually develops on the second or third day in a previously well infant. In many infants irritability had been noted immediately before the haemorrhage and it was associated with convulsions in some cases.

It is the impression of most neonatologists that this condition has become much less common in recent years. This is probably due to improved standards of both obstetric and neonatal care. It is now a very rare cause of death in premature infants. It has been suggested that continuous positive airway pressure (CPAP) is the best method for treating established haemorrhage.

POLYCYTHAEMIA

This is another well recognised complication of intrauterine growth retardation. Chronic fetal hypoxia due to placental insufficiency appears to be the stimulus for erythropoietin production providing the stimulus for the manufacture of an increased number of red blood cells.

There is no generally agreed definition as to what is polycythaemia but a haematocrit above 65% is widely accepted. The incidence of polycythaemia in SGA babies ranges between 12–50%. There is a loose association between high haematocrit and hyperviscosity and it is this latter condition that is mostly associated with complications. An 18% incidence of hyperviscosity has been reported in a group of SGA infants and a venous haematocrit of 64% was predictive for this condition.[(16)] Twice as many infants in the hyperviscosity group developed symptoms than in the group of SGA infants without this condition. Reduced blood flow due to increased viscosity causes sludging of blood in the arteriolar bed of the brain and bowel which may cause thrombosis. Unfortunately there is no clinical method available to measure blood viscosity.

The clinical features of polycythaemia are plethora, breathlessness, irritability and possibly abdominal distension. If cerebral thrombosis occurs frank convulsions may develop. Necrotising enterocolitis may also develop as the result of polycythaemia.

The management of hyperviscosity is dilutional exchange transfusion. This is recommended in all infants with PCV above 70% and those who are symptomatic with PCV above 65%. A total of 20 ml of plasma per kg should be exchanged for a similar volume of the infant's blood by a procedure similar to exchange transfusion.

CEREBRAL COMPROMISE

The brains of SGA infants have been assessed to investigate whether IUGR has any effect on cerebral function. It is known that SGA infants are more likely to have an abnormal electroencephalogram (EEG) compared with appropriately grown infants. Schulte *et al.*[(17)] compared EEG findings in a group of SGA infants of toxaemic mothers with a group of well grown babies of similar gestational age. The SGA babies had significantly more immature EEG patterns both in active and quiet sleep than their controls. Some infants had definitely abnormal traces for their age which were not due to either asphyxia or hypoglycaemia.

It is of interest that some studies have suggested that IUGR may actually cause accelerated brain maturation. The conduction time of an electrical impulse can be timed through the brain by neurophysiological techniques. The central conduction time from an auditory stimulus reaching the cochlea to the cortex was found to be significantly increased in both preterm SGA[(18)] and full-term growth retarded infants. The cause of this apparent maturation is not known. In a study of immature rats who had suffered experimental intrauterine growth retardation there was depression in the cerebral myelination but no delay in its development.[(20)] The effect of IUGR on the brain does not appear to affect the peripheral nervous system.

Intraventricular haemorrhage

It has been suggested that SGA infants are more at risk of intraventricular haemorrhage (IVH) than infants of normal birthweight[21] but this data was based on autopsy results which do not reflect the full spectrum of disease. Others have suggested that IVH is less common in SGA infants[22] based on a retrospective study with matched controls. The incidence of IVH was 42% in the appropriate-for-gestational-age (AGA) group and 11% in the SGA group.

More recent reports using real-time ultrasound imaging of the brain have failed to find any association between either IVH or periventricular leucomalacia and growth retarded infants. It is reasonable to believe that despite the apparent advanced maturity of the growth retarded infant's brain, this has no measurable effect on the incidence of recognizable pathology occuring in the newborn period. The risk of long-term developmental or neurological sequelae is however increased in some growth retarded infants and this is discussed in the next chapter.

METABOLIC DISORDERS

A variety of metabolic disorders have been reported to occur with increased frequency in growth retarded infants.

Disorders of fluid balance

SGA infants have an elevated plasma volume at birth compared to normally grown babies as well as an expanded extracellular compartment.[23] This appears to be most marked in those infants with severe retardation in their linear measurements. These infants may show peripheral oedema. Despite the increased volume of fluid within SGA babies they actually conserve their fluid better than similarly grown but non-growth retarded infants. This is because their renal function is better able to conserve water and sodium, and their skin is less permeable to transepidermal water loss than infants of the same birthweight but who were AGA. Growth retarded infants require considerably less fluid than AGA infants in the first few days after birth.

Calcium metabolism

Plasma venous calcium is significantly lower and phosphorous levels higher in SGA infants compared with those who are AGA.[24] Cockburn suggested that convulsions were more likely in the growth retarded group due to the hypocalcaemia. These days hypocalcaemic fits are extremely rare and probably benign and this is unlikely to cause significant morbidity.

The bone mineral content of full-term SGA babies has been shown to be significantly less than infants who were born of appropriate birthweight.[25] This may be related to retarded height and bone age seen in older children who had been born growth retarded.

Heat loss

SGA infants have a large surface area to body weight ratio and are therefore more likely to lose heat through their skin. Jones and Roberton[4] found that 23% of SGA infants had a temperature below 36°C, but this figure rose to 35% of infants born below the 2.3rd centile. Only 4% of babies were actually hypothermic with a body temperature below 35°C.

Hypothermia is theoretically a problem in this group but in modern perinatal units no baby should be allowed to become cold, and careful attention must be paid to ways of avoiding cold stress.

INFECTION

The growth retarded infant appears to be more at risk of infection than infants who are AGA. This is related to a number of immunological problems. SGA infants have consistently low levels of immunoglobulins, particularly IgG.[26] This is probably related to impaired transplacental passage due to placental insufficiency. There was little evidence that the IgG levels improve in the first 5 months after birth and these infants appear to be more likely to develop bacterial infections.

These infants also show impairment of humoral immunity. The levels of circulating T-lymphocytes are reduced, but there is no reduction in B-cells. In addition opsonisation, chemotactic activity, bactericidal and phagocytic cellular activity have all been shown to be reduced.[27,28] The abnormality in T-lymphocytes is probably related to the severe thymic hypoplasia that occurs in severely growth retarded infants. There is evidence that the lymphocyte abnormality persists in later life.

Prevention of infection in growth retarded infants is therefore important. This is best achieved by the avoidance of cross-infection particularly in hospital. Scrupulous hand washing is essential and the parents should be advised to avoid their child coming in contact with other children with respiratory tract infections.

REFERENCES

1. Miller HC, Hassanein I. Diagnosis of impaired fetal growth in newborn infants. *Pediatrics* 1971; **48**:511-522.
2. Oakley JR, Parsons RJ, Whitelaw AGL. Standards for skinfold thickness in British newborn infants. *Arch Dis Child* 1977; **52**:287-290.
3. Heinonen K, Matilainen R, Koski H, Launiala K. Intrauterine growth retardation (IUGR) in pre-term infants. *J Perinat Med* 1985; **13**:171-178.
4. Jones RAK, Roberton NRC. Small for dates babies: are they really a problem? *Arch Dis Child* 1986; **61**:877-880.
5. Levene MI, Kornberg J, Williams THC. The incidence and severity of post-asphyxial encephalopathy in full-term infants. *Early Hum Dev* 1985; **11**:21-26.
6. MacDonald HM, Mulligan JC, Allen AC, Taylor PM. Neonatal asphyxia. I. Relationship of obstetric and neonatal complications to neonatal mortality in 38 405 consecutive deliveries. *J Pediatr* 1980; **96**:898-902.
7. Levene MI. Management and outcome of birth asphyxia. In: *Fetal and Neonatal Neurology and Neurosurgery*. Eds. MI Levene, MJ Bennett, J Punt.

Edinburgh: Churchill Livingstone, 1987: pp. 383-392.
8. Cornblath M, Odell CB, Levin EY. Symptomatic neonatal hypoglycaemia associated with toxaemia of pregnancy. *J Pediatr* 1959; **55**:545-562.
9. Járai I, Mestyán J, Schultz, Lázár A, Halász M, Krassy I. Body size and neonatal hypoglycaemia in intrauterine growth retardation. *Early Hum Dev* 1977; **1**:25-38.
10. Pribylová H, Rázová M, Vondrácek J. Glycogen content in subcutaneous adipose tissue of newborns of different birthweights in the first week of life. *Biol Neonate* 1980; **38**:154-160.
11. Collins JE, Leonard JV. Hyperinsulinism in asphyxiated and small-for-dates infants with hypoglycaemia. *Lancet* 1984; **ii**:311-313.
12. Pildes AS, Patel DA, Nitzan M. Glucose disappearance rate in symptomatic neonatal hypoglycemia. *Pediatrics* 1973; **42**:75-82.
13. David R. Neonatal resuscitation: historical perspective and current practice. In: *Clinics in Critical Care Medicine. Neonatal Intensive Care.* Ed. RD Guthrie. New York: Churchill Livingstone, 1988: pp.1-20.
14. Butler NR, Alberman ED (Eds). *Perinatal Problems.* Edinburgh: Churchill Livingstone, 1969 .
15. Sly PD, Drew JH. Massive pulmonary haemorrhage: a cause of sudden unexpected deaths in severely growth retarded infants. *Aust Paediatr J* 1981; **17**:32-34.
16. Hakanson DO, Oh W. Hyperviscosity in the small-for-gestational-age infant. *Biol Neonate* 1980; **37**:109-112.
17. Schulte FJ, Hinze G, Schrempf G. Maternal toxaemia, fetal malnutrition and bioelectric brain activity in the newborn. *Neuropaediatrie* 1971; **2**:439-460 .
18. Kesson AM, Henderson-Smart DJ, Pettigrew AG, Edwards DA. Peripheral nerve conduction velocity and brainstem auditory evoked responses in small for gestational age preterm infants. *Early Hum Dev* 1985; **11**:213 - 219 .
19. Todorovich RD, Crowell DH, Kapuniai LE. Auditory responsivity and intrauterine growth retardation in small for gestational age human newborns. *Electroencephalogr Clin Neurophysiol* 1987; **67**:204-212 .
20. Bourré JM, Morand O, Chanez C, Dumont O, Flexor MA. Influence of intrauterine malnutrition on brain development: alteration of myelination. *Biol Neonate* 1981; **39**: 96-99 .
21. Harcke HT, Naeye RL, Storch A, Blanc WA. Perinatal cerebral intraventricular hemorrhage. *J Pediatr* 1972; **80**:37-42.
22. Procianoy RS, Garcia-Prats JA, Adams JM, Silvers A, Rudolph AJ. Hyaline membrane disease and intraventricular hemorrhage in small for gestational age infants. *Arch Dis Child* 1980; **55**:502-505.
23. Cassady G. Body composition in intrauterine growth retardation. *Ped Clin N Amer* 1970; **17**:79-99.
24. Cockburn F. Some biochemical aspects of intrauterine growth retardation. *Arch Dis Child* 1969; **44**:136.
25. Minton SD, Steichen JJ, Tsang RC. Decreased bone mineral content in small-for-gestational-age infants compared with appropriate-for-gestational-age

infants: normal serum 25-hydroxyvitamin D and decreasing parathyroid hormone. *Pediatrics* 1983; **71**:383-388.
26. Chandra RK. Fetal malnutrition and postnatal immunocompetence. *Am J Dis Child* 1975; **93**: 450-454.
27. Ferguson AC. Prolonged impairment of cellular immunity in children with intrauterine growth retardation. *J Pediatr* 1978; **93**:52-56.
28. Xanthou M. Immunologic deficiencies in small-for-dates neonates. *Acta Paediatr Scand*, Suppl. 1985; **319**:143-149.

Fetal growth: mortality and morbidity

Dr A. Stewart

Mortality and morbidity together have been accepted for many years as the correct outcomes to measure perinatal events and interventions. It is generally believed that factors which affect one will affect the other, and ideally, any effect will be in the same direction.

Birthweight was recognised as the main determinant of neonatal mortality as long ago as 1950. All reported statistics indicate that it remains an important determinant with very low birthweight (VLBW, <1500 g) now accounting for almost half of all neonatal deaths in England and Wales. The contribution of VLBW to childhood morbidity is less clear. Attempts to estimate this have led some to conclude that it is not large[1,2] but there continues to be debate about whether the contribution may be changing as mortality rates fall.

Inspection of the published data on mortality and morbidity in VLBW infants indicates that the relation of VLBW with these two variables may have differed over time. For example, neonatal mortality in VLBW has fallen consistently since the 1960s[3,4] and there has been a similar reduction in mortality among the smallest infants who weigh less than 1000 g, the extremely low birthweight (ELBW) infants.[2-4] By contrast, although morbidity fell initially in VLBW infants,[3,4] there has been little change in published values of the prevalence of serious neurodevelopmental impairments for over 15 years.[3-5] Virtually no change has been reported in the prevalence among ELBW since the earliest report of the outcome of these infants was made in 1972[6] and, calculated as a proportion of the total live births, the prevalence in the ELBW infants is only little greater than that in the VLBW group as a whole.[3] Thus it appears that the relation of birthweight to mortality and morbidity may not be quite as simple as is sometimes assumed.

More than 15 years ago, Lubchenco[7] drew attention to the importance of considering birthweight and gestation together when examining mortality data. Philip *et al.* [8] again emphasised the point when they published figures for mortality for the 1980s, as did Dehan *et al.*[9] when reporting a large study of births in the Paris region in 1985. Nevertheless, there is very little published information on the relation of gestation itself with mortality and/or morbidity. It is often assumed that it has the same effect as birthweight and there is a tendency to make decisions using this assumption because gestation may now be measured more accurately than fetal weight (and hence birthweight), particularly when early ultrasound estimations are available. Here, on the basis of reports published since 1980, the relation of both birthweight and gestation with mortality and morbidity are examined to discover if this assumption is justified. The data are also examined in order to try to understand the principal determinants of outcome when birthweight and gestation are discrepant.

OUTCOME MEASURES

For the purposes of this discussion only two mortality measures will be considered. These are *neonatal mortality*, which includes all deaths of liveborn infants in the first 28 days of life and *total mortality* which refers to neonatal mortality plus deaths up to the end of the first year of life. This category also includes deaths up to discharge from hospital.

Morbidity as an indication of an adverse outcome in survivors is much less clearly or consistently defined in published data. As well as "local" terminology, it depends on several factors including the age of the children and the type of assessment used as the basis for categorising the children into those with a normal or abnormal outcome. The results in the majority of studies are based on the assessment of young children and only consider serious neurodevelopmental impairments causing functional disability ("major" impairments). These neurodevelopmental impairments usually include cerebral movement disorders (often called cerebral palsy), hearing loss, blindness and overall developmental delay (developmental quotient, DQ, < 80) or cognitive defects (intelligence quotient IQ, > 2 standard deviations below the mean for the test). In a few reports, only selected morbidities are considered as, for example, cerebral palsy with or without cognitive deficits. Morbidities of this kind however, require very precise definition, and this is rarely provided. A few reports consider a much wider definition of adverse outcome and include impairments that cause little if any disability at the age of assessment. These less serious ("minor") impairments are rarely well defined. It is often difficult to know exactly what is meant or on what basis they have been identified. For this reason comparison between studies is probably not justified. Trends from individual studies, however, may be meaningful and need to be noted.

The importance of the age of assessment cannot be over-emphasised. In young children under the age of about four years, cognitive defects and those of fine and higher motor skills and of coordination cannot be recognised. Only very crude associations exist between, for example, results of developmental assessment at one year and the level of cognitive functioning or the presence of visuo-motor defects at four years.[10] Thus caution must be exercised in the interpretation of results and, of course, only studies concerning children assessed at similar ages can be compared or their data pooled.

BIRTHWEIGHT

Mortality

All reports published since the 1950s indicate that mortality increases as birthweight decreases and the relation is more or less linear. This applies to all definitions of mortality and to whatever birthweight decrements are chosen. Data are available from national statistics, for example those provided for England and Wales by the Office for Census and Population Studies (OCPS) and from individual population-based studies,[8,11,12] including studies confined to ELBW infants.[13] Data from Saigal *et al.*[13] are shown in Table 1, according to each 100 g from 501 to 1000 g.

Table 1. Mortality among infants weighing < 1000 g at birth (Saigal *et al*).[13]

Birthweight (g)	(n)	Mortality (%)
1000–901	63	29
900–801	50	38
800–701	49	51
700–601	52	69
600–501	41	98

Morbidity

In a recent large population study of infants weighing < 2001 g,[12] outcome judged by the presence of serious, disabling impairments in the pre-school period worsened as birthweight decreased by 500 g decrements. This was true of the total impairments detected and of individual diagnoses. The values for the prevalence of major impairments in individual weight groups correspond closely with the values reported in other studies where only selected weight groups were studied, and ranged from 4.5% in infants weighing 1501–2000 g, through 11% for infants weighing 1001–1500 g, to 15% for those weighing 501–1000 g. Another population study concentrated on infants weighing ≤ 1000 g.[13] Although the overall prevalence of major neurodevelopmental impairment was comparable to that found in infants who weighed < 1001 g in other studies, there was no increase in the prevalence as birthweight decreased in 100 g decrements (Table 2). A similar effect was noted in a referral centre study from Melbourne [14] where the outcome for infants weighing 501–750 g was the same as that for infants weighing 751–1000 g (Table 2). Experience in a London specialist referral centre (University College Hospital) was identical, and the results are also shown in Table 2, although it must be emphasised that these figures were not obtained from a population-based study. Thus in contrast to mortality, there appears to be an important change in outcome as judged by major morbidity at 1000 g, but thereafter there is no further worsening of neurodevelopmental outcome with reduction of birthweight down to the lowest currently compatible with survival.

There are a few studies which report the outcome of VLBW infants at school age. These have recently been reviewed by Fawer and Calame.[5] In general, the prevalence of major impairments is similar to that reported at younger ages and the overall level of cognitive functioning measured by IQ is within normal limits.This is also reported in ELBW infants although there tends to be a very wide range of IQ scores found among these tiniest infants. In spite however, of an apparently normal potential an excess of VLBW children appear to fail in school.[15] This finding has been variously attributed to "developmental disorders" which include visuomotor abnormalities and problems of fine motor skills, language delay, learning

Table 2. Morbidity among infants weighing < 1000 g (McMaster)[13] (Melbourne),[19] (University College Hospital, unpublished)

Birthweight (g)	Major impairment (%)		
	McMaster	Melbourne	UCH
1000–901	17	–	–
900–801	9	–	–
800–701	14	25*	13*
700–601	10	–	–
600–501	0	27+	17+

* 1000–751 g
\+ 750–501 g

disabilities and socio-economic deprivation. Fawer and Calame have suggested that school failure occurs when two or more of these disorders are present in the same child regardless of the overall IQ.[5] Insufficient school-age children have been studied since the introduction of modern perinatal care to be certain of the extent of school failure or to know if the risk increases as birthweight decreases among the smallest infants.

GESTATION

Mortality

There are relatively few studies of the effect of gestation on mortality, presumably because of the difficulty of making accurate assessments of length of gestation. As expected, the available data indicates that mortality increases as gestation decreases.[8, 12] However, there appear to be large changes at ~33 weeks and again at ~27 weeks. The numbers reported with gestation below 26 weeks are very small [16,17] and the data need very cautious interpretation. Table 3 gives examples from two studies, including one based on a whole population, and the experience of a regional referral centre, University College Hospital, London.

Morbidity

There are even fewer published reports of the relation of gestation to morbidity. Two studies consider only infants born before 29 weeks.[16, 17] The results are based on assessment of children aged 2 years or less; both indicate that outcome, as judged by major impairments, worsens at or about 26–27 weeks of gestation and then remains constant (Table 4). This is also the experience at University College Hospital, London (Table 4), but the numbers in these studies are so small that no firm conclusion can be drawn.

Table 3. Mortality among infants born before 29 weeks of gestation (Melbourne)(16) (Dundee)(17) (University College Hospital, unpublished).

Gestation (w)	Mortality (%)		
	Melbourne	Dundee	UCH
28	25	38	36
27	24	–	36
26	40	58*	45
25	74	–	61
24	66	–	69
23	93	89+	100

* 1000–751 g
+ 750–501 g

Table 4. Major neurodevelopmental impairments among infants born before 29 weeks of gestation (Melbourne)(16) (Dundee)(17) (University College Hospital, unpublished)

Gestation (w)	Major impairment (%)		
	Melbourne	Dundee	UCH
28	7	39	9
27	9	–	6
26	20	20 *	6
25	27	–	19
24	8	–	20
23	50	0 +	–

* 1000–751 g
+ 750–501 g

At University College Hospital, London we have been following up a cohort of infants born before 33 weeks since 1979. These infants have been enrolled for study because they had ultrasound brain imaging in the neonatal period and we wished to investigate the relation of lesions identified in this way with long term outcome.[18] Within this cohort the prevalence of major impairments was 8% for the whole group and ranged between 6 and 8% for infants born between 32 and 26 weeks (Table 4). The prevalence appeared to increase to about 20% in infants born at 25–24 weeks but the numbers are too small to interpret. The oldest members of our cohort have been re-examined at four and eight years. At four years, the prevalence of major impairments had increased to 15% for the group as a whole, largely because of deficits of cognitive functioning that could not be detected when the children were younger.[19] At four years 15% also had minor impairments. Almost half of these minor impairments were due to deficits of cognitive functioning.[10] Gestation did not appear to affect the prevalence of either major or minor impairments in the cohort.[19] The prevalence of major impairments was unchanged when the cohort was examined at eight years [20] and the mean IQ (WISC R) was 103 ± 16. Detailed analysis of the results of cognitive testing, however, suggests that there may be subtle problems of cognitive processing that may lead to difficulties with learning and interfere with children's abilities to achieve their full potential, as measured by overall IQ .[20]

WHERE BIRTHWEIGHT DOES NOT CORRESPOND WITH GESTATION.

There are many causes of discrepancy between birthweight and gestation and several different definitions, and there is agreement that such infants form a heterogenous group. Infants whose weight is believed to be inadequate for their period of gestation, defined either according to birthweight centile (below the 10th or even the 3rd) or standard deviation (more than 2 SD below the mean) cause the most concern. They may be referred to as having intrauterine growth retardation or being small for gestational age (SGA). In this discussion they will be referred to as SGA as this does not imply cause. When considering mortality and morbidity several workers have emphasised the importance of excluding infants with lethal congenital malformations.[8, 16] Also, it is likely that the proportion of multiple births will affect these variables, but this is rarely specified.

Mortality

In studies where mortality data are given both according to birthweight and gestation,[8, 12] when birthweight is relatively low, mortality appears to be in accordance with birthweight and not gestation. In studies where comparison is made between infants whose weight is appropriate for the period of gestation (AGA) and SGA infants,[21,22] SGA mortality is either equal to or greater than the mortality of AGA infants of equivalent weight. Infants born at or near term appear particularly disadvantaged. Thus it appears that the factors which determine the relatively low birthweight also determine the mortality and outweigh any possible advantages of a greater maturity.

Morbidity

Where cause is known, as for example in children with a chromosomal defect, the prognosis depends on this diagnosis. For the remainder interpretation of the available data is very difficult. Results of studies appear to differ widely, presumably depending on the distribution of cause within the study group, and even some of the most recent reports concern infants born ten or more years ago,[5] when facilities for early diagnosis were not generally available and attitudes to the care of the SGA infant still tended to be pessimistic. In the most recent report available,[23] outcome at one to two years in SGA infants diagnosed on the basis of several different ultrasound measurements appeared to be directly related to period of gestation and Fawer and Calame came to this same conclusion from their review of the literature,[5] namely that morbidity in SGA infants is determined largely by gestation. The only exceptions appear to be those infants whose birthweight is so profoundly discrepant of gestation that it falls below the 2.3rd centile. These infants appear to have an exceptionally poor prognosis with an excess of serious neuromotor impairments and of deficits of cognitive functioning.[24–26] Fawer and Calame point out that although the overall outcome of SGA infants may be similar to their AGA peers of comparable gestation, the type of impairments detected as they grow older tend to differ.[5,26] For example SGA infants born at term may have an increased risk of minor learning difficulties and school failure, whereas the risk of these problems in pre-term SGA infants is not as great as that of their AGA peers. In a group of SGA infants, Harvey *et al.* [27] found there was good correspondence between performance on cognitive testing at four to five years of age and the duration of slow intrauterine head growth but not birthweight centile.

PREDICTION OF OUTCOME

Mortality and morbidity data are needed for predictive purposes as well as evaluation. From the studies reviewed here it is clear that estimates for risk of mortality and neurodevelopmental morbidity can be made on the basis of both birthweight and gestation. It seems reasonable to use estimates of this kind when making perinatal management decisions, provided it is recognised that they are fairly crude. Attempts to improve prediction by using objective measures such as Doppler ultrasound assessments of blood flow velocity in uterine or fetal vessels, as described elsewhere in this volume, should be welcomed. Before being introduced for general use, these measurements require careful validation by examining their relation with the condition of the surviving infant in the first days of life as well as the intermediate and long term outcomes. Mortality alone is not an adequate outcome for this purpose.

The choice of appropriate outcome measures to evaluate these perinatal investigations — and any subsequent interventions that may be planned — is extremely important.[28] In practical terms there is either the crude approach of a "head count" of infants who do not have disabling impairments and who can be expected to function as satisfactory citizens, which can be made between one and two years; or detailed assessments of all aspects of functioning including those of cognition, which cannot be made until the children are over four years of age. It is only from the more detailed approach that we can answer the question of whether a particular intervention has *any* effect. There is a third option. By considering a "package" which includes early objective measures of brain structure and function and neurological measures it may be possible to predict longer term outcome in fairly considerable detail.[28] There are already data which suggest that this may be feasible. For example, among very preterm infants ultrasound brain scan findings obtained at discharge from hospital and neurological examination at the age equivalent to term together predict normal neurodevelopmental progress with a probability of 98%.[29] Neurodevelopmental status assigned at age one year on the basis of neuromotor, neurosensory and developmental assessment in the same group of infants predicts very accurately neuromotor and neurosensory status at four and at eight years.[10,20] Neurodevelopmental status at one year also predicts children who are at risk of cognitive deficits and of problems of fine and higher motor skills at four years.[10] There is much more information needed before it is reasonable to apply these predictive principles to the evaluation of perinatal events, fetal investigations or interventions, but this information is likely to be obtained if selected long term studies can be carried out.

CONCLUSIONS

Neonatal mortality and deaths during the first few months of life appear to be directly related to both birthweight and gestation; the smaller or less mature the infant, the higher the mortality. Although neurodevelopmental outcome in survivors also worsens as birthweight or gestation decrease, this relationship does not appear to hold at the lower end of either distribution. Thus there is no worsening in long term prognosis as birthweight decreases below 1000 g or gestation shortens below 26 weeks. Data are very limited and those that are available may be subject to many selection biases, but until better information becomes available it must not be assumed that the smaller or less mature the infant, the worse the long term outlook for the survivors. In SGA infants in whom there is no clear reason why their birthweight is less than the tenth centile for gestation, in very general terms, mortality depends on birthweight and long term outcome in survivors is related to gestation. This relationship holds both for the prevalence and the type of impairments which are diagnosed as the children grow older. Thus, both birthweight and gestation must be considered when evaluating perinatal events, fetal investigations and interventions. Of equal importance is the need for precisely defined outcome measures when investigating these factors. Those currently available range from crude "head counts" of young children with or without major impairments to the results of detailed assessments of all aspects of functioning which can only be carried out in older children. Alternatively, it may be possible to predict long term outcome on the basis of objective measures of brain structure and function made in the early days of life in association with neurological assessments made throughout the first year of life. Preliminary results suggest that this approach may be feasible.

ACKNOWLEDGEMENTS

This work was supported by The Medical Research Council.

REFERENCES

1. Alberman E. The epidemiology of congenital defects: a pragmatic approach. In: *Paediatric Research: a Genetic Approach*. Eds. M Adinolfi, P Benson, F Giannelli, M Seller. London: Heinemann, 1982: pp.1–12.
2. Stewart A. The baby under 1000g: outcome. In: *The Baby Under 1000g*. Eds. D Harvey, RWI Cooke, G Levitt. Potters Bar: John Wright, 1988; In press.
3. Stewart A, Reynolds EOR, Lipscomb AP. Outcome for infants of very low birthweight: survey of world literature. *Lancet* 1981; **i**:1038–1041.
4. McCormick MC. The contribution of low birth weight to infant mortality and childhood morbidity. *N Engl J Med* 1985; **312**: 82–90.
5. Fawer C–L, Calame A. Assessment of neurodevelopmental outcome. In: *Fetal and Neonatal Neurology and Neurosurgery*. Eds. MI Levene, MJ Bennett, J Punt. Edinburgh: Churchill Livingstone, 1988: pp. 71–88.
6. Alden ER, Mandelkorn T, Woodrum DE, Wennberg RP, Parks CR, Hodson WA. Morbidity and mortality of infants weighing less than 1000 g in an intensive care nursery. *Pediatrics* 1972; **50**: 40–49.
7. Lubchenco LO. *The High Risk Infant*. Philadelphia: WB Saunders, 1976.
8. Philip AGS, Little GA, Polivy DR, Lucey JF. Neonatal mortality risk for the eighties: the importance of birth weight/gestational age groups. *Pediatrics* 1981; **68**: 122–130.
9. Dehan M, Goujard J, Vodovar M, Crost M, Gautier JP, Benisvy C, Rougeot C, Plissier M, Voyer M. Enquête sur les prématurés de moins de 33 semaines d'âge gestationnel nés en 1985 dans la région parisienne: mortalité, devenir à 1 et 2 ans. In: *Société Française de Médecine Périnatale: dix-huitièmes journées nationales* (proceedings), 1988: pp.151–159.
10. Stewart AL, Costello AM, Hamilton PA, Baudin J, Townsend J, Bradford BC, Reynolds EOR. Relation between neurodevelopmental status at one and four years in very preterm infants, *Dev Med Child Neurol* 1989; In press.
11. Pharoah POD, Alberman ED. Mortality of low birthweight infants in England and Wales 1953 to 1979. *Arch Dis Child* 1981; **56**: 86–89.
12. Powell TG, Pharoah POD, Cooke RWI. Survival and morbidity in a geographically defined population of low birthweight infants. *Lancet* 1986; **i**: 539–543.
13. Saigal S, Rosenbaum P, Stoskopf B, Sinclair JC. Outcome in infants 501 to 1000 gm birth weight delivered to residents of the McMaster Health Region. *J Pediatr* 1984; **105**: 969–976.
14. Orgill AA, Astbury J, Bajuk B, Yu VY. Early development of infants 1000 g or less at birth. *Arch Dis Child* 1982; **57**: 823–827.
15. Klein N, Hack M, Gallagher J, Fanaroff AA. Pre school performance of children with normal intelligence who were very low-birth-weight infants. *Pediatrics* 1985; **75**: 531–537.
16. Yu VYH, Loke HL, Bajuk B, Szymonowicz W, Orgill AA, Astbury J. Prognosis for infants born at 23 to 28 weeks' gestation. *Br Med J* 1986; **293**: 1200–1203.
17. Walker EM, Patel NB. Mortality and morbidity in infants born between 20 and 28 weeks gestation. *Br J Obstet Gyaecol* 1987; **94**: 670–674.

18. Stewart AL, Reynolds EO, Hope PL, Hamilton PA, Baudin J, Costello AM, Bradford BC, Wyatt JS. Probability of neurodevelopmental disorders estimated from ultrasound appearance of brains of very preterm infants. *Dev Med Child Neurol* 1987; **29**: 3–11.
19. Costello AM, Hamilton PA, Baudin J, Townsend J, Bradford BC, Stewart AL, Reynolds EO. Prediction of neurodevelopmental impairment at four years from brain ultrasound appearance of very preterm infants. *Dev Med Child Neurol* 1988; **30**: 711–722.
20. Baudin J, Lloyd B, Edwards D, Townsend J, Stewart A, Reynolds EO. Abnormal cognitive and processing skills in very preterm infants at 8 years of age. *Pediatr Res* 1988; **24**: 267 (abstract).
21. Starfield B, Shapiro S, McCormick M, Bross D. Mortality and morbidity in infants with intrauterine growth retardation. *J Pediatr* 1982; **101**: 978–983.
22. Teberg AJ, Walther FJ, Pena IC. Mortality, morbidity, and outcome of the small-for-gestational age infant. *Sem Perinatol* 1988; **12**: 84–94.
23. Amiel-Tison C, Llado J, Bréart G, Tchobroutsky C. Le prognostic vital et neuro-psychique évalué avant la naissance sur les caractéristiques du retard de croissance intra-utérin. In: *Société Française de Médicine Périnatale: dix-huitièmes journées nationales* (proceedings), 1988; pp.100–107.
24. Jurgens-van der Zee AD, Bierman-van Eedenburg MEC, Fidler VJ, Olinga AA, Visch JH, Touwen BC, Huisjes HJ. Preterm birth, growth retardation and acidemia in relation to neurological abnormality of the newborn. *Early Hum Dev* 1979; **3**: 141–154.
25. Huisjes HJ. Intrauterine growth retardation: a question of definition. In: *Aspects of Perinatal Morbidity*. Ed. HJ Huisjes. Groningen: Universitaire Boekhandel Nederland B.V., 1981; pp.54–60.
26. Rantakillio P. A 14-year follow-up of children with normal and abnormal birth weight for their gestational age. A population study. *Acta Paediatr Scand* 1985; **74**: 62–69.
27. Harvey D, Prince J, Bunton J, Parkinson C, Campbell S. Abilities of children who were small-for-gestational-age babies. *Pediatrics* 1982; **69**: 296–300.
28. Stewart AL. Prediction of long-term outcome in high-risk infants: the use of objective measures of brain structure and function in the neonatal intensive care unit. In: *Baillière's Clinical Obstetrics and Gyaecology: Antenatal and Perinatal Causes of Handicap.* Vol 2. Ed: N Patel. London: Baillière Tindall, 1988; pp.221–236.
29. Stewart AL, Hope PL, Hamilton PA, Costello AM, Baudin J, Bradford BC, Amiel-Tison C, Reynolds EO. Prediction in very preterm infants of satisfactory neurodevelopmental progress at 12 months. *Dev Med Child Neurol* 1988; **30**: 53–63.

Discussion

Chairman: Professor P.W. Howie

HAN: As a paediatrician I think that we are still confusing ourselves like the obstetricians. I would like to highlight what Professor Levene and Dr Stewart have just said. I think that we are talking about two different disease entities. Professor Levene has talked about an SGA infant which is near term or at term, and Dr Stewart has told us what has happened with premature babies, low birthweight babies. We have to define what we are going to talk about. Are we talking about SGA, or are we talking about premature babies, or are we talking about a combination of the two of them?

LEVENE: I think that is absolutely right. The vast majority of growth retarded fetuses are born close to term and it is a small minority who are extremely premature. When you look at the literature on follow-up of SGA it is extremely confusing. The general conclusions are that if you are born at full term and growth retarded you are likely to catch up both in terms of growth and intellectually. If you are born preterm and growth retarded you are less likely to catch up and you are more likely to have intellectual deficits. I think that we have to exclude cerebral palsy because I do not believe that there is any direct relationship between SGA and cerebral palsy. We are talking about intellectual deficit presumably because the brain has been restricted in growth. Intervention is the most important area. What we want to know is about getting the baby out earlier, and once the baby is born, not whether he lives or dies (because he is almost certainly going to live), but whether we can improve his subsequent intelligence by getting him out and feeding him as compared with leaving him in and letting his brain continue to be restricted. The intervention control studies are extremely important. Dr Lucas in Cambridge has done some studies looking at milk feeding in premature babies and has shown that your intelligence is significantly higher if you are fed one type of milk compared with another. These studies do not take that long to do, but I would say that a year is too short. You have got to look at intelligence, and I do not believe that you can measure intelligence until the child is at least 3 years old.

MILNER: When you talk about morbidity, Dr Stewart, are you talking about neurodevelopmental morbidity and not the totality of morbidity to which I alluded?

STEWART: Yes, I was talking specifically about "head" in that particular context.

MILNER: When you, Professor Levene, referred to the Lucas paper you said "he suggests that...". I would argue slightly differently. The type of study from which Lucas has made these deductions is unlikely to be repeated. You are going to have to accept his utterance, because he certainly believes that he has demonstrated it, and then accepting his database, acknowledge that he has made a most important breakthrough. All our beliefs on the relationship between neonatal hypoglycaemia and subsequent neurodevelopment stem from the Cornblath and Schwartz database[1] going back into the mid-sixties and the concepts of symptomatic/non-symptomatic hypoglycaemia. We then come on to the very strong association between so-called symptomatic hypoglycaemia and subsequent neurodevelopmental deficit. Paediatricians across the board have been working possibly or probably in the delusion that asymptomatic hypoglycaemia was not a worry. I think that the importance of the Lucas paper will certainly come out in our discussion.

What we are debating here is a matter of very profound public health importance. The ethos of the MRC in the past decade has been more towards what it perceived as "science". You have to fight harder if you are coming in with a public health label on your research project than if you come in with a scientific label.

HOWIE: The remarks that you are making are perfectly appropriate and I do not think that just the Medical Research Council needs to be identified in these terms. I think that the funding bodies as a whole find technologically-based research which has relatively short term objectives a much more attractive prospect. Yet without the kind of patience required for long term studies, the conclusions are always going to be limited in terms of their practical value.

BRUDENELL: The Birthright Scientific Committee should also be pointed in the direction of more long term studies.

RUSH: Long term studies are useful to improve and refine one's methodology in child assessment, but it is irrelevant unless it is also built around structured useful intervention. The absence of obstetric input into considerations of long term studies is tragic. Everything we have heard cries out for structured intervention. I was particularly interested in Professor Levene's data. Your syntax almost implied that you considered that those events were aetiologically related, that there may have been causal relationships in the frequency of abnormality in the group that you were seeing. We have to be very careful in saying what we think are causal and what are still a "soup" of associations, in which causality and therefore intervention is at a primitive stage of understanding.

LEVENE: My point was that it represents the high risk group. No direct causal relationship was implied.

STEWART: One of the things that I would have gone on to say was: which of the two parameters by which we judge SGA has the dominant role in dictating outcome? If you look at the literature it looks as though birthweight probably has the dominant role in mortality, and gestation has the dominant role in determining outcome. But there is always a payoff between those two things. The payoff in terms of more maturity seems to be almost lost in terms of mortality.

Professor Levene, one of the reviews in your book has come up with the conclusion that it looks like it is gestation which determines outcome in the SGA liveborn infant rather than anything else. The reviewers made the point that in terms of SGA, although group for group they may have the same overall level of morbidity, the type of morbidity is different. They make the point that the term SGA child is not particularly at risk of major problems, but they are particularly at risk of minor problems, and perhaps more failure later on. By comparison the preterm infants are not at such risk of later minor deficits. You have got to take both things into consideration.

HOWIE: If what you say is true it is of enormous importance because it would suggest that even a quite modest prolongation of gestation may have quite extraordinary implications in terms of outcome and eventual public health policy.

STEWART: It may be that there is a point at which there is a shout for help because the fetus is not very comfortable, then there is a point at which he is much better off out than in. To actually define this may be very important.

ALBERMAN: I would like to take issue with Dr Stewart on that one, and I would like to come back to the point I made earlier. It is a point that the people working with cerebral palsy are making so loudly that one cannot ignore it. There is usually a reason for being SGA, and certainly among the SGA children there is an excess of children who have been damaged or who have an inherent intrinsic abnormality from way back. In those particular children, and I do not know what proportion it is nor who they are, prolonging gestation or keeping them alive is probably only going to increase their morbidity if the morbid antecedents were there before the delivery and are the reason for the SGA. In the series that I have followed up there are a whole host of syndromes and abnormalities which nothing one did at delivery or during the neonatal period would have altered. That is the group which must be treated with care. One of the reasons that we are in this mess is that people have been so bad at recording even what little gestation they are sure about. On a national or geographical scale people are very good about recording birthweight, but gestation has never been recorded so we cannot do the large scale studies that we have been doing on birthweight. Regarding the UK, the National Birthday Trust data sets in theory give the possibility of doing this, except that the Department of Health in their wisdom decided to do it by place of birth and not by place of residence which makes life extremely difficult. If we can as a profession push very hard to get what we can out of the Birthday Trust data sets and out of the child health systems that are now growing everywhere, then as well as Dr Stewart's and Professor Levene's superb work, we will be able to look at the public health issues.

CLAPP: Speaking from an obstetrical point of view, this is important in terms of helping the obstetrician decide the right thing to do in a given case. In terms of central nervous system function in early postnatal life we ought to be able to detect the infant who is going to demonstrate long term minor abnormality very early on. If one were to design a long term follow-up study, what the obstetrician needs is a test that can dissect out what is related to before birth versus what happens after birth in terms of long term outcome. I would make a strong plea for the inclusion in any long term evaluation of an extremely detailed immediate neonatal evaluation. The plasticity of the developing central nervous system being what it is, as time goes on you are liable to lose these very sensitive markers. The discriminators are not fine enough in terms of what you want that citizen ultimately to be, perhaps. As an obstetrician it would be extemely helpful to have some immediate follow-up data that you then could use to go back and change interventions and use that as your point of outcome rather than the Apgar scores, survival or seizures.

COCKBURN: From Scotland, in a current MRC supported study, there will be data which will identify gestational age as well as birthweights. The stillbirth information is all there. They have already been followed up at 10 months and 2 years. This is a $4^1/_2$ year study. Once you get to this stage the data becomes sullied because there are postnatal events to take into consideration. I want to remind you of some work that Winnock reported many years ago in which he indicated intrauterine growth retardation alone, in a group of human studies as well as animal studies, decreased the total brain cell number to about 90% of normal. Similarly if he took small numbers of postnatally starved children but who had grown well *in utero*, again he got a reduction at about 18 months or 2 years to about 90% of normal. Where he had intrauterine growth retardation plus neonatal starvation or poor nutrition the brain cell number was reduced to 40% of normal. This equates in some ways to what Dr Stewart has been describing, in that intrauterine growth retardation on its own may not create severe deficits in brain cell number or structure. But if you have postnatal malnutrition associated with it, as you may do in the low birthweight infants, you may then have significant deficits. You have got to look not only at the prenatal events but also carefully document what happened postnatally in terms of growth and development, particularly during the first year.

HALL: The Scottish national data set has had gestational age for many years and the study that Leslie Much is going to continue has already been going with a very good follow-up of all the very low birthweight children born in Scotland. There is also a Dutch national study of low birthweight and low gestation deliveries which has just been published.(2)

STEWART: The idea of having a package of assessment is very good. We have been looking at objective measures of brain structure and function at University College with Osmond Reynolds. One of the strong pieces of information that is coming out of that is that there are "horses for courses". There are certain measurements which you can make during the immediate perinatal period or at a particular age which give you very important information, but no one measurement tells you everything. We are going to have to design a package of observations. What we have already shown is that if you add just one objective measurement and a neurological examination together you immediately get more information in terms of picking out the "undamaged" infants. I think that sort of approach is going to be much more widely looked into. Also, there has got to be more work on relating one assessment, say the term total package of results, with 1 year, with 2 years, with 3 years, with 4 years and with 8 years. Then perhaps we are going to understand just exactly how strong and how precise our prediction can be. We know we have got good crude prediction, but can we get it much more precise? If we look at a child at 10 years and discover that he has problems of functioning, the origin of that could be anywhere along the line.

HOWIE: The combination of neurology and ultrasound — did you get your figures from just the small baby group or was that from a wider group?

STEWART: We originally realised that the specificity of an abnormal scan and an abnormal neurological examination was actually 99% while the sensitivity was very low. So we started all over again and did a prospective study of all the deliveries for one year. Those were the results I showed you.

HOWIE: Was this across a wide birthweight spectrum?

STEWART: It is a cohort of children who were born before 33 weeks' gestation. It is in the preterm ones where the ultrasound is going to be relevant.

LEVENE: I disagree with that. You are looking at a very highly selected group of very high risk babies born in a tertiary referral centre in the middle of London. That tells you nothing of what is happening in a geographical area, and that is what we need to know. We do not need to know about the ones who are highly selected that everybody knows about. What we want to know is what can obstetricians detect before the baby is born? What interventions can we make in order to try and reduce morbidity or even improve intelligence later on? We must be planning geographically based studies where this information can be obtained. Where ultrasound is not relevant, detailed neurological examinations are not relevant, because they do not give you the information you want. The majority of these babies are full term. But at the same time you then need to do intervention studies in a controlled clinical setting on babies where you can intervene, and then have a control group where there is no intervention. That is the only way we are going to find out whether we can produce subtle reductions in impairment of intelligence.

WIGGLESWORTH: I have a list of seven ways in which the brain can go wrong or be wrong in our enormous disparate group of small-for-dates babies. It is fairly critical that anyone who is planning any sort of study should know something about the basic things that can go wrong. The brain is not a mystical object. Firstly an asymmetric growth retarded baby may have a brain of something like 18–20% of body weight. So that in itself puts the baby at all sorts of risks. Apart from that, specific growth retarding mechanisms may cause specific abnormalities of brain development such as fetal alcohol syndrome with neuronal dysplasias, etc. You must know about those and recognise the syndromes. Secondly, there is a group of growth retarding conditions which may also be associated with episodic acute intrauterine damage. This is the type where, for instance, you have twins which come into the growth retarded group, with the twin-twin transfusion syndrome. Then we have the classic kind of uteroplacental damage growth retardation which may give an obvious increased tendency to intrapartum asphyxia because of the reduction in reserve. These are the ones who have an increased tendency to the classic type of perfusion intrapartum asphyxia. There is a sub-group to that because, of course, some get cranial trauma. We have got the relatively big head in that group and the relatively poor, thin skull, and so there may be a traumatic component. Then we have the group of postnatal problems of the growth retarded babies, such as hypoglycaemia. Also if they are growth retarded plus premature they are then obviously in the IVH/PVL* type range. The next group includes the extemely growth retarded babies of any type in which inevitably the brain growth must be impaired; that is a fairly small group. Finally we have the whole of the

* IVH/PVL: intraventricular haemorrhage/periventricular leucomalacia

background socioeconomic interactions, where if there are problems beforehand and the baby is born into a low socioeconomic group there may be later impairment. Anyone who is doing any sort of study on developmental impairment must not become fixed in trying to follow up one specific idea; there will be a disparate group of problems to deal with.

RUSH: This country has the world's most intensive and valuable experience in the national cohort follow up studies of 1946, 1958 and 1970. They do not exist anywhere else in the world. They have been enormously valuable. But I will assert that the problems that this group is facing are not going to be addressed by population-based follow-up studies. These only identify risk groups; they only raise hypotheses; they demonstrate where problems are. Professor Alberman's point about aetiology in cerebral palsy really raises the issue precisely. What you do need are intervention trials in order to refine your clinical activities. We have generated enough hypotheses in these discussions to keep us busy for the next half century. I hear from this group not the need for large scale population follow-up studies, nor even refinement of technology for child assessment, but rather a fairly urgent need to see whether therapies currently being used and now being promulgated in some centres but not others actually have any long term effect.

STEWART: That is an extremely helpful comment. The whole question of the interaction of the two kinds of study is something that we must not lose sight of. I would like to respond to Professor Levene. When I talk about attempting to design a package of evaluation, it is not the fact that it is being designed on a particular cohort in an intensive care unit, or whatever, that is relevant. That is irrelevant to the design of the package. The package has got to be designed and then we can apply it to the population data. Until we have got the methodology to handle the wider population we will continue to make a mess of the population studies. We have got to have much tighter methodology. That is where there are problems, because the sort of neurological observations that one can make, and which appear to be extremely predictive and extremely meaningful, are actually very simple. The essential part is that they are very structured and very disciplined. Then we finally can do what you very rightly have suggested that we should do.

We keep hearing about the effect on IQ and the effect on cognitive function. We must be very cautious because IQ measurements are actual measurements, but there is some question of whether they are an appropriate end point for what we are likely to want to know. One piece of statistics which has come out of our 4-year-old assessment is that if you take the IQ as measured conventionally at 4 years of age, and you look at how it relates to other problems, out of 171 children who all had ultrasound brain scans, all born before 33 weeks and all followed serially (so we know what their neurological situation is as well as their ultrasound scan) there are 11 whose IQ is below 80. According to the test that we are using, that is immediately out with acceptable standards. In those children, completely unrecognised at 1 year, their low IQ is the only isolated problem. They had no evidence of impaired neurological or fine motor skills, etc. at 4 years of age. Their ultrasound scans were normal. Their term neurological examination was normal and at the age of 1 year their neurological examination was normal and their developmental quotient was within the normal range. They are a very interesting group, but I think that we have to be very careful if we are going to talk about IQ as an outcome measure, because it is probably fairly insensitive.

REFERENCES

1. Cornblath MK, Schwartz R. *Disorders of Carbohydrate Metabolism in Infancy*. 2nd edition. Philadelphia: WB Saunders, 1976: pp.372-374.
2. Verloove-Vanhorick SP, Verwey SA, Brand R, Benneboek GJ, Kierse MJNC. Neonatal mortality risk in relation to gestational age and birth weight. *Lancet* 1986; **i:** 55–57.

CONCLUSIONS

NORMAL FETAL GROWTH

Size at birth

Animal studies reveal effects of both embryonic and maternal genotypes on normal fetal growth and birthweight. The evidence suggests the maternal effect operates late in gestation, whereas embryonic and early fetal growth is determined solely by the embryonic genetic contribution.

Experiments were described using the mouse embryo, in which either increase or decrease of the early embryonic mass resulted in undergrowth or overgrowth respectively, up to or during the time of organogenesis when the fetus self-corrected towards normality.

Particularly interesting was the description of long term effects on postnatal mice of disturbances in early embryonic size, which include absolute overgrowth of the limbs, behavioural and motor neuropathy and reduced fertility.

Human fetal growth curves

In analysing fetal growth both cross-sectionally and longitudinally, pitfalls were illustrated which may come from accepting cross-sectional fetal growth charts as representative of normal biology. Careful longitudinal study of growth in the last trimester showed this to be linear and with a constant variance, estimated from ultrasound measurements made between 18 and 20 weeks.

Placental control of fetal metabolism

Our perception of the classes of nutrients which the fetus uses as energy sources was expanded. In particular, the flexibility of amino acids as energy sources as well as building blocks was highlighted.

Placenta as an endocrine regulator

The placenta as an endocrine regulator was considered particularly against the clinical background of early pregnancy failure and pregnancy complicated by diabetes mellitus. Maternal serum levels of progesterone, oestradiol, human chorionic gonadotrophin and human placental lactogen did not appear to have any clinical value in assessing early pregnancy outcome or infant birthweight.

Control of cellular multiplication and differentiation

A review of the interplay of factors (endocrine, paracrine, nutritional and genetic) involved in fetal growth control revealed an area of intense research and great interest. On balance, the macro-molecules encoded by the fetal genome appear to be important mediators of cellular growth and differentiation. The interplaying factors noted above appear to be more modulatory than controlling.

Maternal diet and fetal substrate provision

Successful reproduction in the human takes place within a wide range of energy intakes.

Basal metabolic rates in pregnant individuals may be related to pre-pregnancy body stores.

Short-term manipulations of maternal diet can have significant effects on the substrate mix through altered insulin sensitivity.

FETAL OVERGROWTH

The review of overgrowth illustrated how the more common clinical example, infant of a diabetic mother (IDM), has been more fully analysed, and is more clearly understood, than the less common clinical syndromes such as nesidioblastosis and Beckwith-Wiedemann syndrome (BWS).

Genetic factors play a part in the aetiology of these syndromes which require much further study.

Most examples of generalised fetal overgrowth so far recognised are associated with fetal hyperinsulinaemia or vascular disturbance.

There is no clear definition of fetal macrosomia.

It is clear that in creating clinically useful definitions of macrosomia attention must be paid to:

i) birthweight and length by gestational age;
ii) neonatal subcutaneous fat measurement;
iii) ultrasonographic estimation of fetal growth velocity.

The last is particularly important since a stable velocity only slightly greater than average will result in macrosomia.

Further, it is difficult to predict reliably the macrosomic fetus with current technology.

There does not appear to be any way of avoiding occasional catastrophic obstetric accidents resulting from shoulder dystocia.

FETAL UNDERGROWTH

Epidemiology

The need for a clear definition of fetal undergrowth was reiterated.

Birthweights at 40 weeks' gestation are not normally distributed, showing an excess of smaller babies in most published series.

This excess could be explained by environmental factors such as smoking, drinking alcohol and short or long-term nutritional deficits.

Such factors account for some, but not all the consistent differences between birthweight distributions in different ethnic groups.

Genetic contributions to these differences should be taken into account.

The robustness of population-specific birthweight distributions may be contributed to by intergenerational influences in birthweight which, with some exceptions, tend to perpetuate the inheritance of small or large birthweights.

Aetiology

The three components which determine fetal growth retardation were discussed: namely, fetal disease, placental abnormalities and maternal disease. The question of placental compensatory changes was discussed.

Nutritional variations in pregnancy and fetal growth

Severe acute nutritional deprivation will lead to lowered birthweight, especially in the third trimester, and this loss is reversible by re-feeding in the third trimester.

Iatrogenic nutritional deprivation can produce lowered birthweight, especially if protein intake is increased. Such intervention can lead to decreased stature in childhood.

Chronic deprivation is difficult to study in the human. Effects appear to be only partly reversed with supplementary feeding during pregnancy.

Well-designed supplementation trials suggest:

i) Protein-dense supplements are toxic and are associated with low birthweight;
ii) Normal protein density supplementation produced small increases in birthweight;
iii) It is unknown whether these small increases are associated with reduced mortality and better long-term function.

The United States "WIC" ("Women, Infants and Children") nutritional programme was associated with increased birthweight, longer gestational age and reduction in fetal mortality after 28 weeks' gestation. There was evidence of decreased maternal fat stores in late pregnancy and increased inappropriate newborn head size. The long-term implications of these effects have not been estimated.

Animal experimental studies of utero-placental blood supply in fetal growth

Both placental and fetal size are limited by utero-placental blood flow.

Fetal growth rate appears to be quite sensitive to the minor reductions in flow which restrict growth without metabolic compromise. This down-regulation of fetal growth rate to match the substrate supply has obvious survival value. Data point to the placenta as a regulator of the reduction in fetal growth.

A decrease in placental perfusion and/or substrate delivery may induce the placental release of one or more peptide moieties which inhibit the effect of multiple growth factors, and thereby suppress the rate of fetal and placental growth.

Clinical implications of fetal undergrowth

Serial symphysis–fundal height measurements compare fairly well with a single fetal abdominal circumference measurement made by ultrasound, but would only identify some 75% of small-for-gestational-age (SGA) babies.

A majority of the participants felt that an ultrasound scan at 18–20 weeks not only helps to estimate the dates but is of value for the diagnosis of structural fetal abnormalities, and the later SGA fetus.

The accuracy of the weight prediction formulae using ultrasound measurements is improved by using all four parameters, namely, biparietal diameter, abdominal circumference, head circumference and femur length.

The benefits, in terms of improvement in fetal outcome, of routine scanning at any of the stages of pregnancy have yet to be established.

Fetal biometry does not predict the degree of fetal hypoxia.

It is possible to measure blood flow parameters in the uterine and umbilical vessels, and in the fetal circulation using Doppler ultrasound. Whilst velocity waveform measurements of umbilical blood flow are easy to perform, errors can occur due to technological problems and methodology.

Fetal blood flow is known to be affected by fetal breathing, fetal activity state and drugs, and further studies are needed to identify other features that may affect fetal circulation.

Doppler blood flow velocity measurements during pregnancy need to be further investigated before their value can be determined in routine clinical practice.

Most biochemical tests carried out in pregnancy are unreliable for diagnosis of fetal health.

The role of maternal serum alphafetoprotein measurements in identification of fetal neural tube defects is well established. Its role in conjunction with other biochemical tests in identifying chromosomal abnormalities needs to be established.

Most placental function tests correlate well with placental mass.

If ultrasound measurements are not available then placental function tests can be used to pick up 40–50% of cases of SGA babies.

If accurate and routine ultrasound is available, then routine use of placental function tests is not justified.

The combination of pulsed Doppler/realtime ultrasound makes it possible to estimate blood flow in large fetal vessels. In SGA fetuses the aortic and umbilical flow is lower than in appropriate-for-gestational-age (AGA) fetuses. Technical development improving the accuracy of estimating flow is necessary before possible application in the clinical context.

The waveform of the fetal arterial velocity changes in a characteristic way in SGA fetuses developing hypoxia: the end diastolic velocity decreases and eventually disappears. More complex evaluation of the waveform with emphasis on its end-diastolic phase provides more useful information than the mathematical indices, for example, ponderal index, A/B ratio.

Clinical dating and assessment

A value for gestational age, using completed weeks, should be attributed to every woman, with an indication of its certainty.

Where good menstrual data exist, gestational age should normally be calculated from this using Naegele's rule.

Where menstrual data are inadequate or suspect, ultrasound scan assessment of size should be used, and is more reliable the earlier the gestation.

The normal duration of pregnancy is not known precisely.

Clinical risk factors (e.g. obstetric history, maternal size, maternal weight gain, maternal smoking, fundal height measurement) should be used to identify possible smallness for gestational age requiring further evaluation by ultrasound investigation.

Ultrasound scan assessment of fetal size in early pregnancy is often helpful in confirming gestational age estimated from menstrual data, and will itself provide an accurate assessment of gestational age where menstrual data are unreliable.

Ultrasound scanning at 18–20 weeks' gestation can detect a considerable proportion of cases of fetal malformation. Because biological variation in fetal size is greater at that time than in early pregnancy, estimation of gestational age based on fetal size may be less reliable than in early pregnancy. Measurement of fetal size may however be useful as a baseline for future measurements of fetal growth.

A scan in the late second and third trimester identifies most unusually small or unusually large fetuses.

In the opinion of some of the participants, the benefits in terms of improvement in fetal outcome of routine ultrasound scanning at any of these stages of pregnancy have yet to be established.

Therapy in IUGR

There are no controlled trials of potential therapies.

Potential approaches to the therapy of IUGR include steps to improve:

i) maternal condition, e.g. stopping smoking and treatment of maternal disease;
ii) fetal condition, e.g. by hyperalimentation;
iii) blood flow, e.g. by the use of betamimetic and antithrombotic drugs.

Cordocentesis gives an insight into the pathology and adaptations of the SGA baby. Some SGA fetuses are chromosomally abnormal. Cordocentesis studies have shown that some SGA fetuses are hypoxaemic, hypercapnaeic, acidotic, and have abnormalities in their carbohydrate, lipid, and amino acid metabolism.

There is a relationship between blood flow and acid base studies in cord blood which can be corrected by maternal oxygenation.

Fetal activity and biophysical evaluation

Fetal behaviour may reflect central nervous system maturation.

Few data exist on the effect of hypoxia on fetal behavioural activity.

Fetal activity scanning systems effectively select out those babies in good condition.

Data on the use of scanning systems in the evaluation of the IUGR baby are sparse.

The ability to repeat the evaluation daily is attractive.

Reductions in fetal activity may indicate with reasonable accuracy that the baby is becoming acidotic.

There is a need for prospective studies to establish the worth of the biophysical profile in IUGR.

Intrapartum monitoring in IUGR

SGA babies show a higher incidence of clinical indices of fetal distress in labour.

SGA babies have a reduced buffering capacity to adapt to metabolic stress.

A normal CTG is usually a reassuring feature in the management of SGA babies in labour.

Neonatal management in SGA

There is an urgent need for agreed definitions and endpoints in evaluation of actions.

In addition to low birthweight for gestational age, ponderal index can be a useful measure of the wasted infant.

The risk of mortality in the SGA baby is not increased over AGA babies of the same gestational age.

Some postnatal complications of the.SGA baby are maturity related. RDS has a reduced incidence.

Asymptomatic hypoglycaemia may be related to subsequent neurodevelopmental disability and this deserves further evaluation.

Post-asphyxial encephalopathy may be a useful measure of intrapartum compromise.

Mortality and morbidity

The relationship of birthweight and gestation with morbidity differs from the relationship with mortality.

Both pieces of information are therefore needed to evaluate outcome. When birthweight and gestation are discrepant, the published literature indicates that mortality relates to birthweight, and morbidity to gestation.

Outcome measures range from "satisfactory citizen count" to the results of detailed neurodevelopmental and cognitive assessments at specific ages.

Data are already available from studies of very pre-term infants, relating findings from objective measures of brain structure and function and neurological examination at approximately term, 1, 4 and 8 years which allow early prediction of outcome. For example:

a) A favourable ultrasound brain scan at discharge from hospital and a normal neurological assessment is highly correlated with a good outcome in very pre-term infants;

b) Infants with some neurodevelopmental problems at one year of age nearly always have similar problems at 4 years of age.